STUDY GUIDE

to accompany

Potter • Perry

Basic Nursing

Essentials for Practice

STUDY GUIDE

to accompany

Potter • Perry

Basic Nursing

Essentials for Practice

6th Edition

Patricia A. Castaldi, BSN, MSN, RN

Director

Practical Nursing Program

Union County College

Plainfield, New Jersey

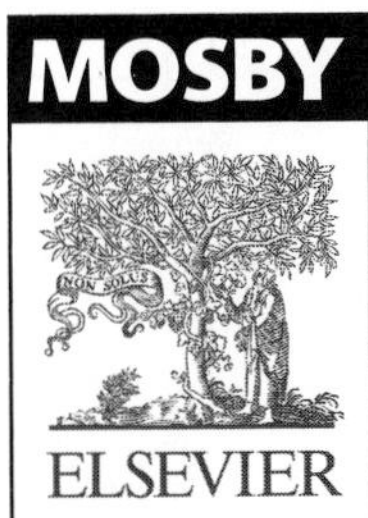

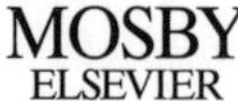

MOSBY
ELSEVIER

11830 Westline Industrial Drive
St. Louis, Missouri 63146

Study Guide to accompany Potter • Perry Basic Nursing: Essentials for Practice

ISBN-13: 978-0-323-04121-8
ISBN-10: 0-323-04121-3

Notice

Knowledge and best practice in this field are constantly changing. As new research and experience broaden our knowledge, changes in practice, treatment, and drug therapy may become necessary or appropriate. Readers are advised to check the most current information provided (i) on procedures featured or (ii) by the manufacturer of each product to be administered, to verify the recommended dose or formula, the method and duration of administration, and contraindications. It is the responsibility of the practitioner, relying on their own experience and knowledge of the patient, to make diagnoses, to determine dosages and the best treatment for each individual patient, and to take all appropriate safety precautions. To the fullest extent of the law, neither the Publisher nor the Author assumes any liability for any injury and/or damage to persons or property arising out or related to any use of the material contained in this book.

The Publisher

ISBN-13: 978-0-323-04121-8
ISBN-10: 0-323-04121-3

Executive Editor: Susan Epstein
Senior Developmental Editor: Robyn L. Brinks
Publishing Services Manager: John Rogers
Senior Project Manager: Beth Hayes

Printed in the United States of America

Last digit is the print number: 9 8 7 6 5 4 3 2 1

To John and Dan for all of your love and support.
Thank you to Rose Currie for your valuable input.

Introduction and Preface

This guide is designed to correspond, chapter by chapter, to *Basic Nursing* (6th edition). Each chapter in this guide contains study aids to assist in learning and applying the theoretical concepts from the text.

The comprehensive chapter review sections allow you the opportunity to evaluate your own level of comprehension after reading the text. Use of the study group questions with fellow students may help in your overall understanding of the nursing content, as well as provide a way to further evaluate your familiarity with that content.

Please note: In this edition of the Study Guide, there are some ***Matching*** exercises that have more choices than are necessary. This is to allow you to discriminate between the choices and apply your knowledge of the terminology. There are also more short answer and multiple response questions to promote your preparation for classroom examinations and the NCLEX®. You may find that there are questions that require you to apply information from other chapters or use other reference sources to answer them.

General study tips to use while reading, taking classroom notes, and preparing for and taking examinations are also included in this guide. Other students have found these ideas to be helpful in their nursing course experiences.

A skills performance checklist has been provided for each of the major skills and procedural guidelines presented in the text. These checklists may be used by faculty members to evaluate your ability to perform the techniques, as well as offer their comments and recommendations for improvement. The checklists represent generally accepted nursing principles and practice. You may need to adapt these skills in order to meet a patient's special needs or follow the particular policy of an institution.

Study Charts

While reading through the chapters in the text, you may create study charts to assist you to organize the material that is covered. The charts allow for a comparison of key concepts in the chapter. There are suggestions for charts to create in the chapters of this text. An example follows:

Routes of Injection

The learning activities presented in this study guide should assist in your review of the text material and your application of the nursing concepts to classroom and clinical experiences.

Route	Angle of Insertion/Needle Size/Maximum Amount of Medication
Intradermal	
Subcutaneous	
Intramuscular	

General Study Tips

While reading

- *Read before the scheduled class:* Highlight key points or outline content in the text that will be covered in the classroom.
- *Look up definitions:* Find the meanings of words you do not recognize while you are going through the text. It helps to have a medical dictionary and a regular dictionary handy!
- *Make notes:* Write down a list of topics that you do not understand while you are reading so that you may clarify them with the instructor.
- *Compare notes:* Use notes taken from the book and in class to create a complete picture of the content.
- *Use study/comparison charts:* Put facts and ideas in an organized form so that you can refer easily to them at a later point, such as when studying for an exam.
- *Use references:* Go back to texts and notes used in other courses (such as anatomy and physiology) to help in understanding new material.

In the classroom

- *Make notes:* Do not try to write everything down. Note the essential information from the class. Jot down questions that you may have as you go along, so that you remember to ask them at some point.
- *Ask questions:* Remember to take advantage of the expertise of the instructor. Do not go away from the class without trying to clear up areas of confusion!
- *Audiotape:* Make audiotapes of classroom discussions, only with instructor permission, if:
  1. There is time to listen to them at some time (such as in the car) and not just collect the tapes.
  2. There are positive results from this process, with better understanding of the material and improved exam grades.

On your own

- *Use available resources:* Take advantage of all of the resources at the school, such as the library, computer laboratory, and skill laboratory. Make time to practice nursing techniques, watch DVDs or videos, and complete computer learning programs.
- *Join/create a study group:* Get together with other students in your class to review material. Study groups offer an opportunity to share information, challenge each other, and provide mutual support.
- *Use time management techniques:* Use available time as efficiently as possible. For example, the time that is spent waiting for an appointment or riding on public transportation may be used to read over materials or complete assignments.

Before an exam

- *Try to remain calm:* Easy to recommend, but hard to do! Learn and use relaxation skills. Don't jump immediately into the exam. Relax and get focused first, then start the test.
- *Be prepared:* Check with the instructor to be sure you have covered the content that will be on the exam. Bring the right materials: pencils, pens, erasers, and so on. Leave enough time to get to the exam so that there is no last minute "rushing in."

During the exam

- *Read the questions carefully:* Determine what the question is asking. Stay focused on the actual question without reading into the situations. If allowed to mark the exam paper, underline key words or cross out unnecessary information to assist in getting to the heart of the question.
- *Do not keep changing your answers:* Most of the time, the first answer selected is correct. Do not change an answer unless you have remembered the correct response.
- *Stay focused:* Take brief moments during the exam, if necessary, to stop and use relaxation techniques to compose yourself.

Contents

Health and Wellness 1

Case Study

1. A personal friend has been experiencing severe stomach and intestinal distress for a few months. She is 35 years old and is employed as an advertisement salesperson for a local newspaper. During this past year, she has been pressured to create more income for her department. When you ask her if she has sought medical treatment, she responds that she "doesn't have the time to go to the doctor." In addition to her job responsibilities, she is a single parent of a grade school child who enjoys a number of after-school activities.
   a. What physical and lifestyle factors are present in this situation?
   b. What initial responses/interventions may be helpful for this individual?

Chapter Review

Match the description/definition in Column A with the correct term in Column B.

	Column A	Column B
______	1. A person's definition and interpretation of symptoms and use of the health care system	a. High-level wellness model
______	2. A belief that patients have the authority to be active participants in determining their health and well-being	b. Internal variables
______	3. Longer than 6 months' duration	c. Body image
______	4. A subjective concept of physical appearance	d. Holistic health
______	5. Developmental stage, intellectual background, emotional and spiritual factors	e. Illness behavior
______	6. Short term and severe	f. Acute illness
		g. Chronic illness

Complete the following:

7. Health is the absence of disease.
   True _____ False _____
8. Identify whether the following are internal or external variables that influence health beliefs and practices:
   a. Financial status
   b. Family health behaviors
   c. Cognitive abilities
   d. Cultural values
   e. Ability to cope with stress
9. An example of a positive health behavior is:
10. An example of a negative health behavior is:

Select the best answer for each of the following questions:

11. At the tertiary level of prevention, the nurse would prepare an educational program for a group requiring:
    1. Chemotherapy
    2. Cardiac rehabilitation
    3. Genetic screening
    4. Sex education

12. At the secondary level of prevention, the intervention that the nurse expects to assist with or provide instruction for is:
    1. Immunization
    2. Referral to outpatient therapy
    3. Performance of a biopsy
    4. Parent performance of the newborn's bath
13. The nurse is working with a patient who is experiencing chronic joint pain. To assist the patient to manage or reduce the pain, the nurse decides to use a holistic health approach. With this in mind, the nurse specifically elects to include:
    1. Aroma therapy
    2. Wound care
    3. Hygienic care measures
    4. Analgesic medications
14. The nurse is completing an assessment for the patient who has come to the medical clinic. Variables that influence the patient's health beliefs and practices are being determined. The nurse is aware that an internal variable for this patient is the:
    1. Way in which the patient celebrates family occasions
    2. Manner in which the patient deals with stress on the job and at home
    3. Frequency of the family's visit to the health care agency
    4. Amount of insurance coverage that is provided by the patient's employer
15. The nurse recognizes that primary prevention is a critical aspect in health care. The target group for a program on hand washing that is aimed at this level of prevention is:
    1. Fourth grade children at the local elementary school
    2. Patients in a cardiac rehabilitation program at the medical center
    3. Parents of a child with a congenital heart defect
    4. Diabetic patients coming to the outpatient clinic
16. The nurse is leading a group of community members who are trying to quit smoking. In the precontemplation phase of health behavior change, the nurse anticipates that the group members will respond by:
    1. Discussing prior attempts at quitting
    2. Recognizing the benefits of not smoking
    3. Expressing irritation when the topic of quitting is introduced
    4. Requesting phone numbers of support people who have participated in the group
17. A young adult student has come to the university's health center for a physical examination. The nurse is conducting the initial interview and is looking for possible lifestyle risk factors. The nurse is specifically alerted to the student's:
    1. Mild hypertension
    2. Mountain climbing hobby
    3. Family history of diabetes
    4. Part-time job at the auto factory
18. According to Maslow's hierarchy of needs, the patient's priority should be:
    1. Physical safety
    2. Psychological safety
    3. Self-esteem
    4. Adequate nutrition
19. During the process of changing behaviors, the nurse determines that the patient is in the maintenance stage on the basis of the following response:
    1. "I don't believe I need injections since I feel okay."
    2. "I may need to adjust my diet a little."
    3. "I take my insulin daily as ordered."
    4. "I have been trying to learn the diet plan."
20. The nurse specifically recognizes the environmental risk for illness upon determining that the patient:
    1. Works in a chemical plant
    2. Has a history of heart disease
    3. Admits to intermittent substance abuse
    4. Is over 65 years of age
21. Correct information for the nurse to share with a female patient includes:
    1. Regular varicella immunizations
    2. A cholesterol level determination every year

3. A flu shot yearly after age 50
4. A test for osteoporosis yearly after age 35

Study Group Questions

- What are the different health models and how can they be applied to different patient situations? What are the advantages and disadvantages of each model?
- What are the different internal and external variables that are present in health practices and illness behavior? Give specific examples of the different variables and possible nursing interventions.
- What behaviors may be observed in a patient during illness? What impact may the patient's illness have on the family/significant others?
- How do the levels of prevention relate to the nursing care of patients in different health care settings?

Study Chart

Create a study chart to compare the Levels of Prevention, *identifying both patient and nursing activities associated with each level.*

2 The Health Care Delivery System

Case Studies

1. A neighbor who has just accepted a new job with a different benefits package stops by to ask if you know anything about managed care. He asks you what an HMO is and what it means to him. The neighbor also tells you that he received a "big book" full of hospital and doctor names that is really confusing.
   a. What information can you provide to this individual?
   b. How could you undertake assisting the neighbor to understand his HMO coverage?
2. A 54-year-old male visits the community health screening and is found to be hypertensive and demonstrating signs of depression. He served in the armed forces for 30 years and received an honorable discharge a few years ago. In discussion with this individual, it appears that he does not have any health care insurance as a part-time employee in a small retail store.
   a. What health care benefits may this individual be eligible for because of his background?
   b. Where could this individual receive secondary or tertiary care if his condition warrants further treatment?
3. An 80-year-old female patient has just been diagnosed with an inoperable cancerous growth in the brain. Having been told of the poor prognosis, she opts to refuse chemotherapy.
   a. Where could this individual be referred for terminal care?

Chapter Review

Match the description/definition in Column A with the correct term in Column B.

	Column A	*Column B*
______	1. Nationwide health insurance program that provides benefits to individuals over 65 years of age	a. Medicaid
______	2. Integration of best knowledge, clinical expertise, and patient values	b. Capitation
______	3. Fixed amount of payment for services per enrollee	c. Globalization
______	4. Short-term relief for persons providing care to ill, disabled older adults	d. Managed care
______	5. Income eligibility for coverage below the federal poverty level	e. Utilization review
______	6. Patient responses directly related to nursing care	f. Medicare
______	7. Administrative control over primary health care services for a defined patient population	g. Respite care
______	8. Worldwide in scope	h. Nursing-sensitive outcomes
		i. Evidence-based practice

Complete the following:

9. A(n) ______________________________ is a system of family-centered care designed to allow patients to live with dignity while dealing with a terminal illness.
10. In an acute care setting, discharge planning begins:

11. Technology influences health care delivery by:

12. Select the appropriate health care service level for each of the following:

Primary care	Secondary acute care	Restorative care
Preventive care	Tertiary care	Continuing care

a. Well-baby care

b. Intensive care treatment

c. Cardiac rehabilitation program

d. Visiting nurses

e. Adult day-care center

f. Immunizations

g. Family planning clinic

h. Mental health counseling

i. Appendectomy surgery

j. Assisted living facility

k. CAT scans

l. Sports medicine

13. The role of the case manager is to:

The focus of case management is on:

14. An example of a vulnerable population is:

15. Many patients who require subacute care are termed:

16. Based on the dimensions of patient-centered care, select all of the following that patients want specifically with regard to *access* to health care:
a. To schedule appointments at convenient times without difficulty _______
b. A setting that focuses on the quality of life _______
c. To receive accurate and timely information _______
d. An environment that is clean and comfortable _______
c. To see a specialist when a referral is made _______
d. A competent and caring staff _______
e. To find transportation when going to different health care settings _______

f. To have family members involved in the plan of care _______

Select the best answer for each of the following questions:

17. The daughter of an older woman expresses her concern that while she is at work her mother, recently diagnosed with Alzheimer's disease, has been found wandering around the neighborhood in a disoriented state. This family may benefit from the services of a(n):
    1. Hospice
    2. Subacute care unit
    3. Adult day-care center
    4. Residential community
18. While working in the community health agency, the nurse visits an older adult patient who is having difficulty performing her activities of daily living (ADLs) in her own home. The patient recognizes that she needs some supervision with medications. In discussions with this patient, the nurse refers the patient to a(n):
    1. Subacute care unit
    2. Assisted living facility
    3. Rehabilitation hospital
    4. Primary care institution
19. A patient being discharged from a medical unit and requiring more constant nursing care at a level above a nursing center or extended care facility is referred by the nurse to the:
    1. Subacute care unit
    2. Home health agency
    3. Urgent care center
    4. Rural primary care facility
20. The nurse's next-door neighbor has recently experienced some health problems. The neighbor visits the nurse to ask about Medicaid coverage. The nurse informs the neighbor that this program is:
    1. Catastrophic long-term care coverage for older adults
    2. A fee-for-service plan that provides preventive health care
    3. A two-part federally funded health care program for older adults
    4. A federally funded and state-regulated program for individuals of all ages with low income
21. A graduate of a nursing program is interested in the occupational health field. The graduate nurse decides to pursue a position at:
    1. The local medical center
    2. A car manufacturing plant
    3. An urgent care center
    4. A physician's office
22. A patient is being discharged from the medical unit of the hospital. While working with the patient, the nurse identifies that intermittent supervision will be required. The patient will also need to rent durable medical equipment for use in the home. There is family support for the patient upon discharge. The nurse will refer this patient to:
    1. A subacute care unit
    2. An extended care facility
    3. A home health agency
    4. An urgent care center
23. The family of a patient has requested that the hospice agency become involved with the patient's care. The nurse recognizes that the services provided by hospice for this patient include:
    1. Extensive rehabilitative measures
    2. Daytime coverage for the working caregivers
    3. Residential care with an emphasis on a return to functioning
    4. Provision of symptom management and comfort measures for the terminally ill
24. Health care costs are generally reduced with:
    1. Treatment in an outpatient facility
    2. Use of new technology
    3. Prescription medications
    4. Identification of acuity levels for hospitalized patients
25. An individual has health insurance coverage that offers an extremely limited choice of providers, with one health care organization to use and less access to specialists. The nurse recognizes that this

individual is covered by a(n):
1. Managed care organization (MCO)
2. Preferred provider organization (PPO)
3. Exclusive provider organization (EPO)
4. Private insurance company

26. In a school health setting, the nurse expects to provide which service?
    1. Communicable disease prevention
    2. Physical assessment
    3. Chronic pain management
    4. Respite care

27. The patient lives in a sparsely populated farm area and has developed abdominal pain that requires medical attention. This patient, per the Omnibus Budget Reconciliation Act (OBRA), will have access to a:
    1. Subacute unit
    2. Home care agency
    3. Rural primary care hospital
    4. Restorative care center

28. A resident assessment instrument (RAI) is used for patient assessment in a:
    1. Hospital
    2. Nursing center
    3. Psychiatric treatment center
    4. Rehabilitation facility

Study Group Questions

- What types of health care financing are available, who is eligible, and what services are covered?
- What does managed care mean to patients and health care providers?
- According to the health care services levels, what health care agencies and services are available, and what are the usual roles for nurses in each agency?
- What are some of the key competencies required of nurses today?

Study Chart

Create a study chart to compare the Types of Health Care Delivery Agencies, *identifying the different health care services provided and the nursing roles and activities for each.*

3 Community-Based Nursing Practice

Case Study

1. A nurse lives in a community that has had a steady increase in the number of older adult residents. The nurse has been approached by some of these residents and asked a variety of health-related questions. The nurse decides to investigate the needs of older adults and the resources available to this population.
   a. For the older adult, what problems and needs should the nurse be able to anticipate?
   b. What kind of programs or services may be available or could be offered in this community for the older adult residents?

Chapter Review

Complete the following:

1. One challenge for community-based health care is:

2. People who live in poverty are more likely to:

3. Mentally ill patients in the community are at a greater risk for:

4. Identify the role of the nurse in community-based practice for each of the following examples:
   a. Coordinating the visits of the physical and occupational therapists

   b. Walking a patient through the "system" and helping to fill out insurance forms

   c. Providing crisis intervention at a shelter

   d. Demonstrating the use of an aerosol nebulizer

5. An example of public policy to improve health is:

6. Nurse specialists in public health nursing are prepared at the level of education.

7. High-risk or vulnerable populations include:

8. Identify whether the following statements about the process of change are true or false:
   a. Complex innovations or changes are easier to adopt than simple ones.
      True _______ False _______
   b. Results should be kept confidential.
      True _______ False _______
   c. Success is more likely if it is compatible with existing values and past experiences.
      True _______ False _______

Select the correct answer for the following:

9. The nurse is aware that the homeless population has a higher prevalence of:
   1. Diabetes mellitus
   2. Heart disease
   3. Mental illness
   4. Asthma
10. The nurse is working with a member of a vulnerable population within the community. An appropriate intervention is for the nurse to:
    1. Provide financial advice, if needed
    2. Set the priorities for the patient and family
    3. Focus on keeping the assessment only on the information that is needed
    4. Consider the meaning of the patient's language and behavior
11. In completing an assessment of a community's social system, the nurse will be investigating the:
    1. Schools
    2. Economy
    3. Educational level of the population
    4. Distribution of the population by age
12. For an older adult in the community with a cognitive impairment, the nurse should plan specifically for this individual to:
    1. Provide a well-lighted, glare-free environment
    2. Promote activities that reinforce reality
    3. Make arrangements for a hearing evaluation
    4. Encourage the use of self-help groups

Study Group Questions

- What are the essential functions of public and community health?
- What is the difference between public health and community-based nursing?
- How does the community health nurse care for the community?
- What competencies are required of a community health nurse?
- What roles are assumed by the community health nurse?
- What are the special needs of vulnerable populations?
- How does the nurse approach and care for vulnerable populations?
- What are the factors involved in the process of change?
- What is included in the assessment of the community?

4 Legal Principles in Nursing

Case Studies

1. In preparation for surgery, you are to have the patient sign the consent form for the procedure. The patient, in discussions about the postoperative care, does not appear to understand what will be done during the surgery.
   a. What are your responsibilities in this situation?
2. You are reviewing the doctor's orders for the medications to be given to the patient. One of the medication orders is very difficult to read. The charge nurse tells you that she is sure it is Lasix 40 mg PO.
   a. What should you do in this circumstance?
   b. What legal implications may be involved if the order is incorrect?
3. A child arrives in the emergency department in critical condition. His parents are divorced.
   a. What issues concerning consent for treatment may be involved in this child's case?
4. You have been observing a nursing colleague on your unit, and she appears to be taking narcotics from the medication cart. There have been occasions where her behavior has been erratic.
   a. What, if any, are your legal responsibilities regarding this colleague's behavior?

Chapter Review

Match the descriptions/definitions in Column A with the correct term in Column B.

	Column A	*Column B*
______	1. A law concerned with the relationships among people and the protection of a person's rights	a. Tort
______	2. Any willful attempt or threat to harm another person	b. Negligence
______	3. A civil wrong or injury for which remedy is in the form of money damages	c. Living wills
______	4. A crime of a serious nature that usually carries a penalty of imprisonment	d. Statutory law
______	5. Limitation of liability for health care professionals offering assistance at the scene of an accident	e. Good Samaritan law
______	6. Conduct that falls below the standard of care	f. Assault
______	7. Any intentional touching of another person's body without consent	g. Common law
______	8. A form of contemporary law created by elected legislative bodies	h. Malpractice
______	9. Documents instructing physician's to withhold or withdraw life-sustaining procedures	i. Battery
______	10. A form of contemporary law created by judicial decision in court when cases are decide	j. Civil law
		k. Felony

Complete the following:

11. A nurse may avoid being liable for negligence by:

12. Identify two areas where standards of care are defined.

13. Informed consent requires that the patient:

14. A 9-year-old boy arrives at the hospital following a fall from a tree. He will need emergency surgery. The 25-year-old brother who has brought him to the hospital may give legal consent.
    True ________ False ________
15. Professional negligence is termed:

16. The ____________________________ laws offer legal immunity to a nurse who stops at the scene of an accident and acts without gross negligence.
17. A verbal or telephone order from a physician usually needs to be signed within ____________________________ hours.
18. The two standards for determination of death are:

19. Proof of negligence requires:
    a. ____________________________
    b. ____________________________
    c. ____________________________
    d. ____________________________
20. The coroner is notified if the patient's death is: ____________________
21. Advance directives act to:

22. Health care workers are required to report:

Select the best answer for each of the following questions:

23. A clinical experience is planned for an acute care facility. The student nurse recognizes that his or her liability for patient care includes:
    1. No individual responsibility for actions while being supervised
    2. A shared responsibility with instructor, staff member(s), and health care agency
    3. Activities performed while working in another capacity, such as a nursing assistant
    4. Accountability for information and techniques that will be learned in the school
24. There has been a serious flu epidemic among the staff at the medical center. Upon arriving to work on the medical unit, the nurse discovers that all of the other nursing staff members have called in sick and there are no other nurses available in the facility. In this situation, the nurse should:
    1. Not accept the assignment and leave the unit
    2. Accept the assignment and identify the poor staffing in each patient's record
    3. Document the situation and provide a copy to nursing administration
    4. Inform the hospital administration that nursing responsibilities have been delegated to other personnel
25. While the nurse is preparing to administer medication, the patient states that he or she refuses the medication. The nurse knows that the medication is important for the patient and proceeds with the injection of the medication. This is considered:
    1. Invasion of privacy
    2. Negligence
    3. Assault
    4. Battery

26. The urgent care center in town is busy this evening. There are many walk-in patients of different ages waiting for treatment. The nurse recognizes that in a nonemergency situation the individual who may give consent for a treatment is:
    1. A 16-year-old student
    2. The grandparent of a minor
    3. A teenage parent
    4. The 14-year-old brother of a patient
27. The nurse observes the following actions and recognizes that an invasion of patient privacy is evident when another nurse:
    1. Shares patient data with other agency personnel not involved in the patient's treatment
    2. Withholds the patient's diagnosis from the family members per the patient's request
    3. Provides details of a major scientific advancement to the public relations' department
    4. Reports an incidence of an infectious disease to the health department
28. The nurse enters the room of her patient and observes that an incident has occurred. The situation is appropriately documented as follows:
    1. "Patient fell out of bed. Physician notified and x-rays ordered."
    2. "Patient found on floor. Laceration to forehead."
    3. "Patient given incorrect medication, became dizzy, and slid to the floor."
    4. "Patient got up out of bed without assistance and appeared to have fallen."
29. While working as a receptionist in a physician's office, the student nurse is offered the opportunity to provide an injection to one of the patients. This individual's liability is based upon the:
    1. Job description of a receptionist
    2. Educational level achieved in the nursing program
    3. Physician's willingness to accept responsibility for this individual
    4. Limits of the malpractice insurance held by the physician and this individual
30. The nurse has administered a medication to a patient with a documented allergy to that medication. A standard of care is applied when:
    1. There is a determination of an injury to the patient
    2. An amount of financial compensation is determined
    3. Criminal statutes from the federal government are investigated
    4. The nurse's action is compared to that of another nurse in a similar circumstance
31. Of the following actions, which one is considered to be assault?
    1. The nurse threatens to administer medication to a patient who refuses it.
    2. A surgeon operates on the wrong leg.
    3. A nurse fails to use aseptic technique.
    4. A nursing assistant restrains a confused patient.
32. The National Organ Transplant Act (1984) allows for or requires:
    1. Health care agency removal of organs with the family's consent
    2. Donor transplant without the patient's consent
    3. Physicians who certify death to participate in organ removal and transplant
    4. Health care providers to ask family members to consider organ and tissue donation

Study Group Questions

- What are the sources and types of laws?
- What are intentional and unintentional torts?
- How may intentional torts be applied to nursing situations?
- What criteria are necessary for negligence/malpractice to occur?
- How are the standards of care defined and applied?
- Which individuals may give consent for treatment?
- What is the role of the nurse in obtaining consent?

- What is the role of the nurse in situations related to death and dying, employment contracts, and organ and tissue donation?
- How can the nurse minimize his/her liability?
- What situations require reporting by the nurse?
- How is the profession and practice of nursing influenced by legal issues?
- What are some of the legal concerns for nurses working in specialty areas, such as obstetrics?

Study Chart

Create a study chart describing how to Minimize Liability, *identifying the nursing actions to reduce possible liability for the following situations: short staffing, floating, patient occurrences, and reporting/recording.*

5 Ethics

Case Study

1. You are the home care nurse for a 42-year-old male patient, Mr. R., who has severe multiple sclerosis. He tells you on several occasions that he is tired of living this way, not being able to do anything for himself. Mr. R. says that he has read about individuals who have been "helped to die," and he asks if you can assist him in finding out more about this procedure.
   a. Apply the steps for processing an ethical dilemma to this situation.
   b. What is the role of the nurse in this situation?

Chapter Review

Match the description/definition in Column A with the correct term in Column B.

	Column A	Column B
______	1. Supporting the patient's right to informed consent	a. Ethics
______	2. Considering the patient's best interest	b. Fidelity
______	3. Avoiding deliberate harm	c. Justice
______	4. Keeping promises	d. Morals
______	5. Determining the order in which patients should be treated	e. Bioethics
______	6. Consideration of standards of conduct	f. Autonomy
______	7. Ethics within the field of health care	g. Beneficence
______	8. udgment about behavior	h. Accountability
______	9. Personal beliefs about the worth held for an idea or object	i. Nonmaleficence
		j. Values

Complete the following:

10. In accordance with the Health Insurance Portability and Accountability Act of 1996 (HIPAA), access to a patient's medical record by a family member requires:

11. One of the major factors contributing to the nursing shortage today is:

12. Identify an end-of-life issue that has ethical implications for nurses.

13. Identify the ethical theory for each of the following descriptions:
    a. Proposes that actions are right or wrong based on the essence of right and wrong in the principles of fidelity, truthfulness, and justice.
    b. Discusses how ethical decisions affect women.
    c. Proposes that the value of something is based on its usefulness.

d. Discusses nursing, gender, and ethical dilemmas.

14. For the following areas, provide a specific example of how ethical concerns may be involved:
    a. Cost containment

    b. Cultural sensitivity

Select the best answer for each of the following questions:

15. A professional code of ethics includes:
    1. Legal standards for practice
    2. Extensive details on moral principles
    3. Guidelines for approaching common ethical dilemmas
    4. A collective statement of group expectations for behavior
16. By administering medication to a patient on a unit in an extended care facility, the nurse is applying the ethical principle of:
    1. Justice
    2. Fidelity
    3. Autonomy
    4. Beneficence
17. The nurse has been working with a patient who has had abdominal surgery. The patient is experiencing discomfort and has been calling for assistance quite often. The ethical principle of fidelity is demonstrated when the nurse:
    1. Changes the dressing
    2. Provides a warm lotion back rub
    3. Informs the patient of the actions of the medications administered
    4. Returns to assist the patient with breathing exercises at the agreed-upon times
18. The student nurse is assigned to work with parents who refuse to have essential medical treatment provided to their child. The medical center is pursuing a court order to force the family to accept the treatment plan that will assist the child. The nurse has strong feelings for the family's position, as well as the importance of the medical treatment. The first step for the nurse to take in attempting to resolve this ethical dilemma is to:
    1. Examine personal values
    2. Evaluate the outcomes
    3. Gather all of the facts
    4. Verbalize the problem
19. Application of the deontological ethical theory is illustrated by the following nurse's statement:
    1. "It would never be right to stop providing feedings to a patient."
    2. "I believe that the client was cured because of a divine intervention."
    3. "The loss of his leg in the accident has helped this patient to become a stronger person."
    4. "The surgery did not eliminate the client's problem entirely, but it has helped to reduce the level of discomfort."
20. An example of accountability in nursing practice is:
    1. Documenting care
    2. Giving medication to a patient
    3. Assessing the patient's comfort level
    4. Completing an incident report
21. The last phase in the processing of an ethical dilemma is to:
    1. Evaluate the action taken
    2. Consider treatment options
    3. Negotiate the options and outcomes
    4. Identify the problem

Study Group Questions

- What are ethics and what is the purpose of a code of ethics in a profession?
- What principles are promoted in a profession?
- How can the nurse be a patient advocate?
- What are the basic standards of ethics?
- What are values and how are they developed?
- How do values relate to ethics?

- How does the professional determine that an ethical dilemma exists?
- What are the steps for processing an ethical dilemma?
- What ethical dilemmas may arise in health care and nursing practice?

Study Chart

Create a study chart to identify and compare Responsibility, Accountability, Confidentiality, Competence, Judgment, and Advocacy, *providing examples of nursing behaviors for each.*

Critical Thinking and Nursing Judgment 6

Case Study

1. You are the home care nurse and have been assigned to visit a patient who requires dressing changes for a foot ulceration. When you arrive in the home, you identify that the patient does not have any commercially packaged dressings or saline solution. You have used the last of your supplies and the drive back to the office will take more than 1 hour. The dressing that the patient has on her foot is saturated with purulent drainage.
   a. What options are available to you in this situation?
   b. What further investigation about the patient and her living situation may be necessary?

Chapter Review

Match the description/definition in Column A with the correct term in Column B.

	Column A	Column B
______	1. Process of recalling an event to determine its meaning and purpose	a. Scientific method
______	2. Series of clinical judgments that result in informal or formal diagnoses	b. Decision making
______	3. End point of critical thinking that leads to problem resolution	c. Inference
______	4. Significance or meaning of findings in relation to one another	d. Diagnostic reasoning
______	5. Process that moves from observable facts from an experience to a reasonable explanation of those facts	e. Reflection
		f. Intuition

Complete the following:

6. Identify one example of how critical thinking is used in each step of the nursing process:
   a. Assessment
   b. Nursing diagnosis
   c. Planning
   d. Implementation
   e. Evaluation

7. Identify the level of critical thinking demonstrated by each of the following:
   a. Trusts experts to have the right answers for every problem
   b. Analyzes and examines problems more independently
   c. Makes choices without assistance and accepts accountability

8. Identify the attitude of critical thinking demonstrated for each of the following:
   a. Performing a skill safely and effectively
   b. Questioning an order that appears incorrect
   c. Performing a systematic and thorough pain assessment
   d. Developing a unique way to teach the patient how to change a dressing
   e. Admitting to the nurse manager that a medication was given in error

Select the best answer for each of the following questions:

9. In employing critical thinking, the first step that the nurse should use is:
   1. Evaluation
   2. Decision making
   3. Self-regulation
   4. Interpretation
10. Having worked for a number of years in the acute care environment, the nurse has achieved an ability to use a complex level of critical thinking. The nurse:
    1. Acts solely on his or her own opinions
    2. Trusts the experts to have the answers to problems
    3. Implements creative and innovative options
    4. Applies rules and principles the same way in every situation
11. Clinical care experiences have recently begun for the student nurse. When beginning to work with patients, the student nurse implements critical thinking in practice by:
    1. Asking for assistance if uncertain
    2. Sharing personal ideas with peers
    3. Acting on independent judgments
    4. Relying on standardized, textbook approaches
12. The nurse has an extremely large patient assignment this evening and begins to feel overwhelmed. The priority activity, based on the following choices, is for the nurse to:
    1. Share his or her feelings with colleagues
    2. Call the supervisor and ask for assistance
    3. Review the overall assignment to get his or her bearings
    4. Move right into patient care, starting with the room closest to the nurse's station
13. Orientation for the new nurses has begun. The instructor for the orientation is assembling information on critical thinking and nursing approaches. The instructor recognizes that critical thinkers in nursing:
    1. Make quick, single-solution decisions
    2. Act on intuition instead of experience
    3. Review data in a disciplined manner
    4. Alter interventions for every circumstance
14. The nurse is caring for a patient who is experiencing a respiratory disorder. Intuition is a part of the critical thinking process for the nurse. While caring for the patient, the nurse demonstrates intuition by:
    1. Reviewing the care with the patient in advance
    2. Observing communication patterns
    3. Establishing a nursing diagnosis
    4. Sensing that the patient is not doing as well this morning
15. Upon entering the room at 2:00 AM, the nurse notes that the patient is not in bed; instead the patient is sitting in the chair and states that she is having difficulty sleeping. Employing critical thinking, the nurse responds by:
    1. Assisting the patient back into bed

2. Determining more about the patient's sleep problem
3. Positioning the patient and providing a warm blanket
4. Obtaining an order for a hypnotic medication

16. The nurse has a diverse patient assignment this evening. When reviewing the patients' conditions, the nurse determines that the first individual that should be seen is:
    1. The patient who is hypotensive
    2. The patient receiving a visit from a family member
    3. The patient being treated by the respiratory therapist
    4. The patent waiting for the effects of an analgesic that was given 5 minutes ago
17. In using the critical thinking skill of self-regulation, the nurse will:
    1. Be orderly in data collection
    2. Look at all situations objectively
    3. Use scientific and experiential knowledge
    4. Reflect on his or her own experiences and improve performance
18. The question that the nurse asks himself or herself specifically in the process of reflection is the following:
    1. "What could I have done differently?"
    2. "What's going on right now?"
    3. "How can the patient's status change?"
    4. "What should I do to communicate this information?"
19. The nurse personally believes that substance abuse is a serious problem with negative consequences for patients and families. The nurse, however, provides excellent care to the patient who is admitted with this problem. The nurse is displaying the critical thinking attitude of:
    1. Integrity
    2. Fairness
    3. Discipline
    4. Perseverance

Study Group Questions

- How is critical thinking integrated into nursing practice?
- What attitudes are needed by the nurse in order to be a critical thinker?
- How are the competencies of critical thinking applied in clinical practice?
- Why is critical thinking important throughout the nursing process?

7 Nursing Process

Case Studies

1. Mr. B., a 47-year-old male patient, has come to the annual community health fair. During a routine blood pressure screening, it is determined that his blood pressure is significantly above normally expected levels.
   a. What additional assessment data should be obtained from the patient and family?
   b. What limitations exist in this situation for completing an assessment?
2. Mr. B. returns for a follow-up visit at the medical center's adult health clinic. Mr. B. is diagnosed with hypertension and an antihypertensive medication is prescribed, but he appears unsure about how and when he should take the prescription. Mr. B. also identifies that his father died from a heart attack at 54 years of age.
   a. Identify the relevant assessment data for this patient.
   b. Based upon this information, identify two nursing diagnoses.
3. During Mr. B.'s appointment at the adult health clinic, he was found to have high blood pressure, and antihypertensive medication was prescribed. Mr. B. did not have any prior knowledge of or experience with either hypertension or hypertensive medication. In addition, it was found that Mr. B.'s father died at age 54 of a heart attack.
   a. Based on the nursing diagnoses that were developed, identify one long-term or short-term goal for each diagnosis and at least one expected outcome for each goal.

Nursing diagnoses	Long-term or short-term goals	Expected outcomes
1.		
2.		

   b. Identify two nursing interventions that may be appropriate in assisting the patient to achieve the expected outcomes and goals.
4. At his next visit to the adult health clinic, Mr. B. tells the nurse that he is taking the antihypertensive medication that was ordered by the physician "when he remembers." He says that he is trying to use the relaxation techniques that he was taught during his last visit, but he does not use them regularly.
   a. What nursing implementation methods should take priority at this time?
   b. What, if any, alterations need to be made in the original plan of care designed with Mr. B.?
5. Mr. B. returns to the adult health clinic for evaluation of his status. His blood pressure is lower than before, but remains slightly above normal limits. He exercises once or twice a week, and states that this is making him feel better. Mr. B. shows the nurse a calendar where he has marked down the times for taking his medication. Mr. B. relates that he has been trying very hard to use the relaxation techniques when he starts to feel anxious or overwhelmed. He identifies that he cannot control all of his "destiny," but he is going to try to do things that may help him to avoid what happened to his father.
   a. In accordance with previously identified outcomes, what nursing evaluation may be made on this patient's status?
   b. What areas, if any, may require reassessment?

Chapter Review

Match the description/definition in Column A with the correct term in Column B.

	Column A	Column B
________	1. Unintended effect of a medication, diagnostic test, or intervention	a. Subjective data
________	2. Observations or measurements made by the nurse during assessment	b. ADLs
________	3. Comparing data with another source to determine accuracy and relevancy	c. Concept map
________	4. Multidisciplinary, outcome-based care plan	d. Critical pathway
________	5. Clinical judgment about patient responses to health problems or life processes	e. Nursing diagnosis
________	6. Information obtained through the senses	f. Cue
________	7. Activities performed in the course of a normal day	g. Objective data
________	8. Support for why a specific nursing action is chosen	h. Scientific rationale
________	9. Interpretation of cues	i. Inference
________	10. Information provided by the patient verbally	j. Validation
		k. Adverse reaction

Complete the following:

11. The three phases of an interview are:

12. Identify at least one goal, one expected outcome, and one nursing intervention for the following nursing diagnoses:
    a. *Deficient knowledge related to the need for postoperative care at home*
       Goal:
       Expected outcome:
       Nursing intervention:
    b. *Constipation related to lack of physical activity*
       Goal:
       Expected outcome:
       Nursing intervention:

13. Identify whether the following are examples of *cognitive*, *interpersonal*, or *psychomotor* skills in patient care:
    a. Preparing and administering an injection
    b. Completing a health history
    c. Providing emotional support to a family member
    d. Changing a surgical dressing
    e. Recognizing the patient's need for nutritional instruction

14. Before implementing standing orders, the nurse should check:

15. Based on the following data clusters, identify possible nursing diagnoses:
    a. Abdominal pain, three loose liquid stools per day, hyperactive bowel sounds:
    b. Fatigue, weakness, tachycardia upon activity, exertional dyspnea:

16. The steps of the implementation phase of the nursing process are:

17. During interactions with the patient, the nurse gathers more data and identifies a new patient need. The nurse should:

18. A patient with diabetes mellitus comes to the outpatient center for care. There is a written plan for diet counseling, medication, and follow-up care. These specific procedures are termed a _______________ for care.
19. An example of an indirect nursing intervention is:

20. Identify all of the following that may usually be delegated to unlicensed assistive personnel:
    a. Skin care _______
    b. Tracheostomy care _______
    c. Hygienic care _______
    d. Personal grooming _______
    e. Urinary catheterization _______
    f. Administration of IV medications _______
    g. Assistance with ambulation _______
21. Specify how the following patient outcomes may be improved:
    a. Erythema will be less noticeable
    b. Pulse rate will be normal
    c. Patient's calorie intake will increase

Select the best answer for each of the following questions:

22. The new graduate is preparing to work with patients on the medical unit. The nursing process is applied as a:
    1. Method for processing the care of many patients
    2. Tool for diagnosing and treating patients' health problems
    3. Guideline for determining the nurse's accountability in patient care
    4. Logical, problem-solving approach to providing patient care
23. Upon admission, the nurse begins to assess the patient. The patient appears uncomfortable, stating that she has severe abdominal pain. The nurse should:
    1. Inquire specifically about the discomfort
    2. Let the patient rest, returning later to complete the assessment
    3. Perform a complete physical examination immediately
    4. Ask the family about the patient's health history
24. The following nursing diagnoses are proposed for patients on the medical unit. The diagnostic statement that contains all of the necessary components is:
    1. *Impaired gas exchange related to accumulation of lung secretions*
    2. *Imbalanced nutrition related to chemotherapy treatment*
    3. *Ineffective grieving process*
    4. *Pain related to abdominal surgery*
25. The nurse is working with patients who come to the community center for health screenings and educational sessions. An example of a wellness nursing diagnosis label that is appropriate for this group is:
    1. *Risk for impaired skin integrity*
    2. *Readiness for enhanced family coping*
    3. *Altered parent/infant attachment*
    4. *Fluid volume deficit*

26. In reviewing the nursing diagnoses written by the new staff member, the supervisor identifies the correctly written nursing diagnosis as:
    1. *Altered respiratory function related to abnormal blood gases*
    2. *Urinary infection related to long-term catheterization*
    3. *Deficient knowledge related to need for cardiac monitoring*
    4. *Pain related to severe arthritis in finger joints*
27. The nurse is working with a patient who has the following symptoms: dyspnea, ankle edema, weight gain, abdominal distention, hypertension. The nursing diagnosis that is most appropriate for these signs and symptoms is:
    1. *Ineffective tissue perfusion*
    2. *Disturbed body image*
    3. *Impaired gas exchange*
    4. *Excess fluid volume*
28. A patient is to have abdominal surgery tomorrow. The nurse determines that an outcome for this patient that meets the necessary criteria is:
    1. Patient will be positioned every 2 hours
    2. Patient will express fears about surgery
    3. Patient will achieve normal elimination pattern before discharge
    4. Patient will perform active range-of-motion exercises every 2 hours while in bed
29. There are a number of activities that are to be performed by the nurse during the clinical shift. In deciding to perform a nurse-initiated intervention, the nurse:
    1. Administers oral medications
    2. Orders laboratory tests
    3. Changes a sterile dressing
    4. Teaches newborn hygienic care
30. The nurse is implementing a preventive nursing action when:
    1. Immunizing patients
    2. Assisting with hygienic care
    3. Inserting a urinary catheter
    4. Providing crisis intervention counseling
31. The nurse has been working with the patient in the rehabilitative facility for 2 weeks. The nurse is in the process of evaluating the patient's progress. During the evaluation phase, the nurse recognizes that:
    1. Nursing diagnoses always remain the same
    2. Time frames for patient outcomes may be adjusted
    3. Evaluative skills differ greatly from those for patient assessment
    4. The number of nursing diagnoses and outcomes is most important
32. An expected outcome for a patient is the following: "Pulse will remain below 120 beats/minute during exercise." If the patient's pulse rate exceeds 120 beats per minute one out of every three exercise periods, the nurse appropriately evaluates the patient's goal attainment as:
    1. Patient has achieved desired behavior
    2. Patient requires further evaluation of progress
    3. Patient's response indicates need for elimination of exercise
    4. Patient does not comply with therapeutic regimen
33. The nurse is caring for a patient who has been medically stable. During the change-of-shift report, the nurse is informed that the patient is experiencing a slight arrhythmia. To avoid complications during the implementation of care, the nurse plans to:
    1. Evaluate the patient's vital signs
    2. Ask about the patient's prior diagnoses
    3. Contact the physician immediately
    4. Tell the nursing assistant to perform the usual care for the patient
34. For a patient in the acute care facility, the nurse identifies several interventions. The statement that best communicates the activity of the nurse is:
    1. Assist with range-of-motion exercises
    2. Take the patient's vital signs
    3. Refer the patient to a physical therapist
    4. Provide 30 ml of water with the nasogastric tube feedings every 4 hours

35. The nurse is working with a patient who has diabetes mellitus. The nursing diagnosis that the nurse identifies is: *Deficient volume fluid related to osmotic diuresis.* An appropriate patient outcome, based on this nursing diagnosis, is:
    1. Patient will have an increased urinary output
    2. Patient will decrease the amount of fluid intake over 24 hours
    3. Patient will demonstrate a decrease in edema in the lower extremities
    4. Patient will have palpable peripheral pulses and good capillary refill
36. The nurse is working with a patient who is experiencing abnormal breath sounds and thick secretions. The nurse identifies a nursing diagnosis of:
    1. *Deficient fluid volume*
    2. *Ineffective airway clearance*
    3. *Risk for altered mucous membranes*
    4. *Dysfunctional ventilatory weaning response*
37. In completing a health history, the nurse obtains psychosocial information from the patient that includes the:
    1. Reason for seeking health care
    2. Past health problems
    3. Primary language spoken
    4. Physical safety status
38. The patient tells the nurse that she feels she may not be using the crutches correctly when ambulating. The best way for the nurse to validate this information is to:
    1. Ask the family about the patient's ambulation
    2. Ask the physician how the patient was taught
    3. Discuss the problem with the other staff members
    4. Observe the patient using the crutches
39. An example of the most appropriately written nursing diagnosis is:
    1. *Acute pain related to surgery*
    2. *Shortness of breath related to immobility*
    3. *Anxiety related to lack of knowledge about cardiac monitoring*
    4. *Recurrent infection related to improper catheterization procedure*
40. In determining which one of the following patients on the medical unit to visit first, the nurse selects the patient with which one of the following diagnoses?
    1. *Imbalanced nutrition: less than body requirements*
    2. *Ineffective tissue perfusion*
    3. *Deficient knowledge regarding home care resources*
    4. *Impaired physical mobility*
41. An example of a physician-initiated intervention is:
    1. Teaching the patient about the therapeutic diet
    2. Assessing the patient's skin
    3. Providing emotional support
    4. Preparing the patient for a diagnostic test

Study Group Questions

- What is involved in patient assessment, and what priorities does the nurse have in completing an assessment?
- How does the patient assessment fit into the nursing process?
- Why does an error in the assessment phase influence the remaining implementation of the process, and how may the nurse avoid errors?
- What methods may be used to obtain patient data and what type of data is obtained with each method?
- What is involved in a patient interview?
- How may the nurse optimize the environment for a patient interview?
- How may the nurse use different communication strategies to obtain data during patient assessment?
- What is a nursing diagnosis?
- What are the components of a nursing diagnosis?
- How are actual and potential nursing diagnoses different?
- How are medical and nursing diagnoses different?
- What errors are possible in formulating nursing diagnoses, and how may they be avoided?
- Which nursing diagnoses become priorities in planning patient care?

- How are long-term and short-term goals different from one another?
- How are goals and expected outcomes different from one another?
- What are the guidelines for formulating goals and outcomes?
- In selecting nursing interventions, what are three essential nurse competencies?
- How are the three types of nursing interventions different from one another?
- What factors should be considered when selecting nursing interventions?
- What is the purpose of the care plan, and what types are available for use?
- How does the critical pathway differ from the "traditional" care plan?
- How does the consultation process begin, and who and what may be involved in the process?
- What is the focus of the implementation phase of the nursing process?
- What are standing orders and protocols, and how are they used in patient care situations?
- What are the five preparatory nursing activities that are completed before implementing the care plan?
- What are the nursing implementation methods?
- How is nursing implementation communicated to other members of the health care team?
- How is evaluation incorporated into the nursing process?
- How is evaluation used in patient situations, and in nursing practice and health care delivery settings?
- What circumstances would lead to a modification of the care plan?

Study Chart

Create a study chart to compare the Steps of the Nursing Process, *identifying the different activities involved in each step.*

8 Documentation and Reporting

Case Studies

1. Mrs. Q. has just been transferred to her room from the post-anesthesia care unit (PACU) following right hip replacement surgery. She was accompanied by a nurse from PACU. Vital signs were taken upon transfer and found to be within expected limits. A dressing is in place on the patient's right hip. Mrs. Q. does not appear to be having any difficulty at the moment.
   a. What information should be provided by the PACU nurse to the primary nurse on the surgical unit when Mrs. Q. is transferred to her room?
   b. What additional information may Mrs. Q.'s primary nurse want to obtain from the PACU nurse?
2. The primary nurse begins to plan and provide care for Mrs. Q. Upon entering the patient's room, Mrs. Q. is found to be grimacing and moaning in pain. She says that she is having intense pain in her right hip area. The dressing to her hip is dry and intact. Mrs. Q. says that she does not want to move because it really hurts. The primary nurse helps Mrs. Q. to get into a more comfortable position, and begins to prepare the pain medication ordered by the physician. The primary nurse administers the pain medication, and after about one-half hour, Mrs. Q. states that the pain has been reduced. Using SOAP or DAR methods, document the nursing interaction with Mrs. Q.

Chapter Review

Match the description/definition in Column A with the correct term in Column B.

	Column A	Column B
______	1. An oral or written exchange of information between health care providers	a. Record
______	2. Information about patients only provided to appropriate personnel	b. POMR
______	3. Permanent written communication with patients' health care management	c. Acuity recording
______	4. Structured method of documentation with emphasis on the patient's problems	d. Report
______	5. Documentation that requires staff to identify interventions and allows patients to be compared to one another	e. Confidentiality

Complete the following:

6. The following are guidelines for documentation. Indicate the correct action to be taken by the nurse for each guideline.
   a. Never erase entries or use correction fluid, and never use pencil.
   b. Do not write retaliatory or critical comments about patients.
   c. Avoid using generalized, empty phrases.
   d. Do not scratch out errors.
   e. Do not leave blank spaces.
   f. Do not speculate or guess.
   g. Do not record "physician made error."
   h. Never chart for someone else.
   i. Do not wait until the end of shift to record important information.
7. HIPAA (Health Insurance Portability and Accountability Act of 1996) has new regulations that require written consent for disclosure of all patient information.
   True _____ False _____
8. Standards for health care agencies and documentation are set by the:
9. For each of the following, identify an example of how the patient record is used:
   a. Communication:
   b. Financial:
   c. Educational:
   d. Research:
   e. Auditing/monitoring:
10. Provide an example of a malpractice issue related to charting:
11. The best time for the nurse to complete patient documentation is:
12. Subjective statements made by the patient are best documented by:
13. Demonstrate how a student nurse should sign a written patient record:
14. Identify what is wrong with the following notations and how they can be corrected:
    a. "Ate some breakfast."
    b. "Voided an adequate amount."

15. Identify the information that should be included in the patient record for teaching instructions on self-injection of insulin:

16. Provide two items that should be included in a discharge summary:

17. Home care documentation is completed both for quality control and as the basis for:

18. Completion of narrative notes only when there are abnormal patient findings is part of the concept of:

Select the best answer for each of the following questions:

19. The nurse is working in a facility that uses computerized documentation of patient information. To maintain patient confidentiality with the use of computerized documentation, nurses should:
    1. Delete any and all errors made in the record
    2. Only give their password to other nurses working with the patient
    3. Log off of the file or computer when not using the terminal
    4. Remove sensitive patient information, such as communicable diseases, from the record
20. The nurses on the medical unit in an acute care facility are meeting to select a documentation format to use. They recognize that there will be less fragmentation of patient data if they implement:
    1. Source records
    2. Focus charting
    3. Charting by exception
    4. Clinical pathways
21. While caring for a patient on the surgical unit, the nurse notes that the patient's blood pressure has dropped significantly since the last measurement. The nurse shares this information immediately with the health care provider in a(n):
    1. Flow sheet record
    2. Incident report
    3. Telephone report
    4. Change-of-shift report
22. Documentation of patient care is reviewed during the orientation to the facility. The new graduate nurse understands that the method for written documentation that is acceptable is:
    1. Using red ink to chart patient entries
    2. Charting all of the patient care at the end of the shift
    3. Beginning each entry with the time of the treatment or observation
    4. Leaving space at the end of the notations to allow for additional documentation
23. The nurse has been very busy during the shift trying to get all of the patient care activities completed. While documenting one of the patient's responses to a pain medication, the nurse mistakenly writes on the wrong patient's chart. The nurse:
    1. Notes the error at the bottom of the page
    2. Erases the error and completes the entry on the correct chart
    3. Uses a dark color marker to completely cover the error
    4. Draws a straight line through the note and initials the error
24. The nurse is caring for a patient who has had abdominal surgery. Accurate and complete documentation of the care provided by the nurse is evident by the following notation:
    1. "Vital signs taken."
    2. "Tylenol with codeine given for pain."
    3. "Provided adequate amount of fluid."
    4. "IV fluids increased to 100 ml/hr according to protocol."
25. The nurse has been involved in patient care in an agency that uses military time

for documentation. Which of the following represents 4:00 PM?
1. 0400
2. 0800
3. 1400
4. 1600

26. The nurse would **not** expect to find which one of the following in a problem-oriented medical record?
1. Progress notes
2. Narrative notes
3. SOAP notes
4. PIE notes

27. An appropriate action by the student nurse is demonstrated by:
1. Accessing records of other students' patients
2. Writing the patient's name and room number on assignments
3. Copying patient records for review and preparation of care plans
4. Reading the patient's record in preparation for clinical care

28. The nurse enters the patient's room and discovers a yellow pill on the bed under the patient's pillow. The patient receives Lasix 40 mg daily. Which one of the following notations is appropriate to include on an incident or occurrence report?
1. "Patient refused to take Lasix at 10 AM."
2. "Yellow pill found on bed under pillow."
3. "Lasix not administered by primary nurse."
4. "Patient did not receive 10 AM diuretic."

29. Which one of the following statements made by the new staff nurse during change-of-shift report requires correction?
1. "The patient is uncooperative about doing his stoma care."
2. "Oxygen is needed after ambulation. This is a change in priorities."
3. "Ms. Q is a 62-year-old with diabetes mellitus."
4. "The abdominal surgical wound is healing slowly, with no drainage noted."

Study Group Questions

- What is the purpose of documentation and reporting?
- What are the legal guidelines for documentation?
- How do the guidelines influence nursing documentation and reporting?
- What methods are available for documentation of patient data?
- How do the different types of documentation (for example, SOAP, DAR, and narrative) compare to one another?
- How does written documentation compare to computerized systems, and what are the advantages and disadvantages of each method?
- What types of forms are used for patient documentation?
- How does patient documentation change in different health care settings?
- What information is necessary when doing change-of-shift, telephone, transfer, and incident reports?

9 Communication

Case Study

1. For the following patient situations, identify the communication techniques that may be most effective in establishing a nurse-patient relationship:
   a. An older adult patient who has a moderate hearing impairment
   b. The Russian-speaking parents of a young child who has been brought into the emergency department after being involved in a bicycle accident
   c. A young adult patient who is blind and requires daily insulin injections
   d. A 60-year-old Hispanic woman who will be having her first internal pelvic examination

Chapter Review

Match the description/definition in Column A with the correct term in Column B.

	Column A	**Column B**
______	1. Person who initiates interpersonal communication	a. Therapeutic communication
______	2. Information sent or expressed by the sender	b. Metacommunication
______	3. Means of conveying messages	c. Sender
______	4. Person to whom the message is sent	d. Intonation
______	5. Indicates whether the meaning of the sender's message was received	e. Feedback
______	6. Motivates one person to communicate with another	f. Connotations
______	7. Shades or interpretations of a word's meaning rather than different definitions	g. Channels
______	8. Tone of the speaker's voice that may affect a message's meaning	h. Message
______	9. A message within a message that conveys a sender's attitude toward the self and toward the listener	i. Receiver
______	10. Development of a working, functional relationship by the nurse with the patient, fulfilling the purposes of the nursing process	j. Referent
		k. Environment

Complete the following:

11. Determine what level of communication the following examples are:
    a. Talking to oneself
    b. "He looks uncomfortable, and I want to show him that I'm concerned about his discomfort."
    c. The ability to speak to consumers on health-related topics

12. Individuals maintain distances between themselves during interactions. Identify the zone (Intimate, Personal, Social, or Public) that is being used in each of the following examples:
    a. Speaking to a group of students in a classroom

b. Conducting a small group therapy session

c. Performing a physical examination

d. Making patient rounds with a physician

e. Changing a wound dressing

f. Testifying at a hearing

g. Completing a change-of-shift report

13. For the older adult with impaired communication, identify all of the appropriate communication techniques:
   a. Maintain a quiet environment that is free of background noise.

   b. Shift from subject to subject during the conversation.

   c. Let the person know if you are having difficulty understanding him or her.

   d. Use explorative questions to facilitate conversation.

   e. Use long sentences to explain subject matter.

14. The following are examples of inappropriate communication by the nurse. Specify which effective strategy is not being used, and how the nurse may correct the situation.
   a. Calling the patient "Honey"

   b. Reporting to a nursing colleague about the "gallbladder in room 214"

   c. Talking about the patient to other nurses in the elevator

   d. Running into the patient's room to administer medications and then leaving immediately

   e. Informing the patient that the physician will be performing an abdominal hysterectomy and she should expect a midline incision of approximately 10 centimeters

15. For the following examples, write a question that the nurse could ask that would be more appropriate and obtain better information from the patient:
   a. "You're feeling okay today, right?"

   b. "You don't take any medication at home, do you?"

   c. "Are you having any lymphedema?"

   d. "The physician will be doing a paracentesis today. He said he explained it to you."

16. Identify the communication strategy that is being used for each of the following examples:
   a. Sitting with a patient who is crying

   b. Showing interest in the patient who is discussing concerns or sharing family information

c. Saying "Go on" or "Tell me more"

d. Asking the patient to verify the meaning of statements made

e. Directing the attention of the patient to a particular idea in the discussion

17. For the nursing diagnosis *Impaired verbal communication related to aphasia,* identify at least two nursing interventions to promote communication with the patient.

18. Nurses on a medical unit are discussing issues related to their work schedules. Identify the examples of positive responses:
    a. "There's nothing we can do about the staffing situation."

    b. "Don't talk to me like that!"

    c. "What do you think we can do to improve this situation?"

    d. "I want to hear what your concerns are."

19. The nurse takes into account the cultural considerations related to touch. Identify the appropriate action(s):
    a. Stroking the head of a Southeast Asian patient

    b. Assigning a female staff member to care for a female Amish patient

20. For the acronym SOLER, identify the skills for attentive listening:
    S:
    O:
    L:
    E:
    R:

Select the best answer for each of the following questions:

21. The patient tells the nurse that he feels anxious and afraid. The nurse responds by saying, "I will stay here with you." The nurse is using the principle of effective communication known as:
    1. Empathy
    2. Courtesy
    3. Availability
    4. Encouragement
22. Mr. J. states that he believes he may have cancer. The nurse tells him, "I wouldn't be concerned Mr. J. I'm sure that the tests will be negative." The response by the nurse demonstrates the use of:
    1. Assertiveness
    2. False reassurance
    3. Professional opinion
    4. Hope and encouragement
23. The nurse is assigned to a young adult male patient. Gender sensitivity is demonstrated when the nurse:
    1. Uses sexual innuendo
    2. Engages in gender-oriented joking
    3. Stereotypes male and female roles
    4. Uses direct and indirect communication according to gender
24. The patient regularly visits the medical clinic. The nurse is establishing a helping relationship with the patient. During the working phase of a helping relationship, the nurse:
    1. Encourages and helps the patient to set goals
    2. Reminisces about the relationship with the patient
    3. Anticipates health concerns or issues
    4. Identifies a location for the interaction
25. The nurse is interviewing a patient who is in the outpatient area. The nurse uses paraphrasing communication with the statement:
    1. "This is your blood pressure medication. It will help to lower your

blood pressure to the level where it should be."
2. "Do you mean that the pain comes and goes when you walk?"
3. "I would like to return to our discussion about your family."
4. "If I understand you correctly, you are primarily concerned about your dizzy spells."

26. The patient tells you that there are other people in the room that are watching her from under the bed. The nurse employs therapeutic communication when he or she:
1. Identifies that there are no people under the bed
2. Tells the patient that he or she will help look for the other people
3. Asks the patient why other people are watching her
4. Reassures the patient that he or she will tell the people to go away

27. While speaking with a female patient, the nurse notes that she is frowning. The nurse wants to find out about possible concerns by:
1. Asking why the patient is unhappy
2. Telling the patient that everything is fine
3. Identifying that the patient is frowning
4. Asking if the patient is angry about the health care problem

28. The patient's condition has deteriorated and he has been transferred to the intensive care unit. The roommate asks the nurse what is wrong with the patient. The nurse should respond to the roommate by stating:
1. "The patient's condition is no concern of yours."
2. "Everything is fine. Don't worry. He'll be okay."
3. "I recognize your interest in the patient, but I cannot share personal information with you without his permission."
4. "Your roommate's condition worsened overnight and he had to be moved to the intensive care unit for observation."

29. The patient is experiencing aphasia as a result of a CVA (cerebral vascular accident, or stroke). To promote communication, the nurse plans to:
1. Speak louder
2. Use more questions
3. Use visual clues, such as pictures and gestures
4. Refer to a speech therapist to communicate with the patient

30. The patient is talking endlessly about problems in the past with arthritic pain, but the nurse needs to get specific information for the admission assessment. The nurse's best response is:
1. "You seem to have had difficulty managing the arthritis. What are you doing now for the pain?"
2. "You can tell me more at another time. We need to move on to other information now."
3. "You've given me a lot of information, but I have to ask you something else."
4. "Are you taking medication for the arthritis?"

31. The nurse enters the room and finds the patient crying. The best action by the nurse is to:
1. Ask the patient why he or she is crying
2. Tell the patient that things will get better
3. Let the patient know that you will come back later
4. Sit quietly with the patient

32. The patient has a visual impairment. In communicating with this patient, the nurse should:
1. Use flash cards
2. Use simple sentences
3. Caution the patient before any physical contact
4. Speak very loud and slow

33. The nurse tells the patient's family that recovery may be "difficult." This may lead to an issue with:
1. Pacing
2. Clarity
3. Relevance
4. Connotation

34. A cultural group that may perceive continuous eye contact as intrusive or threatening is:
    1. Asian
    2. Hispanic
    3. African American
    4. Northern European
35. The nurse is working with a preschool-age child. An appropriate communication technique to use with an individual in this age-group is to:
    1. Speak loudly and forcibly
    2. Communicate directly with the parents to determine the child's needs
    3. Sit or kneel down to be on the same level as the child
    4. Use medical terms when speaking with the parents so the child will not understand
36. The patient's blood sample was dropped on its way to the lab. The patient asks the nurse why blood needs to be drawn again for the same test. The nurse's best response is:
    1. "One of the vials was dropped and broken by mistake. We will make sure that this sample gets to the lab safely."
    2. "We just have to do the test again."
    3. "Someone didn't do their job right the first time."
    4. "This kind of thing happens. It won't take long."
37. The nurse is evaluating the communication skills used during an interaction with a newly admitted patient. Of all of the statements made, the nurse responded therapeutically with:
    1. "Why aren't you able to keep taking the prescribed medications?"
    2. "We need to move quickly through the rest of the interview because it will be time for your therapy."
    3. "I can understand why you don't like that physician. I think you need to find another one."
    4. "I noticed that you didn't eat any of the lunch. Is there something that is bothering you?"

Study Group Questions

- What is therapeutic communication?
- What are the basic elements of communication?
- How do nurses and patients communicate verbally and nonverbally?
- What factors may influence communication?
- How may a patient's physical, psychosocial, and developmental status influence communication with the nurse?
- How is a helping relationship established with a patient?
- What are the principles/techniques of effective communication?
- How are the principles/techniques used by the nurse in a caring relationship?
- How is communication used within the steps of the nursing process?
- What are some of the barriers to effective communication and how may they be overcome by the nurse?

Study Chart

Create a study chart to compare the Components of Verbal and Nonverbal Communication, *identifying how each one may influence the nurse-patient interaction (e.g., intonation).*

Patient Education 10

Case Study

1. Your patient is Ms. T., a 47-year-old married woman who has come to the medical clinic for evaluation. She has been diagnosed with hypertension and placed on an antihypertensive medication. Ms. T. has no prior knowledge or experience with the diagnosis or the medication. There is a family history of coronary disease, as her father died of a heart attack at 54 years of age.
   a. What information about Ms. T. may affect her motivation to learn?
   b. Formulate a teaching plan for Ms. T., including goals and teaching strategies.

Chapter Review

Match the description/definition in Column A with the correct term in Column B.

	Column A	*Column B*
________	1. Expression of feelings, attitudes, opinions, and values	a. Cognitive learning
________	2. Mental state that allows for focus and comprehension of material	b. Motivation
________	3. Acquiring skills	c. Attentional set
________	4. Intellectual behaviors, including knowledge and understanding	d. Affective learning
________	5. Desire to learn	e. Return demonstration
		f. Psychomotor learning

Complete the following:

6. Part of the Joint Commission on Accreditation of Healthcare Organizations (JCAHO) standards is determination of the academic educational needs of children in health care facilities.
   True _____ False _____
7. From the following, select the appropriate topics for health education related to *Health maintenance and promotion and Illness prevention:*
   a. First aid _______
   b. Occupational therapy _______
   c. Implications of noncompliance with therapy _______
   d. Hygiene _______
   e. Origin of symptoms _______
   f. Immunizations _______
   g. Self-help devices _______
   h. Surgical intervention _______
8. Teaching activities for an infant include:

9. The learner may find it difficult to concentrate in the presence of:

10. When selecting an environment for teaching, the nurse needs to consider:

11. Written materials used for patient teaching are usually presented at the ____________ grade level.
12. Teaching sessions that are usually tolerated best last for _______ minutes. In planning the teaching session, essential information should be taught: ________________

13. For the nursing diagnosis *Noncompliance with medication regimen related to insufficient knowledge of purpose and actions*, identify possible learning goals and outcomes, and nursing interventions.

14. For the following, identify the domain of learning:
    a. Self-injection of insulin
    b. Coping with care of a family member
    c. Complications to be aware of after a heart attack
    d. Response of the family to a member's substance abuse
    e. Sterile dressing technique
    f. Signs and symptoms of hypoglycemia

15. Identify an instructional technique that may be used in each of the following situations:
    a. A small group of patients in a cardiac rehabilitation group who need dietary information
    b. A patient with a leg cast who will be using crutches
    c. Students learning therapeutic communication skills to be used on a mental health unit

16. Explaining how a test will feel before the procedure is performed is an example of:

17. According to national reports, almost _____% of adults in the United States have difficulty reading and understanding health information.

Select the best answer for each of the following questions:

18. The nurse is preparing to teach a group of new parents about infant care. The nurse recognizes that learning can be enhanced with a:
    1. Prior unfamiliarity with the topic area
    2. Fear of health outcomes
    3. Moderate discomfort
    4. Mild anxiety level
19. The patient who most likely has the greatest motivation to learn is the individual who is:
    1. Waiting for the results of diagnostic tests
    2. Hypertensive, but has no symptoms
    3. Dealing with a family conflict
    4. Recovering from reconstructive surgery
20. While preparing a teaching plan for a group of patients with diabetes, the nurse integrates the basic principle of education that:
    1. Material should progress from complex to simpler ideas
    2. Prolonged teaching sessions improve concentration and attentiveness
    3. Learning is improved when more than one body sense is stimulated
    4. Prior knowledge of a topic area interferes with the acquisition of new information
21. During a teaching session for a patient with heart disease, the nurse uses reinforcement to stimulate learning. An example of reinforcement for this patient is:
    1. Allowing the patient to manage self-care needs
    2. Teaching about the disease process while delivering nursing care
    3. Outlining the exercise plan and providing explicit instructions

4. Complimenting the patient on his or her ability to identify the action of prescribed medications

22. After about 20 minutes have passed in the educational session, the nurse notices that the patient is slightly slumped over in the chair and is no longer maintaining eye contact. The nurse should:
    1. Reposition the patient in the chair
    2. Move the patient to a cooler, brighter room
    3. Reschedule the remainder of the teaching for another time
    4. Continue with the teaching session in order to cover the necessary content

23. When preparing to teach the self-injection technique to a patient, the nurse begins with:
    1. Having the patient demonstrate the procedure
    2. Discussing the procedure and the equipment used
    3. Providing written materials and having the patient practice the technique
    4. Demonstrating to the patient how to perform the procedure correctly

24. After teaching the patient about a cerebral vascular accident (CVA/stroke), the nurse prepares to evaluate the patient's psychomotor domain of learning. This is accomplished by:
    1. Observing the patient use a cane to ambulate
    2. Asking the patient about the basic etiology of a stroke
    3. Determining the patient's attitudes about the treatment regimen
    4. Having the patient complete a written schedule for daily activities at home

25. When the teaching session has been completed, the nurse evaluates the patient's cognitive domain of learning to see if there are areas that require additional instruction. The nurse evaluates the patient's ability to:
    1. Perform the range-of-motion exercises independently
    2. Identify the equipment necessary for surgical wound care
    3. Demonstrate the proper use of crutches to ambulate up and down stairs
    4. Discuss concerns about the difficulty in maintaining accurate records of the treatments

26. Which patient appears to be demonstrating the greatest readiness to learn? The patient who says:
    1. "There's nothing wrong with me."
    2. "I think the doctor made a mistake."
    3. "I can manage on my own."
    4. "What do I need to know about this?"

27. A type of reinforcer that works well with children is:
    1. Material
    2. Social
    3. Activity
    4. Negative

28. The nurse recognizes that the most effective teaching strategy for the patient in the acceptance stage is to:
    1. Share small bits of information
    2. Introduce only reality
    3. Provide simple explanations while doing care
    4. Focus on future skills and knowledge

Study Group Questions

- What are the standards (e.g., JCAHO) for patient education?
- How does patient education promote, maintain, and restore health?
- What are the principles of teaching and learning?
- What factors may influence a patient's ability to learn?
- How does an individual's developmental status influence the selection of teaching methodologies?
- How does the teaching process compare with the communication and nursing processes?
- How does the nurse develop a teaching plan for a patient?
- What teaching approaches and instructional methods may be used by the nurse?
- How is patient education documented?

11 Infection Control

Case Studies

1. Your patient is an 86-year-old woman in an extended care facility. She has a urinary catheter attached to a drainage system.
   a. What precautions should be taken for this patient to prevent a urinary tract infection?
2. The patient is a 45-year-old man who had abdominal surgery yesterday. He has a large midline abdominal incision covered by a sterile dressing. He will require dressing changes twice daily.
   a. What precautions should be taken for this patient to prevent wound infection?

Chapter Review

Match the description/definition in Column A with the correct term in Column B.

	Column A	*Column B*
______	1. Arises from microorganisms outside of the patient	a. Exudate
______	2. Cellular response to injury or infection	b. Aseptic technique
______	3. Microorganisms that cause another infection because they are resistant to antibiotics	c. Health care–associated infection
______	4. Infection developed that was not present at the time of patient admission	d. Sterilization
______	5. Methods to reduce or eliminate disease-producing microorganisms	e. Colonization
______	6. Microorganisms that do not cause disease, but help to maintain health	f. Inflammation
______	7. Process that eliminates all forms of microbial life	g. Flora
______	8. Disease-producing microorganism	h. Pathogen
______	9. Substance formed through the inflammatory process that may ooze from openings in the skin or mucous membranes	i. Endogenous infection
______	10. Microorganism grows but does not cause disease	j. Supra Infection
______	11. Ability of microorganisms to produce disease	k. Exogenous Infection
______	12. Being more than normally vulnerable to a disease	l. Virulence
		m. Susceptibility

Complete the following:

13. Identify whether the following are performed using clean or sterile technique in an acute care environment:
    a. Hand hygiene
    b. Postoperative dressing change
    c. Urinary catheter insertion
    d. Barrier precautions
    e. Intramuscular injection
14. An outcome for a patient with a 3-cm-diameter wound is:

15. Immunizations are available for which of the following?
    a. Hepatitis B _______
    b. Diphtheria _______
    c. Rubella _______
    d. Tuberculosis _______
    e. AIDS _______
    f. Varicella _______

16. The nurse is preparing to complete a dressing change and notices the sterile package is torn. The nurse should:

17. Identify specific actions that the nurse can implement to interrupt the chain of infection:
    a. Control or eliminate the infectious agent:
    b. Control or eliminate the reservoir:
    c. Control the portals of exit:
    d. Control transmission:
    e. Control susceptibility of host:

18. What results would be expected for the following laboratory studies in the presence of an infection?
    a. WBC count
    b. Erythrocyte sedimentation rate
    c. Iron level
    d. Neutrophils
    e. Basophils

19. The major cause of health care–associated infections is:

20. A patient's gastrointestinal defenses against infection are altered by:

21. Select the appropriate techniques for isolation precautions from the following:
    a. Wash hands in the clean utility room after patient care: _______
    b. Provide for the patient's sensory needs during care: _______
    c. Prevent visitors from entering the patient's room: _______
    d. Keep face mask below the level of eyeglasses or goggles: _______
    e. Place disposable items in paper bags: _______
    f. Maintain each patient's personal protective equipment (PPE) within the patient's room: _______
    g. Keep PPE at the door to the room or in an anteroom area: _______

22. Handling of biohazardous waste includes:

23. Specify the order in which the following PPE should be applied before entering an isolation room:
    a. Mask _______
    b. Gloves _______
    c. Gown _______

24. If a mask, gown, and gloves are worn into an isolation room, the first item of PPE that is removed when exiting the room is/are the:

25. Select from the following where appropriate asepsis or contamination has occurred:
    a. Handling a sterile dressing with clean gloves _______
    b. Holding a sterile bowl above waist level using sterile gloves _______
    c. Keeping the hands above the elbows after a surgical scrub _______
    d. Turning away from and placing one's back to the sterile field _______
    e. Talking or coughing over the sterile field _______
    f. Discarding sterile packages that are wet _______
    g. Placing objects up to the edge of the sterile field _______
    h. Discarding a small amount of solution before pouring the remainder into a sterile container on the fiel _______

26. For the nursing diagnosis *Impaired skin integrity, related to 2-inch-diameter pressure ulcer on sacrum,* identify a patient goal, objectives, and nursing interventions.

27. Number the flaps on the sterile package in the figure according to which one should be opened first, second, and last.

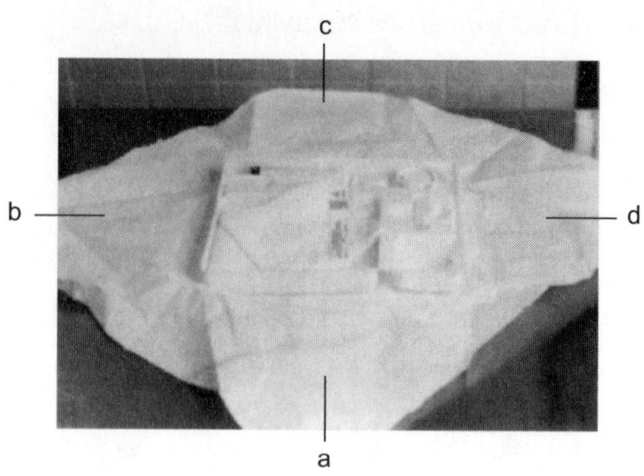

Select the best answer for each of the following questions:

28. At the community health fair, the nurse is asked by one of the residents about the influenza vaccine. The nurse responds to the resident that the influenza vaccine is recommended for individuals who are:
    1. Health care workers
    2. Traveling to other countries
    3. Less than 6 years of age
    4. Between 40 and 65 years of age
29. The nurse is preparing a room for a patient with tuberculosis. The specific aspect for this tier of Standard Precautions that is different from tier 1 is that the care should include:
    1. A private room with negative air flow
    2. Hand hygiene after gloves are removed
    3. Eye protection if splashing is possible
    4. Disposal of sharps in a puncture-resistant container
30. The nurse is preparing a teaching plan for patients about the hepatitis B virus. The nurse informs them that this virus may be transmitted by:
    1. Mosquitoes
    2. Droplet nuclei
    3. Blood products
    4. Improperly handled food
31. The nurse is working on a unit with a number of patients who have infectious diseases. One of the most important methods for reducing the spread of microorganisms is:
    1. Sterilization of equipment
    2. The use of gloves and gowns
    3. Maintenance of isolation precautions
    4. Hand hygiene before and after patient care

32. The assignment today for the nurse includes a patient with tuberculosis. In caring for a patient on droplet precautions, the nurse should routinely use:
    1. Regular masks and eyewear
    2. Regular masks, gowns, and gloves
    3. Surgical hand hygiene and gloves
    4. Particulate filtration masks and gowns
33. The nurse is caring for a patient who has a large abdominal wound that requires a sterile saline soak and dressing. While performing the care, the nurse drops the saline-soaked 4 × 4 gauze near the wound on the patient's abdomen. The nurse:
    1. Discontinues the procedure at this time
    2. Throws the gauze away and prepares a new 4 × 4
    3. Picks up the 4 × 4 with sterile forceps and places it on the wound
    4. Rinses the 4 × 4 with saline and places it on the wound using sterile gloves
34. The nurse is checking the laboratory results of a male patient admitted to the medical unit. The nurse is alerted to the presence of an infectious process based on the finding of:
    1. Iron—80 g/100 ml
    2. Neutrophils—65%
    3. Erythrocyte sedimentation rate (ESR)—13 mm/hr
    4. White blood cells (WBC)—16,000/mm^3
35. The nurse is working with a patient who has a deep laceration to the right lower extremity. To reduce a possible reservoir of infection, the nurse:
    1. Wears gloves and a mask at all times
    2. Isolates the patient's personal articles
    3. Has the patient cover the mouth and nose when coughing
    4. Changes the dressing to the extremity when it becomes soiled
36. The nurse implements droplet precautions for the patient with:
    1. Pulmonary tuberculosis
    2. Varicella
    3. Rubella
    4. Herpes
37. A patient who has had a transplant will require:
    1. Contact isolation
    2. Airborne isolation
    3. Droplet isolation
    4. Protective isolation
38. For a patient with hepatitis A, the nurse is aware that the disease is transmitted through:
    1. Feces
    2. Blood
    3. Skin
    4. Droplet nuclei
39. A sign that is indicative of a systemic infection resulting from a wound is:
    1. Redness
    2. Drainage
    3. Edema
    4. Fever
40. The nurse is aware that older adults are more susceptible to infection as a result of:
    1. Thickening of the dermal and epidermal skin layers
    2. Increased production of T lymphocytes
    3. Increased production of digestive juices
    4. Drying of the oral mucosa

Study Group Questions

- What is the nature of the infectious process?
- What are the components of the chain of infection?
- What are the body's normal defenses against infection?
- What is a health care–associated infection, who are the patients at risk, and how may the nurse prevent this infection?
- How is the nursing process applied to infection control in the acute, extended care, and home care environments?
- What nursing measures may be implemented to prevent or control the spread of infection?
- What is included in Standard Precautions?
- What information may be taught to the patient and the patient's family for prevention or control of infectious processes?
- How does the nurse perform the procedures that are important for infection control?

Name ____________________ Date __________ Instructor's Name __________________________

Procedural Guidelines 11-1 Hand Hygiene

	S	U	NP	Comments
1. Inspect surface of hands for breaks or cuts in skin or cuticles.	_____	_____	_____	__________________
2. Note condition of nails. Nail tips should be less than 1/4-inch long and free of artificial nail extenders. Avoid artificial nails and long or unkempt nails that may harbor microbial loads. Your agency may ban these depending upon their policy. Report and cover any skin lesions before providing patient care.				
3. Inspect hands for visible soiling.	_____	_____	_____	__________________
4. Push wristwatch and long uniform sleeves above wrists. Avoid wearing rings. If rings are worn, remove before hand washing.	_____	_____	_____	__________________
5. Hand antisepsis using an instant alcohol waterless antiseptic rub				
A. Dispense ample amount of product into palm of one hand.	_____	_____	_____	__________________
B. Rub hands together, covering all surfaces with antiseptic.	_____	_____	_____	__________________
C. Rub hands together until the alcohol is dry. Allow hands to dry before applying gloves.	_____	_____	_____	__________________
6. Hand washing using regular lotion soap or antimicrobial soap and water				
A. Be sure fingernails are short, filed, and smooth.	_____	_____	_____	__________________
B. Stand in front of sink, keeping hands and uniform away from sink surface. (If hands touch sink during hand washing, repeat.)	_____	_____	_____	__________________
C. Turn faucet on or push knee pedals laterally, or press pedals with foot to regulate flow and temperature.	_____	_____	_____	__________________
D. Avoid splashing water against uniform.	_____	_____	_____	__________________
E. Regulate flow of water so that temperature is warm.	_____	_____	_____	__________________
F. Wet hands and wrists thoroughly under running water. Keep hands and forearms lower than elbows during washing.	_____	_____	_____	__________________
G. Apply a small amount of soap or antiseptic lathering thoroughly. Soap granules and leaflet preparations are an option.	_____	_____	_____	__________________

	S	U	NP	Comments
H. Perform hand hygiene using plenty of lather and friction for at least 15 seconds. Interlace fingers and rub palms and back of hands with circular motion at least 5 times each. Keep fingertips down to facilitate removal of microorganisms.	_____	_____	_____	____________________
I. Areas under fingernails are often soiled. Clean them with the fingernails of other hand and additional soap, or clean orangewood stick.	_____	_____	_____	____________________
J. Rinse hands and wrists thoroughly, keeping hands down and elbows up.	_____	_____	_____	____________________
K. Dry hands thoroughly from fingers to wrists and forearms with paper towel, single-use cloth, or warm air dryer.	_____	_____	_____	____________________
L. If used, discard paper towel in proper receptacle.	_____	_____	_____	____________________
M. To turn off hand faucet, use clean, dry paper towel, avoiding touching handles with hands. Turn off water with foot or knee pedals (if applicable).	_____	_____	_____	____________________
N. Apply lotion to hands.	_____	_____	_____	____________________

Name ____________ Date ________ Instructor's Name ____________

Procedural Guidelines 11-2 Caring for a Patient on Isolation Precautions

	S	U	NP	Comments
1. Assess isolation indications.	____	____	____	____________
2. Review agency policies and precautions and nursing considerations for the specific isolation system.	____	____	____	____________
3. Review nurses' notes or confer with colleagues regarding patient's emotional state and adjustment to isolation.	____	____	____	____________
4. Perform hand hygiene, and prepare all equipment to be taken into patient's room.	____	____	____	____________
5. Prepare for entrance into isolation room:				
a. Apply either surgical mask or respirator around mouth and nose.	____	____	____	____________
b. Apply eyewear or goggles snugly around face and eyes (when needed).	____	____	____	____________
c. Apply gown, being sure it covers all outer garments. Pull sleeves down to wrists. Tie securely at neck and waist.	____	____	____	____________
d. Apply disposable gloves (NOTE: Unpowdered, latex-free gloves. Bring glove cuffs over edge of gown sleeves.	____	____	____	____________
6. Enter patient's room. Arrange supplies and equipment. (If equipment will be removed from room for reuse, place on clean paper towel.)	____	____	____	____________
7. Explain purpose of isolation and necessary precautions to patient and family. Offer opportunity to ask questions. Assess for evidence of emotional problems caused by being in isolation.	____	____	____	____________
8. Assess vital signs.				
a. If patient is infected or colonized with a resistant organism. Avoid contact of stethoscope or blood pressure cuff with infective material.	____	____	____	____________
b. If you reuse the stethoscope, clean diaphragm, bell, and ear pieces with 70% alcohol. Set aside on clean surface.	____	____	____	____________

	S	U	NP	Comments
c. Use individual or disposable thermometers.	_____	_____	_____	_____
9. Administer medications:				
a. Give oral medication in wrapper or cup.	_____	_____	_____	_____
b. Dispose of wrapper or cup in plastic-lined receptacle.	_____	_____	_____	_____
c. Administer injection, being sure to wear gloves.	_____	_____	_____	_____
d. Discard syringe and uncapped needle or sheathed needle into special container.	_____	_____	_____	_____
e. If you do not wear gloves and hands contact contaminated article or body fluids, wash hands immediately.	_____	_____	_____	_____
10. Administer hygiene.				
a. Avoid allowing gown to become wet.	_____	_____	_____	_____
b. Remove linen from bed. If excessively soiled, avoid contact with gown. Place in leak-proof linen bag.	_____	_____	_____	_____
c. Change gloves and perform hand hygiene as necessary.	_____	_____	_____	_____
11. Collect specimens:				
a. Place specimen containers on clean paper towel in patient's bathroom.	_____	_____	_____	_____
b. Follow procedure for collecting specimen of body fluids.	_____	_____	_____	_____
c. Transfer specimen to container without soiling outside of container. Place container in plastic bag and place label on outside of bag or as per facility policy.	_____	_____	_____	_____
12. Dispose of linen and trash bags as they become full:				
a. Use sturdy, moisture-impervious single bags to contain soiled articles.	_____	_____	_____	_____
b. Tie bags securely at top in knot.	_____	_____	_____	_____
13. Resupply room as needed.	_____	_____	_____	_____
14. Leave isolation room.				
a. Remove gloves. Remove one glove by grasping cuff and pulling glove inside out over hand. Discard glove. With ungloved hand, tuck finger inside cuff of remaining glove and pull it off, inside out.	_____	_____	_____	_____

	S	U	NP	Comments
b. Untie *top* mask strings, hold strings while untying bottom strings, pull mask away from face and drop into trash receptacle. (Do not touch outer surface of mask.)	____	____	____	____
c. Untie waist and neck strings of gown. Allow gown to fall from shoulders. Remove hands from sleeves without touching outside of gown. Hold gown inside at shoulder seams and fold inside out; discard disposable gown in trash receptacle or linen gown in laundry bag.	____	____	____	____
d. Remove eyewear or goggles.	____	____	____	____
e. Perform hand hygiene.	____	____	____	____
f. Explain to patient when you plan to return to room. Ask whether patient requires any personal care items, books, or magazines.	____	____	____	____
g. Leave room and close door, if necessary. (Close door if patient is on airborne precautions.)	____	____	____	____
h. Dispose of all contaminated supplies and equipment in a manner that prevents spread of microorganisms to other persons (see agency policy).	____	____	____	____

Name ______________________ **Date** __________ **Instructor's Name** ____________________________

Procedural Guidelines 11-3 Donning a Surgical Mask

	S	U	NP	Comments
1. Find top edge of mask. Pliable metal fits snugly against bridge of nose.	_____	_____	_____	____________________________
2. Hold mask by top two strings or loops. Tie the two top ties at top of back of head, with ties above ears. (*Alternative:* slip loops over each ear.)	_____	_____	_____	____________________________
3. Tie two lower strings snugly around neck with mask well under chin.	_____	_____	_____	____________________________
4. Gently pinch upper metal band around bridge of nose.	_____	_____	_____	____________________________

NOTE: Change mask if it is wet, moist, or contaminated.

Name ____________ Date ________ Instructor's Name ____________

Procedural Guidelines 11-4 Putting on Sterile Gloves

	S	U	NP	Comments
1. Consider the procedure you will perform, and consult agency policy on use of gloves.	____	____	____	____________
2. Inspect hands for cuts, open lesions, or abrasions. Cover with an occlusive dressing before gloving.	____	____	____	____________
3. Assess if the patient or health care worker has a known allergy to latex.	____	____	____	____________
4. Determine correct glove size and type of glove material you will use.	____	____	____	____________
5. Examine glove package to ensure package is not wet, torn, or discolored.	____	____	____	____________
6. Perform thorough hand hygiene.	____	____	____	____________
7. Remove outer glove package wrapper by carefully separating and peeling apart sides.	____	____	____	____________
8. Grasp inner package and lay it on clean, flat surface just above waist level. Open package, keeping gloves on wrapper's inside surface.	____	____	____	____________
9. Identify right and left gloves. Each glove has a cuff approximately 5 cm (2 inches) wide. Glove dominant hand first.	____	____	____	____________
10. With thumb and first two fingers of nondominant hand, grasp edge of cuff of the glove for the dominant hand. Touch only glove's inside surface.	____	____	____	____________
11. Carefully pull glove over dominant hand, leaving a cuff and being sure the cuff does not roll up wrist. Be sure thumb and fingers are in proper spaces.	____	____	____	____________
12. With gloved dominant hand, slip fingers underneath second glove's cuff. Carefully pull second glove over nondominant hand. Do not allow fingers and thumb of gloved dominant hand to touch any part of exposed nondominant hand. Keep thumb of dominant hand abducted.	____	____	____	____________
13. After second glove is on, interlock hands. Cuffs usually fall down after application. Be sure to touch only sterile sides.	____	____	____	____________

Name ____________________ Date __________ Instructor's Name ____________________________

Procedural Guidelines 11-5 Opening Wrapped Sterile Items

	S	U	NP	Comments
1. Place sterile kit or package containing sterile items on clean, dry, flat work surface above waist level.	_____	_____	_____	____________________
2. Open outside cover, and remove kit from dust cover. Place on work surface.	_____	_____	_____	____________________
3. Grasp outer surface of tip of outermost flap.	_____	_____	_____	____________________
4. Open outermost flap away from body, keeping arm outstretched and away from sterile field.	_____	_____	_____	____________________
5. Grasp outside surface of edge of first side flap.	_____	_____	_____	____________________
6. Open side flap, pulling to side, allowing it to lie flat on table surface. Keep your arm to side and not over sterile surface. Do not allow flaps to spring back over sterile contents.	_____	_____	_____	____________________
7. Repeat steps for second side flap.	_____	_____	_____	____________________
8. Grasp outside border of last and innermost flap.	_____	_____	_____	____________________
9. Stand away from sterile package, and pull flap back, allowing it to fall flat on table.	_____	_____	_____	____________________
10. Use the inner surface of the package (except for the 1-inch border around the edges) as a field to add additional items because it is sterile. Grasp the 1-inch border to move the field over the work surface.	_____	_____	_____	____________________

Name ____________ Date ________ Instructor's Name ______________

Procedural Guidelines 11-6 Preparation of a Sterile Field

	S	U	NP	Comments
1. Perform hand hygiene.	____	____	____	____________
2. Place pack containing sterile drape on work surface and open.	____	____	____	____________
3. Apply sterile gloves (optional, see agency policy).	____	____	____	____________
4. With fingertips of one hand, pick up the folded top edge of the sterile drape along the 1-inch border.	____	____	____	____________
5. Gently lift the drape up from its outer cover and let it unfold by itself without touching any object. Keep it above the waist. Discard the outer cover with the other hand.	____	____	____	____________
6. With the other hand, grasp an adjacent corner of the drape and hold it straight up and away from the body.	____	____	____	____________
7. Holding the drape, first position and lay the bottom half over the intended work surface.	____	____	____	____________
8. Allow the top half of the drape to be placed over the work surface last.	____	____	____	____________
9. Grasp the 1-inch border around the edge to position as needed.	____	____	____	____________

Vital Signs 12

Case Studies

1. You are involved in taking blood pressure (BP) readings at a community health fair.
   a. What types of blood pressure readings indicate that follow-up care should be recommended?
   b. What other information may be obtained from the patient while taking the blood pressure reading?
2. Your patient has bilateral casts on the upper arms.
   a. How will you obtain the patient's pulse rate and blood pressure?
3. You are working in an extended care facility and the nurse reporting off identifies that one of the patents is febrile.
   a. What signs and symptoms do you expect to find with a patient who is febrile?
   b. What interventions are indicated for febrile patients?
4. The patient is being monitored with pulse oximetry. The device does not appear to be working.
   a. What "troubleshooting" can you perform to determine if the pulse oximeter will work properly?

Chapter Review

Match the description/definition in Column A with the correct term in Column B.

		Column A		*Column B*
______	1.	Decrease of systolic and diastolic pressures below normal	a.	Tachypnea
______	2.	Another word for fever	b.	Diffusion
______	3.	Rate and depth of respirations increase	c.	Bradypnea
______	4.	Widening of blood vessels	d.	Hypothermia
______	5.	Pulse rate below 60 beats per minute for an adult	e.	Apnea
______	6.	140/90 mm Hg for two or more readings	f.	Bradycardia
______	7.	Rate of breathing regular but abnormally rapid	g.	Hypotension
______	8.	Decreased body temperature	h.	Hyperventilation
______	9.	Controls body temperature like a thermostat in a home	i.	Hypothalamus
______	10.	No respirations for several seconds	j.	Hypertension
______	11.	Rate of breathing regular but abnormally slow	k.	Vasodilation
______	12.	Movement of oxygen and carbon dioxide between the alveoli and red blood cells	l.	Febrile
______	13.	Normal breathing	m.	Auscultatory gap
______	14.	Temporary disappearance of sounds between Korotkoff sounds	n.	Eupnea

Complete the following:

15. Convert the following temperature readings:
    a. 97° F = _____ ° C
    b. 38.4° C = _____ ° F
    c. 102° F = _____ ° C
    d. 39.4° C = _____ ° F
    e. What readings on Fahrenheit and centigrade thermometers should alert the nurse to an alteration in the patient's temperature regulation?

16. Indicate on the model where the following pulses should be palpated:
    a. Brachial
    b. Radial
    c. Apical

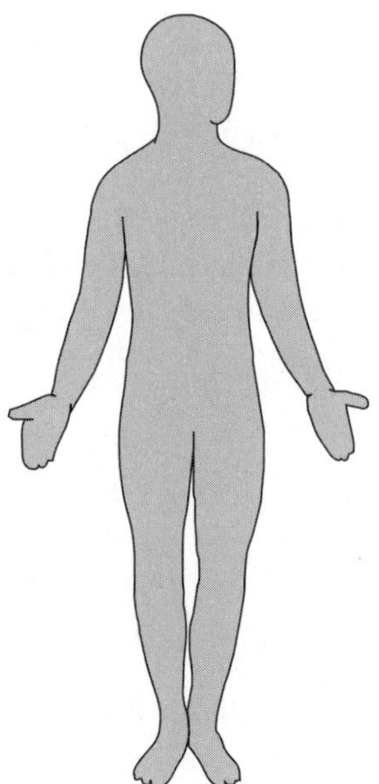

17. Indicate on the aneroid and mercury scales where the following blood pressure readings would be noted:
    a. Korotkoff sounds first heard at 164 mm Hg and inaudible at 92 mm Hg

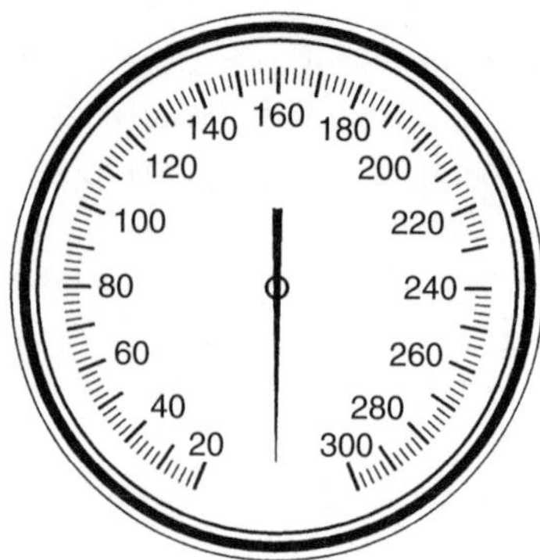

    b. Korotkoff sounds first heard at 112 mm Hg and inaudible at 64 mm Hg

18. Vital sign measurements may not be delegated to unlicensed assistive personnel.
    True _____ False _____

19. Identify the interventions that will reduce body temperature in the following ways:
    a. Conduction:

    b. Convection:

20. The patient is on isolation precautions and temperature measurements are being used to monitor the status of the fever. The thermometer of choice in this situation is a:

21. The patient has bilateral arm casts. The blood pressure should be taken _________________________ and the _________________________ artery should be used.

22. For the patient who has had a right mastectomy, the nurse should take the blood pressure:

23. Vital signs are usually recorded on the:

24. Decreasing hemoglobin levels will _________________________ the respiratory rate.

25. To obtain arterial oxygen saturation for an adult patient, the pulse oximeter may be applied to:

26. The expected SpO_2 level is:

27. Select all of the correct techniques for blood pressure measurement from the following:
    a. The cuff is 40% of the circumference of the limb being used. _______
    b. The bladder encircles 50% of the arm of an adult. _______
    c. The cuff is deflated at a rate of 2 to 3 mm Hg per second. _______
    d. The arm is kept below the level of the heart. _______
    e. The cuff is inflated to 30 mm Hg above the point where the pulse disappears. _______
    f. The systolic blood pressure is identified as the first onset of Korotkoff sounds. _______
    g. A difference of 30 mm Hg is expected between the left and right arm measurements. _______

28. The difference between the radial and apical pulses is a(n):

29. The difference between the systolic and diastolic blood pressure is the:

Select the best answer for each of the following questions:

30. The nurse is working on a pediatric unit and assessing the vital signs of an infant admitted for gastroenteritis. The nurse expects that the vital signs are normally the following (where BP is blood pressure in units of mm Hg, P is pulse rate in units of beats per minute, and R is respirations in units of breaths per minute):
    1. BP = 90/50, P = 122, R = 46
    2. BP = 90/60, P = 80, R = 20
    3. BP = 100/60, P = 140, R = 32
    4. BP = 110/50, P = 98, R = 40

31. While working in the extended care facility, the nurse expects the vital signs of an older adult patient to be:
    1. BP = 98/70, P = 60, R = 12
    2. BP = 120/60, P = 110, R = 30
    3. BP = 140/90, P = 74, R = 14
    4. BP = 150/100, P = 90, R = 25

32. The student nurse is taking vital signs for her assigned patients on the surgical unit. The student is aware that a patient's body temperature may be reduced after:
    1. Exercise
    2. Emotional stress

3. Periods of sleep
4. Cigarette smoking

33. While working in the emergency department, the nurse is carefully monitoring the vital signs of the patients who have been admitted. The nurse is alert to the potential for a decrease in a patient's pulse rate as a result of:
    1. Hemorrhage
    2. Hypothyroidism
    3. Respiratory difficulty
    4. Epinephrine (adrenaline) administration

34. A patient is being treated for hyperthermia. The nurse anticipates that the patient's response to this condition will be:
    1. Generalized pallor
    2. Bradycardia
    3. Reduced thirst
    4. Diaphoresis

35. Several friends have gone on a ski trip and have been exposed to very cold temperatures. One of the individuals appears to be slightly hypothermic. The best initial response by the nurse in the ski lodge is to give this individual:
    1. Soup
    2. Coffee
    3. Cocoa
    4. Brandy

36. When checking the temperature of the patient, the nurse notes that he is febrile. An antipyretic medication is ordered. The nurse prepares to administer:
    1. Digoxin (Lanoxin)
    2. Prednisone (Orasone)
    3. Theophylline (Theo-Dur)
    4. Acetaminophen (Tylenol)

37. The nurse has been assigned a number of different patients today in the long-term care unit. When taking vital signs, the nurse is alert to the greater possibility of tachycardia for the patient with:
    1. Anemia
    2. Hypothyroidism
    3. A temperature of 95° F
    4. A patient-controlled analgesic (PCA) pump with morphine drip

38. While reviewing the vital signs taken by the aide this morning, the nurse notes that one of the patients is hypotensive. The nurse will be checking to see if the patient is experiencing:
    1. Lightheadedness
    2. A decreased heart rate
    3. An increased urinary output
    4. Increased warmth to the skin

39. Vital sign measurements have been completed on all of the assigned patients. The nurse will need to immediately report a finding of:
    1. Pulse pressure—40 mm Hg
    2. Apical pulses—78, 80, 76 beats per minute
    3. Apical pulse—82 beats per minute, radial pulse—70 beats per minute
    4. BP—140/80 mm Hg left arm, 136/74 mm Hg right arm

40. The nurse is preparing to take vital signs for the patients on the acute care unit. A tympanic temperature assessment is indicated for the patient:
    1. After rectal surgery
    2. Wearing a hearing aid
    3. Experiencing otitis media
    4. Following an exercise session

41. Blood pressure monitoring is being conducted on the cardiac care unit. The nurse is determining whether an automatic blood pressure device is indicated for use. This device is selected for the patient with:
    1. An irregular heartbeat
    2. Parkinson's disease
    3. Peripheral vascular disease
    4. A systolic blood pressure above 140 mm/Hg

42. A 34-year-old patient has come to the physician's office for an annual physical examination. The nurse is completing the vital signs before the patient is seen by the physician. The nurse alerts the physician to a finding of:
    1. T—37.6° C
    2. P—120 beats per minute
    3. R—18 breaths per minute
    4. BP—116/78 mm Hg

43. The nurse is assigned to the well-child center that is affiliated with the acute care facility. A mother brings her 1½-year-old son to the center for his immunizations. The nurse assesses the child's pulse rate by checking the:
   1. Radial artery
   2. Apical artery
   3. Popliteal artery
   4. Femoral artery
44. The nurse determines that the patient's pulse rate is significantly lower than it has been over the past week. The nurse reassesses and finds that the pulse rate is still 46 beats per minute. The nurse should first:
   1. Document the measurement
   2. Administer a stimulant medication
   3. Inform the charge nurse or physician
   4. Apply 100% oxygen at a maximum flow rate
45. The most important sign of heat stroke is:
   1. Hot, dry skin
   2. Nausea
   3. Excessive thirst
   4. Muscle cramping
46. The most accurate temperature measurement for an adult patient experiencing tachypnea and dyspnea is:
   1. Oral
   2. Rectal
   3. Axillary
   4. Tympanic
47. The nurse should insert a rectal thermometer into the adult patient:
   1. ½ inch
   2. 1 inch
   3. 1½ inches
   4. 2 inches
48. The patient is showing the nurse how he is taking his temperature at home. During the demonstration, the patient drops and breaks the glass thermometer containing mercury. The first action by the nurse is to:
   1. Remove the patient from the area
   2. Open the windows in the room
   3. Wipe away the mercury with a wet paper towel
   4. Contact the Environmental Protection Agency (EPA) for directions
49. For the patient who is experiencing a febrile state, the nurse should:
   1. Ambulate the patient frequently
   2. Restrict fluid intake
   3. Keep the patient warm
   4. Provide oxygen as ordered
50. It is anticipated by the nurse that bradycardia will be evident if the patient is:
   1. Exercising
   2. Hypothermic
   3. In severe pain
   4. Extremely anxious
51. The nurse anticipates that the patient with hypertension will be receiving:
   1. Diuretics
   2. Antipyretics
   3. Narcotic analgesics
   4. Anticholinergics
52. To determine the arterial blood flow to the patient's feet, the nurse should assess the:
   1. Radial artery
   2. Brachial artery
   3. Popliteal artery
   4. Dorsalis pedis artery
53. The nurse anticipates an increase in blood pressure for the patient who is:
   1. Sleeping
   2. Overweight
   3. Taking narcotics
   4. Hemorrhaging
54. Prehypertension is classified as an average of repeated readings of:
   1. Systolic 120 to 139 mm Hg, diastolic 80 to 89 mm Hg
   2. Systolic 140 to 159 mm Hg, diastolic 90 to 99 mm Hg
   3. Systolic 160 to 179 mm Hg, diastolic 90 to 99 mm Hg
   4. Systolic above 180 mm Hg, diastolic above 100 mm Hg

Study Group Questions

- What are the guidelines for measurement of vital signs?
- When should vital signs be taken?
- How does the nurse determine which sites and equipment to use for measurement of vital signs?
- What body processes regulate temperature?

- What factors influence body temperature?
- How is the temperature measurement converted from centigrade to Fahrenheit and vice versa?
- What sites and equipment are used for temperature measurement?
- What nursing interventions are appropriate for increases and decreases in the patient's body temperature?
- What factors influence the pulse rate?
- What sites may be used for pulse rate assessment?
- How should the stethoscope be used in pulse rate assessment?
- What changes may occur in the pulse rate and rhythm?
- What nursing interventions are appropriate for alterations in the pulse rate?
- What is blood pressure?
- What factors may increase or decrease blood pressure?
- What are abnormal alterations in blood pressure?
- What equipment is used for blood pressure measurement?
- What nursing interventions are appropriate for increases and decreases in blood pressure?
- What body processes are involved in respiration?
- How are respirations assessed?
- What alterations may be noted in the patient's respirations?
- How does pulse oximetry function and what is its purpose?
- What are the procedures for assessment of temperature, pulse rate, respirations, blood pressure, and pulse oxygen saturation?
- What should be included in patient and family teaching for measurement and evaluation of vital signs?

Study Chart

Create a study chart to compare the Vital Signs Across the Life Span, *identifying expected temperature, pulse rate, respiration, and blood pressure for each age-group.*

Name ____________ Date ____________ Instructor's Name ____________

Performance Checklist: Skill 12-1 Measuring Body Temperature

	S	U	NP	Comments
Assessment				
1. Assess for signs and symptoms of temperature alterations and for factors that influence body temperature.	____	____	____	____________
2. Determine any previous activity that would interfere with accuracy of temperature measurement. Wait 20 to 30 minutes before measuring oral temperature if patient has smoked or ingested hot or cold liquids or food.	____	____	____	____________
3. Determine appropriate site and measurement device to be used.	____	____	____	____________
Planning				
1. Explain route by which you will take temperature and importance of maintaining proper position until reading is complete.	____	____	____	____________
Implementation				
1. Perform hand hygiene.	____	____	____	____________
2. Assist patient in assuming comfortable position that provides easy access to route through which you will measure temperature.	____	____	____	____________
3. Obtain temperature reading.				
A. **Oral Temperature Measurement With Electronic Thermometer**				
(1) Apply disposable gloves (*optional*).	____	____	____	____________
(2) Remove thermometer pack from charging unit. Attach oral probe (blue tip) to thermometer unit. Grasp top of probe stem, being careful not to apply pressure on the ejection button.	____	____	____	____________
(3) Slide disposable plastic probe cover over thermometer probe stem until cover locks in place.	____	____	____	____________
(4) Ask patient to open mouth; then gently place thermometer probe under tongue in posterior sublingual pocket lateral to center of lower jaw.	____	____	____	____________
(5) Ask patient to hold thermometer probe with lips closed.	____	____	____	____________
(6) Leave thermometer probe in place until audible signal indicates completion and patient's temperature appears on digital display; remove thermometer probe from under patient's tongue.	____	____	____	____________

	S	U	NP	Comments
(7) Push ejection button on thermometer stem to discard plastic probe cover into appropriate receptacle.	_____	_____	_____	_____
(8) Return thermometer probe stem to storage position of recording unit.	_____	_____	_____	_____
(9) If gloves worn, remove and dispose of in appropriate receptacle. Perform hand hygiene.	_____	_____	_____	_____
(10) Return thermometer to charger.	_____	_____	_____	_____
B. Rectal Temperature Measurement With Electronic Thermometer				
(1) Draw curtain around bed and/or close room door. Assist patient to Sims' position with upper leg flexed. Move aside bed linen to expose only anal area. Keep patient's upper body and lower extremities covered with sheet or blanket.	_____	_____	_____	_____
(2) Apply gloves.	_____	_____	_____	_____
(3) Remove thermometer pack from charging unit. Attach rectal probe (red tip) to thermometer unit. Grasp top of probe stem, being careful not to apply pressure on the ejection button.	_____	_____	_____	_____
(4) Slide disposable plastic probe cover over thermometer probe until it locks in place.	_____	_____	_____	_____
(5) Squeeze liberal portion of lubricant onto tissue. Dip probe cover's end into lubricant, covering 2.5 to 3.5 cm (1 to 1½ inches) for adult.	_____	_____	_____	_____
(6) With nondominant hand, separate patient's buttocks to expose anus. Ask patient to breathe slowly and relax.	_____	_____	_____	_____
(7) Gently insert thermometer probe into anus in direction of umbilicus 3.5 cm (1½ inches) for adult. Do not force thermometer.	_____	_____	_____	_____
(8) Once positioned, hold thermometer probe in place until audible signal indicates completion and patient's temperature appears on digital display; remove thermometer probe from anus.	_____	_____	_____	_____
(9) Push ejection button on thermometer stem to discard plastic probe cover into an appropriate receptacle.	_____	_____	_____	_____

	S	U	NP	Comments
(10) Return thermometer stem to storage position of recording unit.	____	____	____	____________
(11) Wipe patient's anal area with tissue or soft wipe to remove lubricant or feces, and discard tissue. Assist patient in assuming a comfortable position.	____	____	____	____________
(12) Remove and dispose of gloves in appropriate receptacle. Perform hand hygiene.	____	____	____	____________
(13) Return thermometer to charger.	____	____	____	____________
C. Axillary Temperature Measurement With Electronic Thermometer				
(1) Draw curtain around bed and/or close room door. Assist patient to supine or sitting position. Move clothing or gown away from shoulder and arm.	____	____	____	____________
(2) Remove thermometer pack from charging unit. Be sure oral probe (blue tip) is attached to thermometer unit. Grasp top of probe stem, being careful not to apply pressure on ejection button.	____	____	____	____________
(3) Slide disposable plastic probe cover over thermometer probe until cover locks in place.	____	____	____	____________
(4) Raise patient's arm away from torso. Inspect for skin lesions and excessive perspiration. Insert probe into center of axilla, lower arm over probe, and place arm across patient's chest.	____	____	____	____________
(5) Once positioned, hold thermometer probe in place until audible signal indicates completion and patient's temperature appears on digital display; remove thermometer probe from axilla.	____	____	____	____________
(6) Push ejection button on thermometer stem to discard plastic probe cover into appropriate receptacle.	____	____	____	____________
(7) Return thermometer stem to storage position of recording unit.	____	____	____	____________
(8) Assist patient in assuming a comfortable position, replacing linen or gown.	____	____	____	____________
(9) Perform hand hygiene.	____	____	____	____________
(10) Return thermometer to charger.	____	____	____	____________

	S	U	NP	Comments
D. Tympanic Membrane Temperature Measurement With Electronic Tympanic Thermometer				
(1) Assist patient in assuming comfortable position with head turned toward side, away from you. If patient has been lying on one side, use upper ear.	____	____	____	____
(2) Note if there is obvious earwax in the patient's ear canal.	____	____	____	____
(3) Remove thermometer handheld unit from charging base, being careful not to apply pressure on the ejection button.	____	____	____	____
(4) Slide disposable speculum cover over otoscope-like tip until it locks into place. Be careful not to touch lens cover.	____	____	____	____
(5) If holding handheld unit with right hand, obtain temperature from patient's right ear; left-handed persons obtain temperature from patient's left ear.				
(6) Insert speculum into ear canal following manufacturer's instructions for tympanic probe positioning.	____	____	____	____
(a) Pull ear pinna backward, up and out for an adult. For children younger than 2 years of age, point covered probe toward midpoint between eyebrow and sideburns.	____	____	____	____
(b) Move thermometer in a figure-eight pattern.	____	____	____	____
(c) Fit speculum probe snugly into canal and do not move, pointing tip toward nose.	____	____	____	____
(7) Once positioned, press scan button on handheld unit. Leave speculum in place until audible signal indicates completion and patient's temperature appears on digital display.	____	____	____	____
(8) Carefully remove speculum from auditory canal.	____	____	____	____

(9) Push ejection button on handheld unit to discard speculum cover into appropriate receptacle. ______ ______ ______ ____________________

(10) If temperature is abnormal or a second reading is necessary, replace speculum cover and wait 2 minutes before repeating the measurement in the same ear. Also you can repeat measurement in other ear or try an alternative measurement site or instrument. ______ ______ ______ ____________________

(11) Return handheld unit to charging base. ______ ______ ______ ____________________

(12) Assist patient in assuming a comfortable position. ______ ______ ______ ____________________

(13) Perform hand hygiene. ______ ______ ______ ____________________

Evaluation

1. Inform patient of reading and record measurement. ______ ______ ______ ____________________
2. If you are assessing temperature for the first time, establish temperature as baseline if it is within normal range. ______ ______ ______ ____________________
3. Compare temperature reading with patient's previous temperature and normal temperature range for patient's age-group. ______ ______ ______ ____________________
4. Record temperature in patient's record. ______ ______ ______ ____________________
5. Report abnormal findings to nurse in charge or physician. ______ ______ ______ ____________________

Name ____________ Date ________ Instructor's Name ____________

Performance Checklist: Skill 12-2 Assessing the Radial and Apical Pulses

	S	U	NP	Comments
Assessment				
1. Determine need to assess radial and/or apical pulse.	____	____	____	____________
2. Assess for factors that influence pulse rate and rhythm.	____	____	____	____________
3. Determine patient's previous baseline pulse rate (if available) from patient's record.	____	____	____	____________
Planning				
1. Explain to patient that you will assess pulse or heart rate.	____	____	____	____________
Implementation				
1. Perform hand hygiene.	____	____	____	____________
2. If necessary, draw curtain around bed and/or close door.	____	____	____	____________
3. Obtain pulse measurement.				
A. Radial pulse				
(1) Assist patient to assume a supine or sitting position.	____	____	____	____________
(2) If supine, place patient's forearm straight alongside or across lower chest or upper abdomen with wrist extended straight. If sitting, bend patient's elbow 90 degrees and support lower arm on chair or on your arm. Slightly extend the wrist with palm down until you note the strongest pulse.	____	____	____	____________
(3) Place tips of first two fingers of your hand over groove along radial or thumb side of patient's inner wrist.	____	____	____	____________
(4) Lightly compress against radius, obliterate pulse initially, and then relax pressure so pulse becomes easily palpable.	____	____	____	____________
(5) Determine strength of pulse.	____	____	____	____________
(6) After you feel pulse regularly, look at watch's second hand and begin to count rate.	____	____	____	____________
(7) If pulse is regular, count rate for 30 seconds and multiply total by 2.	____	____	____	____________
(8) If pulse is irregular, count rate for 60 seconds. Assess frequency and pattern of irregularity.	____	____	____	____________
(9) When pulse is irregular, compare radial pulses bilaterally.	____	____	____	____________

B. Apical pulse

(1) Perform hand hygiene, and clean earpieces and diaphragm of stethoscope with alcohol swab. ____ ____ ____ ________________

(2) Draw curtain around bed, and/or close door. ____ ____ ____ ________________

(3) Assist patient to supine or sitting position. Move aside bed linen and gown to expose sternum and left side of chest. ____ ____ ____ ________________

(4) Locate anatomical landmarks to identify the point of maximal impulse (PMI). Find the angle of Louis just below suprasternal notch between the sternal body and manubrium; feels like a bony prominence. Slip fingers down each side of angle to find the second intercostal space (ICS). Carefully move fingers down the left side of sternum to fifth ICS and laterally to the left midclavicular line (MCL). A light tap felt within an area 1 to 2 cm (1/2 to 1 inch) of the PMI is reflected from the apex of the heart. ____ ____ ____ ________________

(5) Place diaphragm of stethoscope in palm of hand for 5 to 10 seconds. ____ ____ ____ ________________

(6) Place diaphragm of stethoscope over PMI at the fifth ICS, at left MCL, and auscultate for normal S_1 and S_2 heart sounds (heard as "lub dub"). ____ ____ ____ ________________

(7) When S_1 and S_2 are heard with regularity, use watch's second hand and begin to count rate. ____ ____ ____ ________________

(8) If apical rate is regular, count for 30 seconds and multiply by 2. ____ ____ ____ ________________

(9) Note if heart rate is irregular, and describe pattern of irregularity (S_1 and S_2 occurring early or later after previous sequence of sounds; for example, every third or fourth beat is skipped). ____ ____ ____ ________________

(10) Replace patient's gown and bed linen; assist patient in returning to comfortable position. ____ ____ ____ ________________

(11) Perform hand hygiene. ____ ____ ____ ________________

(12) Clean earpieces and diaphragm of stethoscope with alcohol swab routinely after each use. ____ ____ ____ ________________

	S	U	NP	Comments
Evaluation				
1. Discuss findings with patient and record measurement.	_____	_____	_____	__________
2. Compare readings with previous baseline and/or acceptable range of heart rate for patient's age.	_____	_____	_____	__________
3. Compare peripheral pulse rate with apical rate, and note discrepancy.	_____	_____	_____	__________
4. Compare radial pulse equality, and note discrepancy.	_____	_____	_____	__________
5. Correlate pulse rate with data obtained from blood pressure reading and related signs and symptoms.	_____	_____	_____	__________
6. Record pulse rate with assessment site in patient's record.	_____	_____	_____	__________
7. Report abnormal findings to nurse in charge or physician.	_____	_____	_____	__________

Name ____________ **Date** ________ **Instructor's Name** ______________

Performance Checklist: Skill 12-3 Measuring Blood Pressure

	S	U	NP	Comments
Assessment				
1. Determine need to assess patient's BP.	____	____	____	____________
2. Determine best site for BP assessment.	____	____	____	____________
3. Determine previous baseline BP (if available) from patient's record.	____	____	____	____________
Planning				
1. Explain to patient that you will assess BP. Have patient rest at least 5 minutes before measuring lying or sitting BP and 1 minute when standing. Ask patient not to speak when BP is being measured.	____	____	____	____________
2. Be sure patient has not ingested caffeine or smoked for 30 minutes before BP assessment.	____	____	____	____________
3. Have patient assume sitting or lying position. Be sure room is warm, quiet, and relaxing.	____	____	____	____________
4. Select appropriate cuff size.	____	____	____	____________
5. Perform hand hygiene, and clean stethoscope earpieces and diaphragm with alcohol swab.	____	____	____	____________
Implementation				
1. With patient sitting or lying, position patient's forearm or thigh, supported at heart level, if needed, with palm turned up; for thigh, position with knee slightly flexed. If sitting, instruct patient to keep feet flat on floor without legs crossed.	____	____	____	____________
2. Expose extremity (arm or leg) fully by removing constricting clothing.	____	____	____	____________
3. Palpate brachial artery (arm) or popliteal artery (leg). With cuff fully deflated, apply bladder of cuff above artery. Position cuff 2.5 cm (1 inch) above site of pulsation (antecubital or popliteal space). If there are no center arrows on cuff, estimate the center of the bladder and place this center over artery. Wrap cuff evenly and snugly around extremity.	____	____	____	____________
4. Position manometer vertically at eye level. Make sure observer is no farther than 1 m (approximately 1 yard) away.	____	____	____	____________

	S	U	NP	Comments
5. Measure blood pressure.				
A. Two-Step Method				
(1) Relocate brachial pulse. Palpate artery distal to the cuff with fingertips of nondominant hand while inflating cuff. Note point at which pulse disappears and continue to inflate cuff to a pressure 30 mm Hg above that point. Note the pressure reading. Slowly deflate cuff, and note point when pulse reappears. Deflate cuff fully and wait 30 seconds.	____	____	____	____
(2) Place stethoscope earpieces in ears and be sure sounds are clear, not muffled.	____	____	____	____
(3) Relocate brachial artery and place diaphragm of stethoscope over it. Do not allow chestpiece to touch cuff or clothing.	____	____	____	____
(4) Close valve of pressure bulb clockwise until tight.	____	____	____	____
(5) Quickly inflate cuff to 30 mm Hg above patient's estimated systolic pressure.	____	____	____	____
(6) Slowly release pressure bulb valve and allow manometer needle gauge to fall at rate of 2 to 3 mm Hg/sec. Make sure there are no extraneous sounds.	____	____	____	____
(7) Note point on manometer when you hear the first clear sound. The sound slowly will increase in intensity.	____	____	____	____
(8) Continue to deflate cuff gradually, noting point at which sound disappears in adults. Note pressure to nearest 2 mm Hg. Listen for 20 to 30 mm Hg after the last sound and then allow remaining air to escape quickly.	____	____	____	____
B. One-Step Method				
(1) Place stethoscope earpieces in ears, and be sure sounds are clear, not muffled.	____	____	____	____
(2) Relocate brachial artery, and place diaphragm of stethoscope over it. Do not allow chestpiece to touch cuff or clothing.	____	____	____	____
(3) Close valve of pressure bulb clockwise until tight.	____	____	____	____

	S	U	NP	Comments
(4) Quickly inflate cuff to 30 mm Hg above patient's usual systolic pressure.	____	____	____	____
(5) Slowly release pressure bulb valve and allow manometer needle to fall at rate of 2 to 3 mm Hg/sec. Note point on manometer when you hear the first clear sound. The sound will slowly increase in intensity.	____	____	____	____
(6) Continue to deflate cuff gradually, noting point at which sound disappears in adults. Note pressure to nearest 2 mm Hg. Listen for 20 to 30 mm Hg after the last sound and then allow remaining air to escape quickly.	____	____	____	____
6. The JNC recommends the average of two sets of BP measurements, 2 minutes apart. Use the second set as the baseline.	____	____	____	____
7. Remove cuff from extremity unless you need to repeat measurement. If this is the first assessment of patient, repeat procedure on the other extremity.	____	____	____	____
8. Assist patient in returning to comfortable position, and cover upper arm if previously clothed.	____	____	____	____
9. Discuss findings with patient as needed.	____	____	____	____
10. Perform hand hygiene. Clean earpieces, bell, and diaphragm of stethoscope with alcohol.	____	____	____	____
Evaluation				
1. Compare reading with previous baseline and/or acceptable value of blood pressure for patient's age.	____	____	____	____
2. Compare blood pressure measurements in both arms or both legs.	____	____	____	____
3. Correlate blood pressure readings with data obtained from pulse assessment and related cardiovascular signs and symptoms.	____	____	____	____
4. Record blood pressure reading in patient's record.	____	____	____	____
5. Report abnormal findings to nurse in charge or physician.	____	____	____	____

Name ____________________ Date __________ Instructor's Name ____________________________

Performance Checklist: Skill 12-4 Assessing Respiration

	S	U	NP	Comments
Assessment				
1. Determine need to assess patient's respiration.	_____	_____	_____	____________
2. Assess pertinent laboratory values.	_____	_____	_____	____________
3. Determine previous baseline respiratory rate (if available) from patient's record.	_____	_____	_____	____________
4. Assess respirations after pulse measurement for adults.	_____	_____	_____	____________
Planning				
1. Be sure patient is in comfortable position, preferably sitting or lying with the head of the bed elevated 45 to 60 degrees.	_____	_____	_____	____________
Implementation				
1. Draw curtain around bed and/or close door. Perform hand hygiene.	_____	_____	_____	____________
2. Be sure patient's chest is visible. If necessary, move bed linen or gown.	_____	_____	_____	____________
3. Place patient's arm in relaxed position across the abdomen or lower chest, or place your hand directly over patient's upper abdomen.	_____	_____	_____	____________
4. Observe complete respiratory cycle (one inspiration and one expiration).	_____	_____	_____	____________
5. After you observe cycle, look at watch's second hand and begin to count rate.	_____	_____	_____	____________
6. If rhythm is regular, count number of respirations in 30 seconds and multiply by 2. If rhythm is irregular, less than 12, or greater than 20, count for 1 full minute.	_____	_____	_____	____________
7. Note depth of respirations.	_____	_____	_____	____________
8. Note rhythm of ventilatory cycle.	_____	_____	_____	____________
9. Replace bed linen and patient's gown.	_____	_____	_____	____________
10. Perform hand hygiene.	_____	_____	_____	____________
Evaluation				
1. Discuss findings with patient as needed.	_____	_____	_____	____________
2. If you are assessing respirations for the first time, establish rate, rhythm, and depth as baseline if within normal range.	_____	_____	_____	____________
3. Compare respiration with patient's previous baseline and normal rate, rhythm, and depth.	_____	_____	_____	____________
4. Correlate respiratory rate, depth, and rhythm with data from pulse oximetry and arterial blood gases, if available.	_____	_____	_____	____________

	S	U	NP	Comments
5. Record respiratory rate and character in patient's record. Indicate type and amount of oxygen therapy if used by patient during assessment.	____	____	____	____________
6. Report abnormal findings to nurse in charge or physician.	____	____	____	____________

Name ____________________ Date __________ Instructor's Name ____________________

Performance Checklist: Skill 12-5 Measuring Oxygen Saturation (Pulse Oximetry)

	S	U	NP	Comments
Assessment				
1. Determine need to measure patient's oxygen saturation.	____	____	____	____________
2. Assess for factors that normally influence measurement of Spo_2.	____	____	____	____________
3. Review patient's record for health care provider's order. Check agency policy or procedure manual for standard of care for measurement of Spo_2.	____	____	____	____________
4. Determine most appropriate site for sensor probe placement.	____	____	____	____________
Planning				
1. Determine previous baseline Spo_2 (if available) from patient's record.	____	____	____	____________
2. Obtain oximeter and probe and place at bedside.	____	____	____	____________
3. Explain purpose of procedure to patient and how you will measure oxygen saturation. Instruct patient to breath normally.	____	____	____	____________
Implementation				
1. Perform hand hygiene.	____	____	____	____________
2. Position patient comfortably. If finger is chosen as monitoring site, support lower arm.	____	____	____	____________
3. If using the finger, remove fingernail polish from finger with acetone.	____	____	____	____________
4. Attach sensor probe to monitoring site.	____	____	____	____________
5. Once sensor is in place, turn on oximeter by activating power. Observe pulse waveform/intensity display and audible beep. Correlate oximeter pulse rate with patient's radial pulse.	____	____	____	____________
6. Inform patient that oximeter will sound if sensor falls off or if patient moves sensor.	____	____	____	____________
7. Leave probe in place until oximeter readout reaches constant value and pulse display reaches full strength during each cardiac cycle. Read Spo_2 value on digital display.	____	____	____	____________
8. Verify alarm limits and volume for continuous monitoring.	____	____	____	____________
9. Discuss findings with patient as needed.	____	____	____	____________
10. Remove probe and turn oximeter power off for intermittent monitoring.	____	____	____	____________

	S	U	NP	Comments
11. Assist patient in returning to comfortable position.	____	____	____	____________
12. Perform hand hygiene.	____	____	____	____________

Evaluation

	S	U	NP	Comments
1. Compare Spo_2 readings with patient's baseline and acceptable values.	____	____	____	____________
2. Compare Spo_2 with Sao_2 obtained from arterial blood gas measurements if available.	____	____	____	____________
3. Correlate Spo_2 reading with data obtained from respiratory rate, depth, and rhythm assessment.	____	____	____	____________
4. During continuous monitoring, assess skin integrity underneath probe at least every 2 hours, based on patients peripheral circulation.	____	____	____	____________
5. Record Spo_2 value in patient's record, indicating type and amount of oxygen therapy used by patient during assessment. Also record any signs and symptoms of oxygen desaturation.	____	____	____	____________
6. Report abnormal findings to nurse in charge or physician.	____	____	____	____________
7. Record patient's use of continuous or intermittent pulse oximetry. Document use of equipment for third-party payers.	____	____	____	____________

Name ____________________ Date __________ Instructor's Name ____________________

Procedural Guidelines 12-1 Measurement of Temporal Artery Temperature

	S	U	NP	Comments
1. Perform hand hygiene.	____	____	____	____________
2. Ensure that forehead is dry; wipe with towel if needed.	____	____	____	____________
3. Place probe flush on patient's forehead to avoid measuring ambient temperature.	____	____	____	____________
4. Press the red scan button with your thumb. Continuous scanning for the highest temperature will occur until you release the scan button.	____	____	____	____________
5. Slowly slide thermometer straight across forehead while keeping probe flush on skin.	____	____	____	____________
6. Keeping the scan button pressed, lift probe from forehead and touch probe to neck just behind earlobe.	____	____	____	____________
7. While scanning, a clicking sound occurs and stops when peak temperature is reached.	____	____	____	____________
8. Release the scan button; read and record temperature. The reading remains on for 15 seconds after the button is released.	____	____	____	____________
9. Clean probe with alcohol wipe or remove and dispose of probe cover if used.	____	____	____	____________

Name ____________ Date ________ Instructor's Name ____________

Procedural Guidelines 12-2 Preparation of Mercury-in-Glass Thermometer

	S	U	NP	Comments
1. Perform hand hygiene. Apply gloves.	____	____	____	____________
2. Hold end (if color-coded, tip will be blue or red) of glass thermometer with fingertips to reduce contamination of bulb.	____	____	____	____________
3. Read mercury level while gently rotating thermometer at eye level. If mercury is above desired level, grasp tip of thermometer securely, stand away from solid objects, and sharply flick wrist downward. Brisk shaking lowers mercury level in glass tube. Continue shaking until reading is below 35.5° C (96° F). Make sure thermometer reading is below patient's actual temperature before use.	____	____	____	____________
4. Insert thermometer into plastic sleeve cover. Apply lubricant to cover 2.5 to 3.5 cm (1 to 1½ inches) on rectal thermometer.	____	____	____	____________
5. Place thermometer using technique appropriate to oral, rectal, or axillary site.	____	____	____	____________
6. Leave thermometer in place 3 minutes for oral or rectal temperatures, 2 minutes for axillary temperature, or according to agency policy.	____	____	____	____________
7. Remove the thermometer. Carefully discard the plastic sleeve. Wipe off secretions with clean tissue, moving toward the bulb.	____	____	____	____________
8. Read thermometer at eye level, read findings, and store thermometer in storage container. Remove gloves and perform hand hygiene.	____	____	____	____________

Name ____________________ Date __________ Instructor's Name __________________________

Procedural Guidelines 12-3 Measuring Orthostatic Blood Pressure

	S	U	NP	Comments
1. With patient supine, take blood pressure measurement in each arm. Select arm with highest systolic reading for subsequent measurements.	_____	_____	_____	__________________________
2. Leaving blood pressure cuff in place, help patient to sitting position. After 1 to 3 minutes with patient in sitting position, take blood pressure. If orthostatic symptoms occur such as dizziness, weakness, lightheadedness, feeling faint, or sudden pallor, stop blood pressure measurement and help patient to a supine position.	_____	_____	_____	__________________________
3. Leaving blood pressure cuff in place, help patient to standing position. After 1 to 3 minutes with patient in standing position, take blood pressure. If orthostatic symptoms occur, stop blood pressure measurement and help patient to a supine position. In most cases, you will detect orthostatic hypotension within 1 minute of standing.	_____	_____	_____	__________________________
4. Record patient's blood pressure in each position. Note any additional symptoms or complaints.	_____	_____	_____	__________________________
5. Report findings of orthostatic hypotension or orthostatic symptoms to nurse in charge and physician or health care provider. Instruct patient to ask for assistance when getting out of bed if orthostatic hypotension is present or orthostatic symptoms occur.	_____	_____	_____	__________________________

Name ____________________ Date __________ Instructor's Name __________________________

Procedural Guidelines 12-4 Palpating Systolic Blood Pressure

	S	U	NP	Comments
1. Perform hand hygiene.	_____	_____	_____	__________________________
2. Apply BP cuff to the extremity selected for measurement.	_____	_____	_____	__________________________
3. Continually palpate the brachial, radial, or popliteal artery with fingertips of one hand.	_____	_____	_____	__________________________
4. Inflate the BP cuff 30 mm Hg above the point at which you no longer palpate the pulse.	_____	_____	_____	__________________________
5. Slowly release valve and deflate cuff, allowing manometer needle to fall at rate of 2 mm Hg/sec.	_____	_____	_____	__________________________
6. Note point on manometer when pulse is again palpable; this is the systolic blood pressure.	_____	_____	_____	__________________________
7. Deflate cuff rapidly and completely. Remove cuff from patient's extremity unless you need to repeat the measurement.	_____	_____	_____	__________________________
8. Perform hand hygiene.	_____	_____	_____	__________________________

Name ____________________ Date __________ Instructor's Name __________________________

Procedural Guidelines 12-5 Automatic Blood Pressure Measurement

	S	U	NP	Comments
1. Determine the appropriateness of using electronic BP measurement.	____	____	____	____________________
2. Determine best site for cuff placement.	____	____	____	____________________
3. Assist patient to comfortable position, either lying or sitting. Plug in device and place device near patient, ensuring that connector hose, between cuff and machine, will reach.	____	____	____	____________________
4. Locate on/off switch and turn on machine to enable device to self-test computer systems.	____	____	____	____________________
5. Select appropriate cuff size for patient extremity and appropriate cuff for machine. Electronic BP cuff and machine are matched by manufacturer and are not interchangeable.	____	____	____	____________________
6. Expose extremity for measurement by removing constricting clothing to ensure proper cuff application. Do not place BP cuff over clothing.	____	____	____	____________________
7. Prepare BP cuff by manually squeezing all the air out of the cuff and connecting cuff to connector hose.	____	____	____	____________________
8. Wrap flattened cuff snugly around extremity, verifying that only one finger fits between cuff and patient's skin. Make sure the "artery" arrow marked on the outside of the cuff is correctly placed.	____	____	____	____________________
9. Verify that connector hose between cuff and machine is not kinked. Kinking prevents proper inflation and deflation of cuff.	____	____	____	____________________
10. Following manufacturer's directions, set the frequency control of automatic or manual; then press start button. The first BP measurement will pump the cuff to a peak pressure of about 180 mm Hg. After this pressure is reached, the machine begins a deflation sequence that determines the BP. The first reading determines the peak pressure inflation for additional measurements.	____	____	____	____________________

	S	U	NP	Comments
11. When deflation is complete, digital display will provide the most recent values and flash time in minutes that has elapsed since the measurement occurred.	____	____	____	________________
12. Set frequency of BP measurements and upper and lower alarm limits for systolic, diastolic, and mean BP readings. Intervals between BP measurements are set from 1 to 90 minutes.	____	____	____	________________
13. You are able to obtain additional readings at anytime by pressing the start button.	____	____	____	________________
14. If frequent BP measurements are required, leave the cuff in place. Remove cuff every 2 hours to assess underlying skin integrity, and if possible, alternate BP sites. When you are finished using the electronic BP machine, clean BP cuff according to facility policy.	____	____	____	________________
15. Compare electronic BP readings with auscultatory BP measurements to verify accuracy of electronic BP device.	____	____	____	________________

13 Health Assessment and Physical Examination

Case Study

1. You are assigned to assist with physical examinations in the outpatient clinic. On the schedule for today are three patients. One of the patients is a 72-year-old Hispanic woman, another is a 16-year-old female, and the last is a 4-year-old boy.
   a. How can you assist each of these patients to feel more at ease before and during the physical examination?

Chapter Review

Match the description/definition in Column A with the correct term in Column B.

	Column A	**Column B**
________	1. Black, tarry stools	a. Ptosis
________	2. Fluid accumulation, swelling	b. Alopecia
________	3. Loss of hair	c. Edema
________	4. Drooping of eyelid over the pupil	d. Jaundice
________	5. Tiny, pinpoint red spots on the skin	e. Bruit
________	6. Curvature of the thoracic spine	f. Melena
________	7. Yellow-orange discoloration	g. Kyphosis
________	8. Increased gastrointestinal motility; growling sounds	h. Petechiae
________	9. Blowing, swishing sound in blood vessel	i. Nystagmus
________	10. Abnormal eye movements	j. Borborygmi
		k. Lordosis

Complete the following:

11. Identify the five skills used in physical assessment and briefly describe each.

12. Identify the following positions for physical examination.

a.

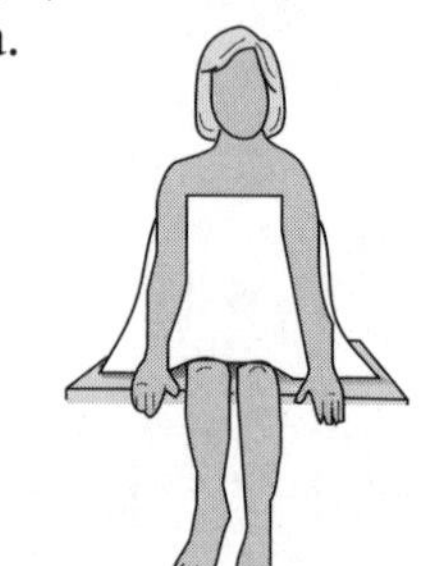

b.

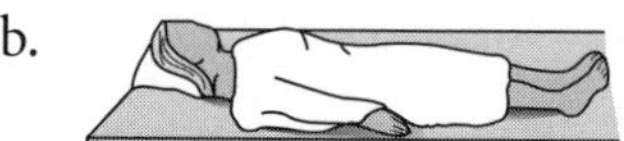

c.

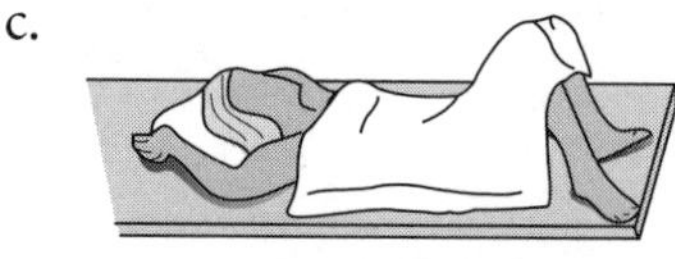

d.

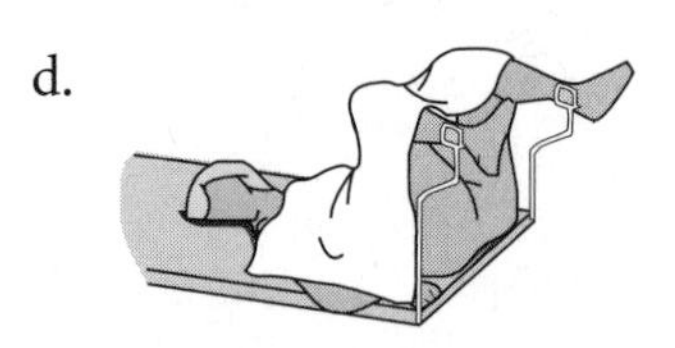

e.

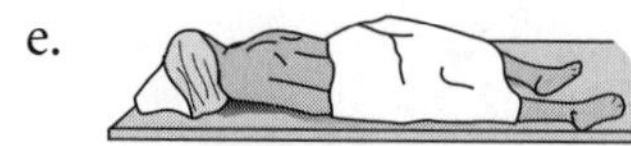

f.

g.

h.

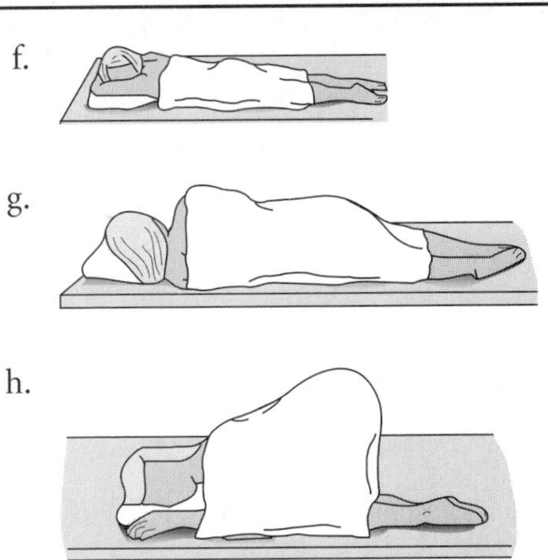

13. Identify which of the pulses is being palpated in each illustration.

a.

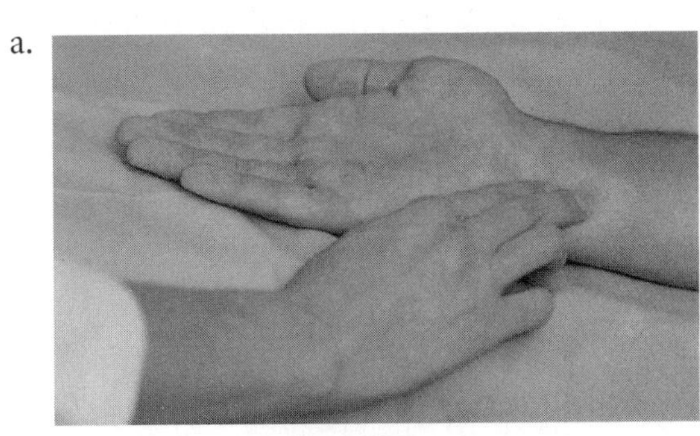

b.

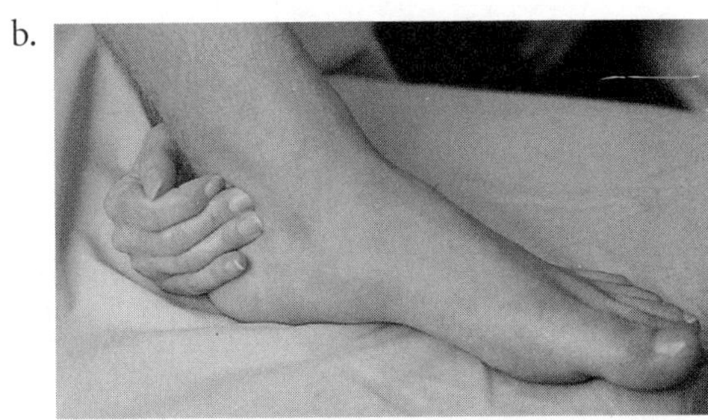

c.

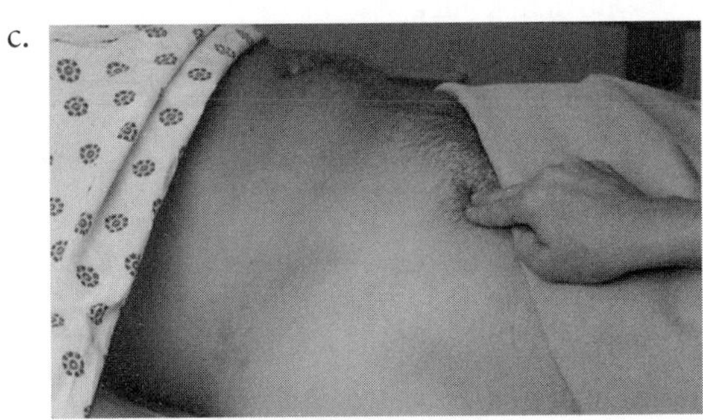

d.

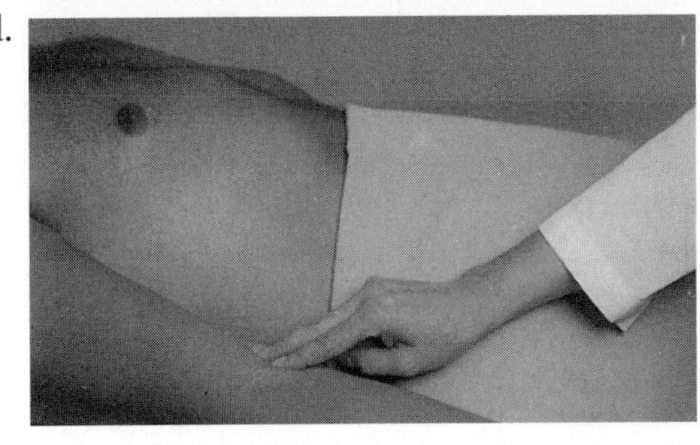

e.

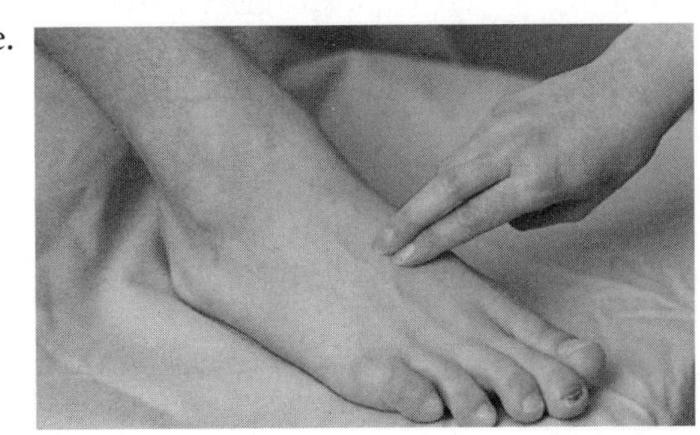

14. Correctly identify the primary skin lesion in each illustration.

a.

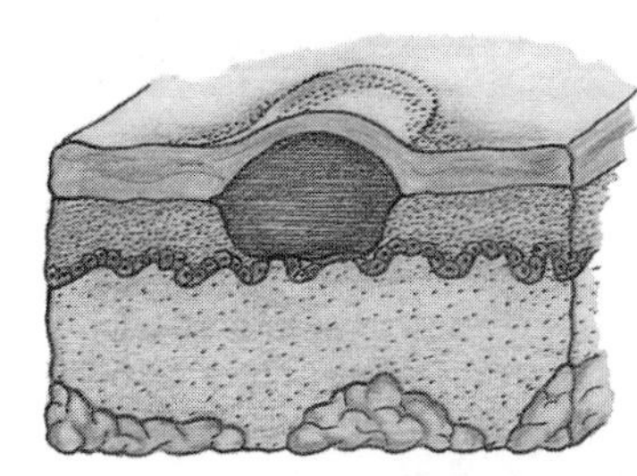

b.

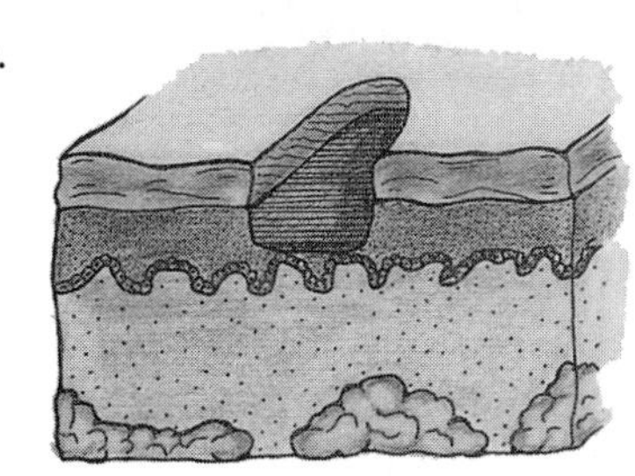

c.

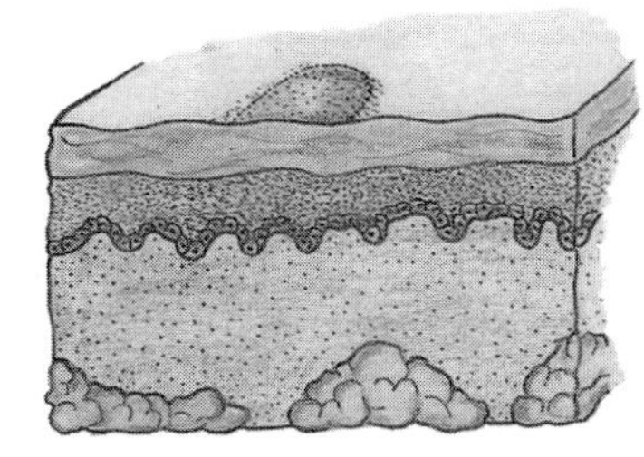

Continued

d.

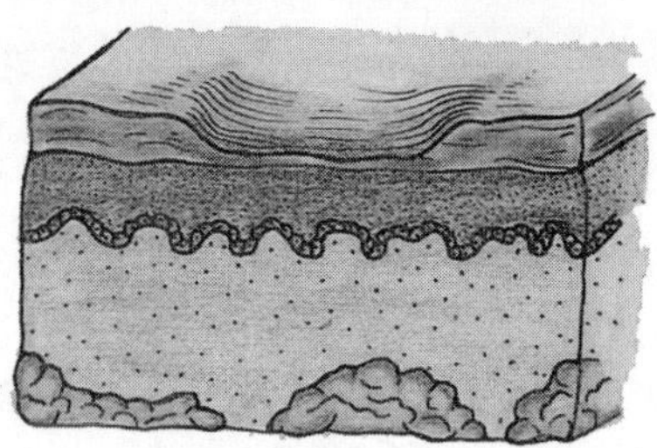

e.

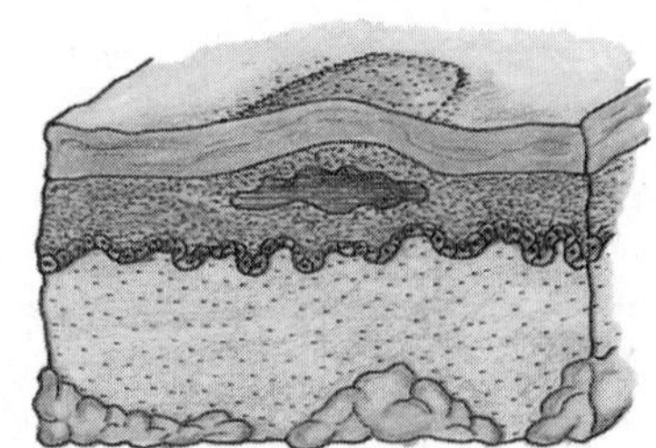

15. Identify on the illustration where the PMI is located.

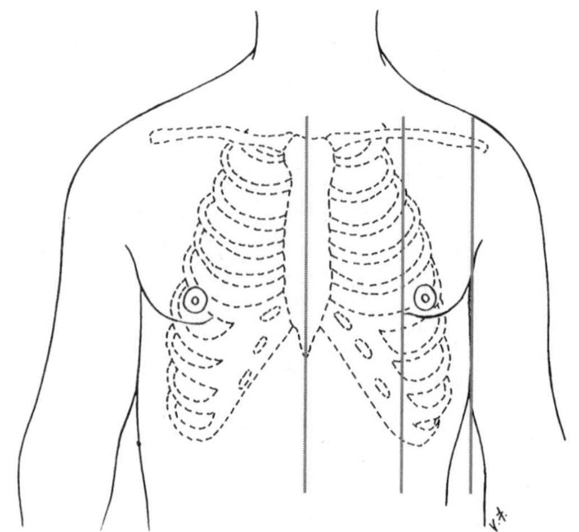

16. Identify a physical and a behavioral finding that may indicate abuse for the following:

	Physical	Behavioral
a. Child sexual abuse		
b. Domestic abuse		
c. Older adult abuse		

17. Identify the abdominal structures that are assessed.

a.

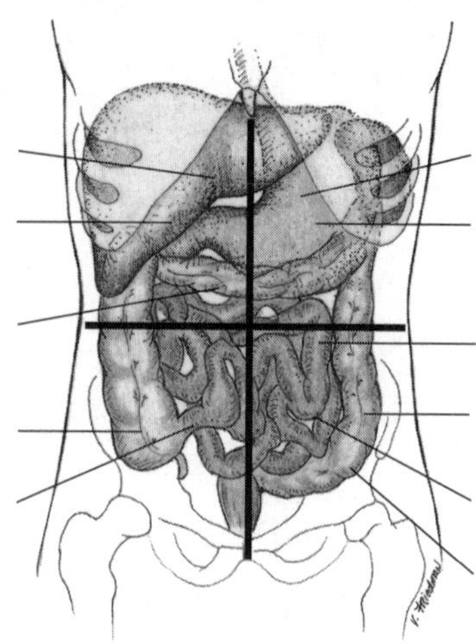

b.

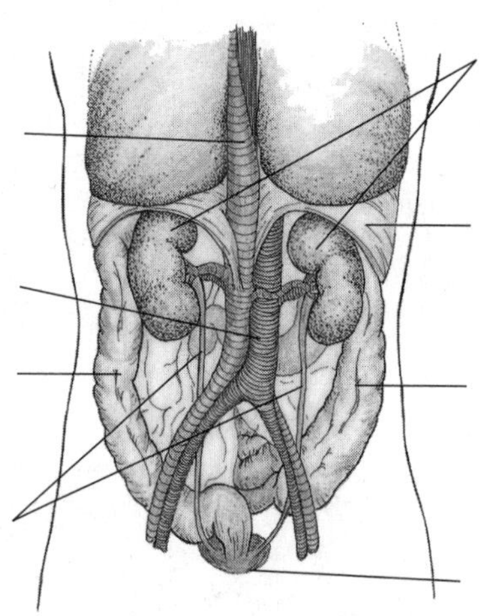

18. Check whether the following physical assessment findings would be expected or unexpected:

	Expected	*Unexpected*
a. Skin lifts easily and snaps back	_____	_____
b. Erythema noted over bony prominences	_____	_____
c. Hair evenly distributed over scalp and pubic area	_____	_____

		Expected	*Unexpected*
d.	Brown pigmentation of nails in longitudinal streaks (dark-skinned patient)	_____	_____
e.	Pallor in face and nail beds	_____	_____
f.	Clubbing of nails	_____	_____
g.	PEERLA	_____	_____
h.	Pupils cloudy	_____	_____
i.	Yellow discoloration of sclera	_____	_____
j.	Eardrum translucent, shiny, and pearly gray	_____	_____
k.	Light brown or gray cerumen	_____	_____
l.	Nasal septum midline	_____	_____
m.	Nasal mucosa pale with clear, watery discharge	_____	_____
n.	Sinuses tender to touch	_____	_____
o.	Teeth chalky white, with black discoloration	_____	_____
p.	Tongue medium red, moist, and slightly rough on top	_____	_____
q.	Soft palate rises when patient says "ah"	_____	_____
r.	Uvula reddened and edematous, tonsils with yellow exudate	_____	_____
s.	Thyroid gland small, smooth, and free of nodules	_____	_____
t.	Lungs resonant to percussion	_____	_____
u.	Costal angle greater than 90 degrees between costal margins	_____	_____
v.	Bulging of intercostal spaces	_____	_____
w.	No carotid bruit present	_____	_____
x.	Extra heart sound noted	_____	_____
y.	Jugular vein distention at 45-degree angle	_____	_____
z.	Dependent edema in ankles	_____	_____

		Expected	*Unexpected*
aa.	Female breasts smooth, symmetrical, without retraction	_____	_____
bb.	Soft, well-differentiated, moveable breast lumps noted	_____	_____
cc.	Bowel sounds active and audible over all four quadrants	_____	_____
dd.	Bulging flanks	_____	_____
ee.	Flat or concave umbilicus	_____	_____
ff.	Rebound tenderness found	_____	_____
gg.	Perineal skin smooth and slightly darker than surrounding skin	_____	_____
hh.	Bartholin's glands palpable, with discharge evident	_____	_____
ii.	Glans penis smooth and pink on all surfaces	_____	_____
jj.	Testes smooth and ovoid	_____	_____
kk.	No crepitus found on range of motion	_____	_____
ll.	Hips and shoulders aligned parallel	_____	_____

mm. Lordosis of spine noted _____ _____

nn. Reflexes symmetrical _____ _____

oo. Able to recall past events, unable to repeat series of five numbers _____ _____

pp. Able to perform rapidly alternating movements _____ _____

19. The patient has an area of discomfort. The nurse will examine this area:
    a. First
    b. Last
20. When using the stethoscope, high-pitched sounds are heard best with the:
    a. Diaphragm
    b. Bell
21. To inspect the adult patient's ear canal, the nurse pulls the auricle:
    a. Up and back
    b. Down and back
22. The position to place the patient in for a genital examination is:

23. The position to place the patient in for an abdominal examination is:

24. In the CAGE questionnaire, the question asked that represents 'A' in the acronym is:

25. A weight gain of 5 lb or 2.2 kg/day indicates:

26. Select all of the following techniques that are correct when assessing patients of different ages:
    a. Speak privately with adolescents about their concerns. _______
    b. Use close-ended questions to increase the speed of the examination. _______
    c. Call children and their parents by their first names. _______
    d. Provide time for children to play. _______
    e. Perform the exam for the older adult near bathroom facilities. _______
    f. Proceed rapidly through the exam of the older adult to finish it as quickly as possible. _______
27. Patients over the age of 65 years should be instructed to have yearly eye exams.
    True _____ False _____
28. The nurse is preparing to perform a skin assessment for an average adult patient. Select all of the following techniques that are correct:
    a. Use fluorescent lighting. _______
    b. Keep the room very warm. _______
    c. Use disposable gloves to inspect lesions. _______
    d. Look for coloration changes by checking the tongue and nail beds. _______
29. A patient with full range of motion with gravity is documented with a grade of _____ and noted as ___________ on the Lovett scale.
30. One example of a test for colorectal cancer is:

31. Select the three best positions that a patient may be placed in for a cardiac assessment:
    a. Prone _______
    b. Supine _______
    c. Lithotomy _______
    d. Sitting _______
    e. Left lateral recumbent _______
    f. Dorsal recumbent _______
    g. Sims' _______

Select the best answer for each of the following questions:

32. The nurse is assessing the patient's nail beds. An expected finding is indicated by:
    1. Softening of the nail bed

2. A concave curve to the nail
3. Brown linear streaks in the nail bed
4. A 160-degree angle between the nail plate and nail

33. An adolescent female arrives at the family planning center for a physical exam. For this patient, the nurse expects to find that the:
1. Breast tissue is softer
2. Nipples project and areolae have receded
3. Areolae are dark and have increased diameter
4. Breasts are elongated and nipples are smaller and flatter

34. The nurse has checked the medical record and found that the patient is experiencing anemia. The presence of anemia is accompanied by the nurse's finding of:
1. Pallor
2. Erythema
3. Jaundice
4. Cyanosis

35. A patient with asthma has come to the urgent care center for treatment. On auscultation of the lungs, the nurse hears rhonchi. These sounds are described as:
1. Dry and grating
2. Loud, low-pitched, and coarse
3. High-pitched, fine, and short
4. High-pitched and musical

36. The patient is admitted to the medical center with a peripheral vascular problem. The nurse is performing the initial assessment of the patient. While assessing the lower extremities, the nurse is alert to a venous insufficiency as indicated by:
1. Marked edema
2. Thin, shiny skin
3. Coolness to touch
4. Dusky red coloration

37. The nurse is performing a complete neurological assessment on the patient following a cerebral vascular accident (CVA/stroke). To assess cranial nerve III, the nurse:
1. Uses the Snellen chart
2. Lightly touches the cornea with a wisp of cotton
3. Whispers into one ear at a time
4. Measures pupil reaction to light and accommodation

38. Student nurses are practicing neurological assessment and determination of cranial nerve functioning. To assess cranial nerve VII, the student nurse should ask the patient to:
1. Say "ah"
2. Shrug the shoulders
3. Smile and frown
4. Stick out the tongue

39. While completing the physical examination, the nurse assesses and reports that the patient has petechiae. The nurse has found:
1. Light perspiration on the skin
2. Moles with regular edges
3. Thickness on the soles of the feet
4. Pinpoint size, flat red spots

40. The nurse reviews the chart and sees that the patient who has been admitted to the unit this morning has a hyperthyroid disorder. The nurse anticipates that an examination of the eyes will reveal:
1. Diplopia
2. Strabismus
3. Exophthalmos
4. Nystagmus

41. In preparation for an examination of the internal ear, the nurse anticipates that the color of the eardrum should appear:
1. White
2. Yellow
3. Slightly red
4. Pearly gray

42. A patient with a history of smoking and alcohol abuse has come to the clinic for a physical examination. Based on this history, the nurse is particularly alert during an examination of the oral cavity to the presence of:
1. Spongy gums
2. Pink tissue
3. Thick, white patches
4. Loose teeth

43. The patient in the physician's office has an increased anteroposterior diameter of the chest. The nurse should inquire specifically about the patient's history of:
1. Smoking
2. Thoracic trauma

3. Spinal surgery
4. Exposure to tuberculosis

44. When auscultating a patient's chest, the nurse hears what appears to be an S_3 sound. This is an expected finding if the patient is:
    1. 10 years old
    2. 35 years old
    3. 56 years old
    4. 82 years old
45. The patient in the medical center has been prescribed bed rest for a prolonged period of time. There is a possibility that the patient may have developed phlebitis. The nurse assesses for the presence of this condition by:
    1. Palpating the ankles for pitting edema
    2. Checking the popliteal pulses bilaterally
    3. Inspecting the thighs for clusters of ecchymosis
    4. Checking the appearance and circumference of the lower legs
46. When teaching the 45-year-old patient in the gynecologist's office about breast cancer, the nurse includes information on recommendations for screening. The patient is informed that a woman her age should have:
    1. Annual mammograms
    2. Biannual CAT scans
    3. Physical exams every 3 years
    4. Breast self-exams every 3 months
47. The patient has been experiencing some lightheadedness and loss of balance over the past few weeks. The nurse wants to check the patient's balance while waiting for the patient to have other laboratory tests. The nurse administers the:
    1. Allen test
    2. Rinne test
    3. Weber test
    4. Romberg test
48. Screenings are being conducted at the junior high school for scoliosis. The nurse is observing the students for the presence of:
    1. An S-shaped curvature of the spine
    2. An exaggerated curvature of the thoracic spine
    3. An exaggerated curvature of the lumbar spine
    4. A bulging of the cervical vertebrae and disks
49. While reviewing the medical record, the nurse notes that the patient has suspected pancreatitis. The nurse assesses the patient for:
    1. Positive rebound tenderness
    2. Midline abdominal pulsations
    3. Hyperactive bowel sounds to all quadrants
    4. Bulging of the flanks with dependent distention
50. An 80-year-old female patient is being assessed by the nurse in the extended care facility. The nurse is assessing the genitalia of this patient and suspects that there may be a malignancy present. The nurse's suspicion is due to the finding of:
    1. Scaly, nodular lesions
    2. Yellow exudates and redness
    3. Small ulcers with serous drainage
    4. Extreme pallor and edema
51. A screening for osteoporosis is being conducted at the annual health fair. To determine the risk factors for osteoporosis, the nurse is assessing individuals for:
    1. Multiparity
    2. A heavier than recommended body frame
    3. An African-American background
    4. A history of dieting and/or alcohol abuse
52. A patient in the rehabilitation facility has experienced a cerebral vascular accident (CVA/stroke) that has left the patient with an expressive aphasia. The nurse anticipates that this patient will:
    1. Be unable to speak or write
    2. Be unable to follow directions
    3. Respond inappropriately to questions
    4. Have difficulty interpreting words and phrases
53. A peripheral pulse that is easily palpable and normal in tension is documented as:
    1. 1+
    2. 2+

3. 3+
4. 4+

54. To assess the patient's visual fields, the nurse should:
    1. Ask the patient to read text
    2. Turn the room light on and off
    3. Move a finger, at arm's length, toward the patient from an angle
    4. Shine a penlight into the patient's eye at an oblique angle
55. The nurse exerts downward pressure on the thigh. This assessment is determining the muscle strength of the:
    1. Triceps
    2. Trapezius
    3. Quadriceps
    4. Gastrocnemius
56. Light palpation involves depressing the part being examined:
    1. 1/2 inch
    2. 1 inch
    3. 1 1/2 inches
    4. 2 inches
57. The nurse teaches the male patient that he should notify a health care provider if he finds the following during a testicular self-examination:
    1. Small, pea-sized lumps on the front of the testicle
    2. Cordlike structures on the top of the testicles
    3. Loose, deeper color scrotal skin with a coarse surface
    4. Smegma under the foreskin
58. The nurse assesses the patient's skin and documents that vesicles are present. This observation is based on the nurse finding:
    1. Flat, nonpalpable changes in skin color
    2. Palpable, solid elevations smaller than 1 cm
    3. Irregularly shaped elevated areas that vary in size
    4. Circumscribed elevations of skin filled with serous fluid

Study Group Questions

- What are the purposes of the physical exam?
- How is physical assessment integrated into patient care?
- How does the nurse incorporate cultural sensitivity and awareness of ethnic physiological differences into the physical exam?
- What are the physical assessment skills, and what information is obtained through their use?
- How does the nurse prepare the patient and environment for the physical exam?
- What similarities and differences exist in the preparation and procedure for a physical exam of a child, adult, and older adult?
- What information is obtained through a general survey?
- What positions and equipment are used for completion of the physical exam?
- What is the usual sequence for performing the physical exam?
- What are the expected and unexpected findings of a complete physical exam?
- What self-screening procedures may be taught to patients?
- How does the nurse report and record the findings of a physical exam?

Study Chart

Create a study chart to compare the Expected vs. Unexpected Findings in a Physical Exam, *working in the sequential order of the exam from the integumentary system through the neurological system.*

14 Administering Medications

Case Studies

1. You are visiting a patient at home who has poor eyesight and occasional forgetfulness. The patient has four oral medications to take at different times of the day.
   a. What strategies may be implemented to assist this patient in maintaining the medication regimen?
2. You are preparing to give medications in the medical center, but the prescriber's handwriting is difficult to read.
   a. What should you do to prevent medication errors?
3. A patient in a long-term care facility is about to receive her medications, but you notice that she does not have an identification band.
   a. What is your next action?
4. You are to administer an injection to a 6-year-old child on a pediatric acute care unit.
   a. What safety measures need to be implemented?
5. You are about to prepare a narcotic medication for administration to your patient. You notice that the previous amount was 24 tablets remaining, but that now there are only 23 tablets left in the box.
   a. What should you do?
6. You are caring for a patient who requires an antipyretic medication that is ordered for oral administration, but the patient has been experiencing severe nausea.
   a. What should you do?

Chapter Review

Match the description/definition in Column A with the correct term in Column B.

	Column A	Column B
_____	1. Placing medication under the tongue	a. Parenteral administration
_____	2. Two medications combined is greater than each given separately	b. Inhalation
_____	3. Secondary effects of the medication, such as nausea	c. Instillation
_____	4. Unpredictable effect of medications	d. Buccal
_____	5. Fluid administered and retained in a body cavity	e. Subcutaneous
_____	6. Injection into tissues below the dermis of the skin	f. Intraocular
_____	7. Severe allergic response characterized by bronchospasm and laryngeal edema	g. Idiosyncratic reaction
_____	8. Inserting medication into the eye	h. Polypharmacy
_____	9. Administering medications through the oral, nasal, or pulmonary passages	i. Sublingual
_____	10. Patient taking many medications	j. Synergistic effect
_____	11. Placing solid medication against the mucous membranes of the cheek	k. Side effects
_____	12. Injecting medication into body tissues	l. Toxic effects
		m. Anaphylactic reaction

Complete the following:

13. Provide an example of how the nurse's professional responsibility in administering medications is controlled or regulated:

14. Identify a strategy for the nurse to implement to avoid errors with medications that appear the same:

15. Provide an example of how each one of the following factors can influence the actions of medications:
    a. Dietary factors:
    b. Physiological variables:
    c. Environmental conditions:

16. Identify the four routes for parenteral administration of medications.

17. For the following medication orders, identify the essential component that is missing. (NOTE: All have been correctly signed by the prescriber.)
    a. Apresoline IM stat
    b. Morphine sulfate 10 mg q3-4h
    c. Vancomycin 1 g IV
    d. Lasix 40 mg bid

18. Identify the six guidelines or "rights" that the nurse uses for administering medications.
    1. ______________________
    2. ______________________
    3. ______________________
    4. ______________________
    5. ______________________
    6. ______________________

19. Place the following steps for mixing two types of insulin in one syringe in the correct sequence:
    a. Using an insulin syringe, inject air, equal to the dose of cloudy insulin you administer, into the cloudy vial. _______
    b. Remove the syringe from the vial of cloudy insulin. _______
    c. Place the needle of the syringe back into the cloudy vial, and withdraw the correct dose. _______
    d. Perform hand hygiene. _______
    e. With the same syringe, inject air, equal to the dose of clear insulin you administer, into the clear vial and withdraw the correct dose into the syringe. _______
    f. Remove the syringe from the clear insulin, and get rid of air bubbles to ensure accurate dosing. _______
    g. Verify insulin labels before preparing the dose to ensure that you give the correct type of insulin. _______
    h. Roll cloudy insulin between the hands to resuspend the insulin preparation. _______
    i. Wipe the tops of both insulin vials with alcohol swabs. _______

20. Identify the form of medication for the following:
    a. Solid dose form for oral use; medication in a powder, liquid, or oil form and encased by a gelatin shell:
    b. Solid dose form mixed with gelatin and shaped in form of pellet for insertion into body cavity:

c. Alcohol or water-alcohol drug solution:

d. Clear liquid containing water and/or alcohol; designed for oral use; usually has a sweetener added:

e. Finely divided drug particles dispersed in a liquid medium; when left standing, particles settle to the bottom of the container:

f. A small, flexible oval consisting of two soft outer layers and a middle layer containing medication:

g. Drug in liquid suspension applied to protect skin:

21. An example of a commonly abused over-the-counter medication is:

22. Noncompliance with or nonadherence to medication therapy may be related to:

23. Identify for each of the following which one of the two has the **faster** absorption or action in the body:

a.	IV _____	or	Oral _____
b.	IM _____	or	Subcutaneous _____
c.	Acidic oral medication _____	or	Alkaline oral medication _____
d.	Tablets _____	or	Solutions _____
e.	Large surface area _____	or	Smaller surface area _____
f.	Less lipid soluble _____	or	Highly lipid soluble _____
g.	Albumin binding _____	or	Non-albumin binding _____

24. The time that it takes for a medication to reach its highest effective concentration is its:

25. Oral medication is contraindicated for a patient with:

26. What is a potential problem with this medication order?
Lasix 40.0 mg

27. Identify the appropriate equivalents for the following:
a. 1 ml = __________ gtt
b. 60 ml = __________ ounces
c. __________ L = 1 quart
d. 3 g = __________ mg
e. 0.25 L = __________ ml
f. _____ ml = 1 teaspoon

28. The Braslow tape uses ______________ to determine safe doses for children in an emergency situation.

29. Verbal orders are usually required to be signed by the prescriber within _________ (time frame).

30. The nurse calculates the medication order and determines that 6 tablets should be given to the patient for each dose. What should the nurse do first?

31. After the patient is given medications, the patient tells the nurse that the medicine looks different from the previous medications. The nurse should:

32. An unopened unit-dose medication that is refused by the patient needs to be discarded.
True _____ False _____

33. Only tablets scored by the manufacturer can be broken in half.
True _____ False _____

34. Crushed medication should be mixed in a large amount of food to mask the taste.
True _____ False _____

35. The nurse is responsible for administering an incorrect medication or dosage.
True _____ False _____

36. An older adult is having difficulty swallowing the pills that are ordered. The nurse should:

37. Identify a technique that may be used to facilitate administration of medications to children:
   a. Oral medications:

   b. Injections:

38. Identify a way that the nurse may minimize the discomfort of an injection.

39. How should a medication that is irritating to the tissues be injected?

40. Identify the correct angle for each of the following illustrations, and the type of injection that is being administered:
a. _________ b. _________ c. _________

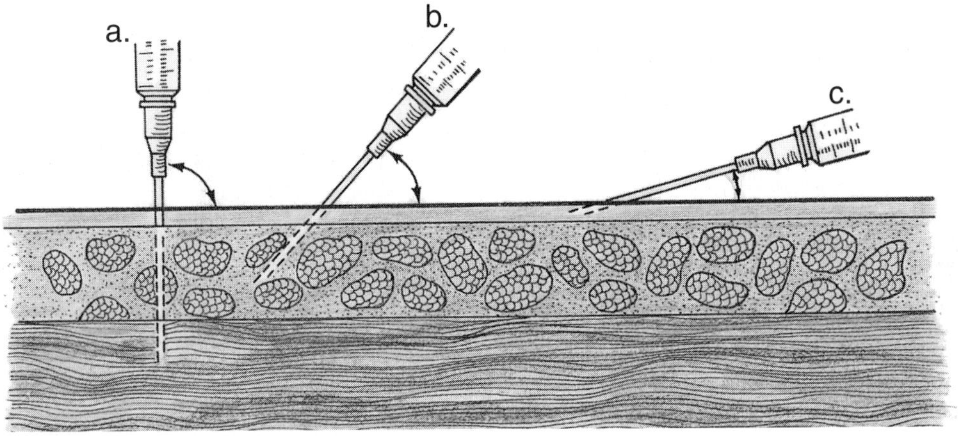

a. b. c.

41. Identify three ways in which medication may be administered intravenously.
1.

2.

3.

42. Identify the following math formulas used for drug dosage calculation:
   a. Solid or liquid adult medications:

   b. Pediatric dosages:

43. Identify the meaning of the following abbreviations:
   a. ac: ______________________________
   b. bid: ______________________________
   c. prn: ______________________________
   d. q4h: ______________________________
   e. stat: ______________________________

44. Calculate the correct dosages for the following medication orders:
   a. Prescriber's order: Synthroid 0.150 mg PO daily
   In stock: Scored tablets labeled 75 mcg
   How many tablets should be given?

b. Prescriber's order: Mellaril 150 mg PO bid
In stock: Mellaril 50 mg/ml
How much of the medication should be given?

c. Prescriber's order: Lasix 20 mg IM stat
In stock: Lasix 10 mg/ml
How much medication should be given?

d. Prescriber's order: Aldomet 250 mg PO bid
In stock: Tablets labeled 125 mg
How many tablets should be given?

e. Prescriber's order: Demerol 75 mg IM prn
In stock: Demerol 25 mg/0.5 ml
How much medication should be given?
Mark the amount to be administered on the syringe.

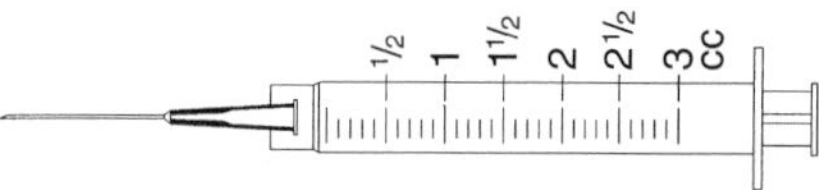

f. Prescriber's order: Regular insulin 24 units
In stock: Regular insulin U-100
How much medication should be administered?
Mark the amount to be administered on the syringe.

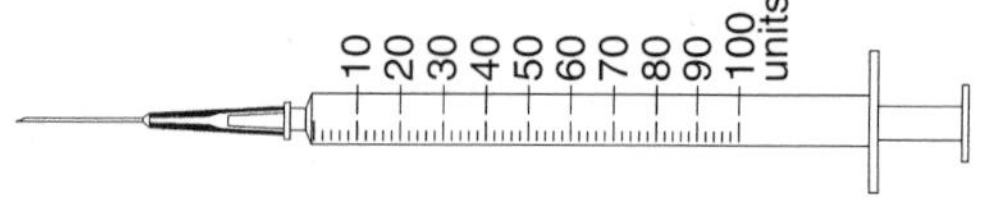

g. Child's body surface area (BSA) = 1.25 m^2
Adult dosage is 25 mg.
How much medication should be given to this child?

45. Identify an area of patient assessment before administration of a parenteral injection:

46. Identify on the figure the sites recommended for subcutaneous injections:

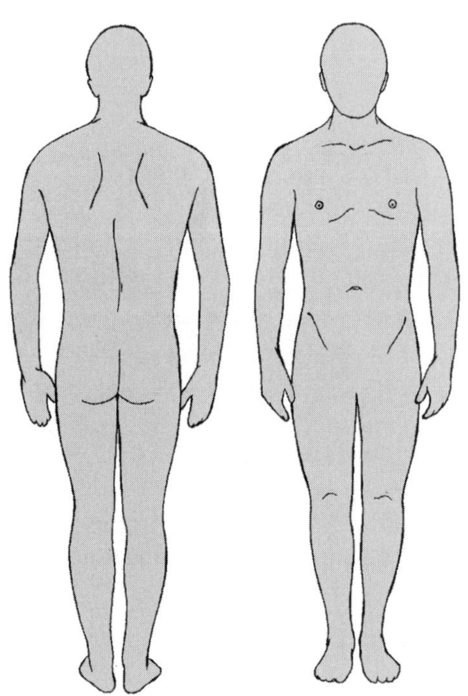

47. Select all of the following actions that are correct for the administration of medications to a patient with dysphagia:
   a. Do not allow the patient to self-administer, even if able. _______
   b. Position the patient upright. _______
   c. Turn the patient's head toward the weaker side to help the patient swallow. _______
   d. Use thinner liquids for the patient to take with the medications. _______
   e. Use a straw for liquids. _______

f. Crush medication and mix with pureed food, if indicated. _______

48. A priority assessment specifically for the patient receiving medication through a nasogastric tube is for the nurse to:

49. Before administration of a topical medication, the nurse needs to:

50. For the administration of ear drops:
   a. Position the patient.

   b. Pull ear pinna backward, up, and out for an adult patient.

   c. Irrigate with _____ ml of __________ temperature fluid.

51. For the use of a metered-dose inhaler:
   a. When the patient has difficulty coordinating the inhaler, a(n) __________ should be used.
   b. The medication order is 2 puffs of the inhaler qid. The canister contains 160 puffs total. How many days will the canister last? _________________

52. The patient should be placed in ____________________ position for the administration of a rectal suppository.

Select the best answer for each of the following questions:

53. The nurse determines the location for an injection by identifying the greater trochanter of the femur, anterosuperior iliac spine, and iliac crest. The injection site being used by the nurse is the:
   1. Rectus femoris muscle
   2. Ventrogluteal area
   3. Dorsogluteal area
   4. Vastus lateralis muscle

54. Upon receiving the assignment for the evening, the nurse notices that two of the patients have the same name. The best way to identify two patients on a medical unit who have the same name is to:
   1. Ask the patients their names
   2. Verify their names with the family members
   3. Check the patients' ID bands
   4. Ask another nurse about their identities

55. The nurse is to administer a subcutaneous injection to an average size adult. The nurse selects a:
   1. 27-gauge, ½-inch needle and 0.5-ml syringe
   2. 25-gauge, ⅛-inch needle and 1-ml syringe
   3. 22-gauge, 1-inch needle and 3-ml syringe
   4. 20-gauge, 1-inch needle and 3-ml syringe

56. The nurse has administered medications to all of the assigned patients on the medical unit. Upon assessing the response of the medications given, the nurse is alert to the possibility of a toxic reaction. This is indicated by the patient experiencing:
   1. Itching
   2. Nausea
   3. Dizziness
   4. Respiratory depression

57. The nursing staff is completing a review of the procedures used for the storage and administration of narcotics. The nurse implements the required procedure when:
   1. Narcotics are kept together with the patient's other medications
   2. Small amounts of medication may be discarded without notation
   3. The narcotic count is checked daily by the medication nurse
   4. A separate administration record is kept in addition to the patient's medication administration record (MAR)

58. An order is written for the patient to receive potassium chloride (KCl) and vitamins intravenously. The nurse goes into the medication room and selects

equipment to provide the medication by a(n):
1. IV bolus administration
2. Tandem administration
3. Piggyback administration
4. Large-volume administration

59. While completing the admission assessment, the nurse discovers that the patient is allergic to shellfish. Later that morning when the nurse is preparing medications for this patient, the nurse will withhold medication that contains:
1. Iodine
2. Alcohol
3. Glucose
4. Calcium carbonate

60. A patient in the nurse practitioner's office is receiving penicillin for the first time. The nurse asks the patient to wait in the office following the administration of the medication. The nurse is observing for a possible anaphylactic response that would be demonstrated by:
1. Drowsiness
2. Pharyngeal edema
3. An increased blood pressure reading
4. A decreased respiratory rate

61. The following order is written for the patient to receive eye medication: 1 gtt OS. The nurse will administer:
1. 1 ml to the right eye
2. 1 drop to the right eye
3. 1 drop to the left eye
4. 1 drop to both eyes

62. A drug that is to be given on a q4h schedule may be administered at:
1. 10 AM and 10 PM
2. 10 AM, 2 PM, and 10 PM
3. 10 AM, 2 PM, 6 PM, and 10 PM
4. 10 AM, 2 PM, 6 PM, 10 PM, and 2 AM

63. A specific assessment that the nurse should make before the administration of an anticoagulant is to check for:
1. An allergy history
2. Evidence of bruising
3. The patient's level of discomfort
4. Increased blood pressure

64. In the event of a mistake in the administration of medications, the first action that the nurse should take is to:
1. Complete an occurrence report
2. Inform the patient of the problem
3. Report the error to the nurse in charge/physician
4. Provide an appropriate antidote for the medication given

65. When preparing to administer the patient's medications, the nurse notes that the prescriber's order is difficult to read. The nurse should:
1. Check with the patient
2. Call the prescriber
3. Call the pharmacist
4. Check with the charge nurse

66. The subcutaneous site that is most commonly used for heparin injections is the:
1. Abdomen
2. Anterior thigh
3. Scapular region
4. Outer aspect of the upper arm

67. The prescriber indicates to the nurse that the patient will be receiving an intermediate-acting insulin. The nurse anticipates that the patient will receive:
1. Insulin glargine (Lantus)
2. Insulin lispro (Humalog)
3. Isophane insulin suspension (NPH)
4. Protamine zinc insulin suspension (PZI)

68. The charge nurse is evaluating the injection technique of the new staff member. The correct technique for a Z-track injection is noted when the new staff member:
1. Uses the deltoid site
2. Pulls the skin 1 to 1½ inches laterally
3. Removes the needle immediately after the injection
4. Releases the skin before the needle is removed

69. For a subcutaneous injection to an average size adult, which one of the following techniques requires correction? The student nurse:
1. Selects a 25-gauge, ⅝-inch needle
2. Injects the needle at a 45-degree angle

3. Recaps the needle after injecting the medication
4. Does not massage the injection site after administration

70. The nurse is aware that a parenteral administration of a concentrated dose of medication in a small amount of fluid is a:
    1. Bolus injection
    2. Piggyback infusion
    3. Volume control infusion
    4. Mini-infuser administration

Study Group Questions

- How are medications named and classified, and what forms of medications are available?
- What legislation and standards guide medication administration?
- How are medications absorbed, distributed, metabolized, and excreted from the body?
- What are the different types of medication actions?
- What are the different routes for medication administration, and what are the advantages, disadvantages, and contraindications for each route?
- What are the systems used for drug measurement, and how are amounts converted within and between the systems?
- How are dosages calculated for oral, parenteral, and pediatric medications?
- What are the roles of the health team members in the administration of medications?
- What are the six "rights" of medication administration?
- What patient assessment data are critical to obtain before administering medications?
- What equipment is used for the administration of medications via the different routes?
- What are the sites/landmarks for parenteral administration?
- What are the procedures for administration of medications?
- How can IV medication be administered?
- How is administration of medications adapted to patients of different ages and levels of health?
- What information is included in patient/family teaching for medication administration?

Study Chart

Create a study chart to compare Parenteral Medication and Preparation, *identifying the equipment, needle gauge, amount of medication, site to be used, and angle of injection for subcutaneous, intramuscular, and intradermal injections.*

Name ____________________ **Date** __________ **Instructor's Name** ________________________

Performance Checklist: Skill 14-1 Administering Oral Medications

	S	U	NP	Comments
Assessment				
1. Check accuracy and completeness of each MAR or computer printout with prescriber's written medication order.				
2. Assess for any contraindications to patient receiving oral medication.				
3. Assess risk for aspiration. Assess patient's swallow, cough, and gag reflexes.				
4. Assess patient's medical history, history of allergies, medication history, and diet history.				
5. Gather and review assessment and laboratory data that influences drug administration.				
6. Assess patient's knowledge regarding health and medication usage.				
7. Assess patient's preferences for fluids. Maintain ordered fluid restriction (when applicable).				
Planning				
1. Determine expected outcomes. Clarify order as necessary.				
2. Recopy or reprint parts of MAR that are difficult to read.				
Implementation				
1. Prepare medications.				
a. Perform hand hygiene				
b. If medication cart is used, move it outside patient's room.				
c. Unlock medicine drawer or cart.				
d. Prepare medications for one patient at a time. Keep all pages of MARs or computer printouts for one patient together.				
e. Select correct drug from stock supply or unit-dose drawer. Compare label of medication with MAR or computer printout.				
f. Check expiration date on all medications.				
g. Calculate drug dose as necessary. Double-check calculation.				
h. When preparing narcotics, check record for previous drug count and compare with supply available.				

	S	U	NP	Comments
i. Prepare solid forms of oral medications.				
(1) To prepare tablets or capsules from a floor stock bottle, pour required number into bottle cap and transfer medication to medication cup. Do not touch medication with fingers. Return extra tablets or capsules to bottle. Break medications that need to be broken to administer half the dosage can be broken using a gloved hand, or cut with a pillating device. Make sure these tablets are prescored.	_____	_____	_____	____________________
(2) To prepare unit-dose tablets or capsules, place packaged tablet or capsule directly into medicine cup. (Do not remove wrapper.)	_____	_____	_____	____________________
(3) Place all tablets or capsules to be given to patient at same time in one medicine cup. Place medications requiring preadministration assessments in separate cups.	_____	_____	_____	____________________
(4) If patient has difficulty swallowing and liquid medications are not an option, use a pill-crushing device, such as a mortar and pestle, to grind pills. If a pill-crushing device is not available, place tablet between two medication cups and grind with a blunt instrument. Mix ground tablet in small amount of soft food (e.g., custard, applesauce).	_____	_____	_____	____________________
j. Prepare liquids:				
(1) Gently shake container. Remove bottle cap from container and place cap upside down or open the unit-dose container. If unit-dose container has correct amount to administer, no further preparation is necessary.	_____	_____	_____	____________________

	S	U	NP	Comments
(2) Hold bottle with label against palm of hand while pouring.	____	____	____	____
(3) Hold medication cup at eye level and fill to desired level. Make sure scale is even with fluid level at its surface or base of meniscus, not edges. For small doses of liquid medications, draw liquid into a calibrated 10-ml syringe without needle.	____	____	____	____
(4) Discard any excess liquid into sink. Wipe lip and neck of bottle with paper towel.	____	____	____	____
(5) Administer liquid medications packaged in single-dose cups directly from the single-dose cup. Do not pour them into medicine cups.	____	____	____	____
k. Compare MAR with prepared drug and container.	____	____	____	____
l. Return stock containers or unused unit-dose medications to shelf or drawer, and read label again.	____	____	____	____
m. Do not leave drugs unattended.	____	____	____	____
2. Administering medications:				
a. Take medications to patient at correct time, and perform hand hygiene.	____	____	____	____
b. Verify patient's identity by using at least two identifiers.	____	____	____	____
c. Compare medication labels with MAR at bedside.	____	____	____	____
d. Explain purpose of each medication and its action to patient. Allow patient to ask any questions about drugs.	____	____	____	____
e. Assist patient to sitting or Fowler's position. Use side-lying position if sitting is contraindicated.	____	____	____	____
f. Administer medication.				
(1) **For tablets:** Patient may wish to hold solid medications in hand or cup before placing in mouth.	____	____	____	____
(2) Offer water or juice to help patient swallow medications. Give cold carbonated water if available and not contraindicated.	____	____	____	____

	S	U	NP	Comments
(3) **For sublingual medications:** Have patient place medication under tongue and allow it to dissolve completely. Caution patient against swallowing tablet whole.	____	____	____	____
(4) **For buccal medications:** Have patient place medication in mouth against mucous membranes of the cheek until it dissolves. Avoid administering liquids until buccal medication has dissolved.	____	____	____	____
(5) Caution patient against chewing or swallowing lozenges.	____	____	____	____
(6) **For powdered medications:** Mix with liquids at bedside, and give to patient to drink.	____	____	____	____
(7) Give effervescent powders and tablets immediately after dissolving.	____	____	____	____
g. If patient is unable to hold medications, place medication cup to the lips and gently introduce each drug into the mouth, one at a time. Do not rush.	____	____	____	____
h. If tablet or capsule falls to the floor, discard it and repeat preparation.	____	____	____	____
i. Stay in room until patient has completely swallowed each medication. Ask patient to open mouth if uncertain whether patient has swallowed medication.	____	____	____	____
j. For highly acidic medications, offer patient nonfat snack if not contraindicated by patient's condition.	____	____	____	____
k. Assist patient in returning to comfortable position.	____	____	____	____
l. Dispose of soiled supplies, and perform hand hygiene.	____	____	____	____
m. Replenish stock such as cups and straws, return cart to medicine room, and clean work area.	____	____	____	____

	S	U	NP	Comments
Evaluation				
1. Evaluate patient's response to medications at times that correlate with the medication's onset, peak, and duration.	____	____	____	____________________
2. Ask patient or family member to identify medication name, purpose, action, schedule, and potential side effects.	____	____	____	____________________
3. Record administration of medication on MAR or computer printout. Return MAR or computer printout to appropriate file for next administration time.	____	____	____	____________________
4. Notify prescriber if patient exhibits a toxic effect or allergic reaction or side effects occur. Withhold further doses.	____	____	____	____________________

Name ____________________ **Date** __________ **Instructor's Name** ______________________________

Performance Checklist: Skill 14-2 Administering Ophthalmic Medication

	S	U	NP	Comments
Assessment				
1. Check accuracy and completeness of each MAR or computer printout with prescriber's written medication order.	_____	_____	_____	____________________
2. Recopy or re-print any portion of MAR that is difficult to read.	_____	_____	_____	____________________
3. Assess condition of external eye structures.	_____	_____	_____	____________________
4. Determine whether patient has any known allergies to eye medications. Also ask if patient has allergy to latex.	_____	_____	_____	____________________
5. Determine whether patient has any symptoms of visual alterations.	_____	_____	_____	____________________
6. Assess patient's level of consciousness and ability to follow directions.	_____	_____	_____	____________________
7. Assess patient's knowledge regarding drug therapy and desire to self-administer medication.	_____	_____	_____	____________________
8. Assess patient's ability to manipulate and hold equipment necessary for eye medication.	_____	_____	_____	____________________
Planning				
1. Determine expected outcomes. Clarify order as necessary.	_____	_____	_____	____________________
2. Recopy or reprint parts of MAR that are difficult to read.	_____	_____	_____	____________________
Implementation				
1. Prepare medication.	_____	_____	_____	____________________
2. Take medications to patient at correct time and perform hand hygiene.	_____	_____	_____	____________________
3. Verify patient's identity by using at least two patient identifiers.	_____	_____	_____	____________________
4. Compare label of medication against MAR for third time.	_____	_____	_____	____________________
5. Explain procedure to patient regarding positioning and sensations to expect.	_____	_____	_____	____________________
6. Arrange supplies and medications at bedside. Apply clean gloves.	_____	_____	_____	____________________
7. Gently roll container.	_____	_____	_____	____________________
8. Ask patient to lie supine or sit back in chair with head slightly hyperextended.	_____	_____	_____	____________________

	S	U	NP	Comments
9. If crust or drainage is present along eyelid margins or inner canthus, gently wash away. Apply damp washcloth or cotton ball over eye for a few minutes to soak crusts that are dried and difficult to remove. Always wipe clean from inner to outer canthus.	____	____	____	____________
10. Hold cotton ball or clean tissue in nondominant hand on patient's cheekbone just below lower eyelid.	____	____	____	____________
11. With tissue or cotton resting below lower lid, gently press downward with thumb or forefinger against bony orbit.	____	____	____	____________
12. Ask patient to look at ceiling.	____	____	____	____________
13. Administer ophthalmic medication.	____	____	____	____________
a. To instill eye drops:				
(1) With dominant hand resting on patient's forehead, hold filled medication eye dropper or ophthalmic solution approximately 1 to 2 cm (1/2 to 1/2 inch) above conjunctival sac.	____	____	____	____________
(2) Drop prescribed number of medication drops into conjunctival sac.	____	____	____	____________
(3) If patient blinks or closes eye or if drops land on outer lid margins, repeat procedure.	____	____	____	____________
(4) After instilling drops, ask patient to close eye gently.	____	____	____	____________
(5) When administering drugs that cause systemic effects, apply gentle pressure with your finger and clean tissue on the patient's nasolacrimal duct for 30 to 60 seconds.	____	____	____	____________
b. To instill eye ointment:				
(1) Ask patient to look at ceiling.	____	____	____	____________
(2) Holding ointment applicator above lower lid margin, apply thin stream of ointment evenly along inner edge of lower eyelid on conjunctiva from inner canthus to outer canthus.	____	____	____	____________
(3) Have patient close eye and roll eye behind closed eyelid.	____	____	____	____________

	S	U	NP	Comments
c. To administer intraocular disc:				
(1) Application:				
(a) Open package containing the disc. Apply gloves. Gently press your fingertip against the disc so that it adheres to your finger. Position the convex side of the disc on your fingertip.	____	____	____	____
(b) With your other hand, gently pull the patient's lower eyelid away from the eye. Ask patient to look up.	____	____	____	____
(c) Place the disc in the conjunctival sac so that it floats on the sclera between the iris and lower eyelid.	____	____	____	____
(d) Pull the patient's lower eyelid out and over the disc.	____	____	____	____
(2) Removal:				
(a) Perform hand hygiene, and put on gloves.	____	____	____	____
(b) Explain procedure to patient.	____	____	____	____
(c) Gently pull down on the patient's lower eyelid.	____	____	____	____
(d) Using your forefinger and thumb of your opposite hand, pinch the disc and lift it out of the patient's eye.	____	____	____	____
14. If excess medication is on eyelid, gently wipe it from inner to outer canthus.	____	____	____	____
15. If patient had eye patch, apply clean patch by placing it over affected eye so entire eye is covered. Tape securely without applying pressure to eye.	____	____	____	____
16. If patient receives more than one eye medication to the same eye at the same time, wait at least 5 minutes before administering the next medication.	____	____	____	____
17. If patient receives eye medication to both eyes at the same time, use a different tissue or cotton ball with each eye.	____	____	____	____

	S	U	NP	Comments
18. Remove gloves, dispose of soiled supplies in proper receptacle, and perform hand hygiene.	____	____	____	____________

Evaluation

	S	U	NP	Comments
1. Note patient's response to instillation; ask if any discomfort was felt.	____	____	____	____________
2. Observe response to medication by assessing visual changes and noting any side effects.	____	____	____	____________
3. Ask patient to discuss drug's purpose, action, side effects, and technique of administration.	____	____	____	____________
4. Have patient demonstrate self-administration of next dose.	____	____	____	____________
5. Record drug, administration, and appearance of eye(s).	____	____	____	____________
6. Record and report any undesirable side effects to nurse in charge or physician.	____	____	____	____________

Name ____________________ Date __________ Instructor's Name ________________________

Performance Checklist: Skill 14-3 Using Metered-Dose Inhalers

	S	U	NP	Comments
Assessment				
1. Check accuracy and completeness of each MAR or computer printout with prescriber's written medication order.	____	____	____	____________
2. Assess respiratory pattern and auscultate breath sounds.	____	____	____	____________
3. If previously instructed in self-administration of inhaled medicine, assess patient's technique in using inhaler.	____	____	____	____________
4. Assess patient's ability to hold, manipulate, and depress canister and inhaler.	____	____	____	____________
5. Assess patient's readiness to learn.	____	____	____	____________
6. Assess patient's ability to learn.	____	____	____	____________
7. Assess patient's knowledge and understanding of disease and purpose and action of prescribed medications.	____	____	____	____________
8. Determine drug schedule and number of inhalations prescribed for each dose.	____	____	____	____________
Planning				
1. Determine expected outcomes. Clarify order as necessary.	____	____	____	____________
2. Check accuracy and completeness of each MAR or computer printout with prescriber's written medication order.	____	____	____	____________
3. Verify patient's identity by using at least two patient identifiers.	____	____	____	____________
4. Perform hand hygiene, and arrange equipment needed.	____	____	____	____________
5. Provide adequate time for teaching session.	____	____	____	____________
Implementation				
1. Prepare medication.	____	____	____	____________
2. Verify patient's identity using at least two patient identifiers.	____	____	____	____________
3. Compare the label of the medication with the MAR one more time at the patient's bedside.	____	____	____	____________
4. Help patient get into a comfortable position, such as sitting in chair in hospital room or sitting at kitchen table in home.	____	____	____	____________

	S	U	NP	Comments
5. Have patient manipulate inhaler, canister, and spacer device. Explain and demonstrate how canister fits into inhaler.	____	____	____	____________
6. Explain what metered dose is, and warn patient about overuse of inhaler and medication side effects.	____	____	____	____________
7. Explain steps for administering inhaled dose of MDI:	____	____	____	____________
a. Insert MDI canister into holder.	____	____	____	____________
b. Remove mouthpiece cover from inhaler.	____	____	____	____________
c. Shake inhaler strongly five or six times.	____	____	____	____________
d. Tell patient to sit up or stand and take a deep breath and exhale.	____	____	____	____________
e. Instruct the patient to position the inhaler in one of two ways:	____	____	____	____________
(1) Close mouth around MDI with opening toward back of throat.	____	____	____	____________
(2) Position MDI 2 to 4 cm (1 to 2 inches) from the mouth.	____	____	____	____________
f. With the inhaler positioned correctly, have patient hold inhaler with thumb at the mouthpiece and the index finger and middle finger at the top.	____	____	____	____________
g. Instruct patient to tilt head back slightly, inhale slowly and deeply through mouth, 3 to 5 seconds, while fully pressing down on the cannister.	____	____	____	____________
h. Have patient hold breath for approximately 10 seconds.	____	____	____	____________
i. Remove MDI, and exhale through pursed lips.	____	____	____	____________
8. Explain steps to administer MDI using a spacer such as an Aerochamber:	____	____	____	____________
a. Remove mouthpiece cover from inhaler and spacer.	____	____	____	____________
b. Insert MDI into end of spacer.	____	____	____	____________
c. Shake inhaler strongly five or six times.	____	____	____	____________
d. Have patient take a deep breath and exhale completely before closing mouth around spacer's mouthpiece.	____	____	____	____________
e. Have patient press medication canister one time, spraying one puff into spacer.	____	____	____	____________

	S	U	NP	Comments
f. Instruct patient to inhale slowly and deeply through mouth for 3 to 5 seconds.	_____	_____	_____	_____
g. Hold full breath for approximately 10 seconds.	_____	_____	_____	_____
h. Remove MDI and spacer before exhaling.	_____	_____	_____	_____
9. Explain steps to administer DPI:				
a. Remove mouthpiece cover. Do not shake DPI.	_____	_____	_____	_____
b. Hold inhaler upright, and turn wheel to the right and then to the left until you hear a click.	_____	_____	_____	_____
c. Exhale away from the inhaler.	_____	_____	_____	_____
d. Position mouthpiece between lips.	_____	_____	_____	_____
e. Inhale deeply and forcefully through the mouth.	_____	_____	_____	_____
f. Hold full breath for 5 to 10 seconds.	_____	_____	_____	_____
10. Instruct patient to wait at least 1 minute between inhalations or as ordered by prescriber.	_____	_____	_____	_____
11. Tell patient not to repeat inhaler doses until next scheduled dose.	_____	_____	_____	_____
12. Explain that patient may feel gagging sensation in throat caused by droplets of medication on pharynx or tongue.	_____	_____	_____	_____
13. Instruct patient on cleaning of inhaler in warm water.	_____	_____	_____	_____
Evaluation				
1. Ask if patient has any questions.	_____	_____	_____	_____
2. Have patient explain and demonstrate steps in use of inhaler.	_____	_____	_____	_____
3. Ask patient to explain medication schedule, side effects, and when to call health care provider.	_____	_____	_____	_____
4. Ask patient to calculate how many days the inhaler will last.	_____	_____	_____	_____
5. After medication instillation, assess patient's respirations and auscultate lungs.	_____	_____	_____	_____
6. Record patient education and patient's ability to perform self-administration.	_____	_____	_____	_____
7. Record medication administration and patient's response.	_____	_____	_____	_____

Name ____________ Date ________ Instructor's Name ____________

Performance Checklist: Skill 14-4 Preparing Injections

	S	U	NP	Comments
Assessment				
1. Check accuracy and completeness of each MAR or computer printout with prescriber's written medication order.	____	____	____	____________
2. Review pertinent information related to medication, including action, purpose, side effects, and nursing implications.	____	____	____	____________
3. Assess patient's body build, muscle size, and weight if giving Sub-Q or IM medication.	____	____	____	____________
Planning				
1. Determine expected outcomes. Clarify order as necessary.	____	____	____	____________
2. Recopy or reprint parts of MAR that are difficult to read.	____	____	____	____________
Implementation				
1. Perform hand hygiene and assemble supplies.	____	____	____	____________
2. Prepare medication. Check medication order or MAR against label on medication.	____	____	____	____________
A. Ampule Preparation:				
(1) Tap top of ampule lightly and quickly with finger until fluid moves from neck of ampule.	____	____	____	____________
(2) Place small gauze pad or unopened alcohol pad around neck of ampule.	____	____	____	____________
(3) Snap neck of ampule quickly and firmly away from hands.	____	____	____	____________
(4) Draw up medication quickly, using a filter needle long enough to reach bottom of ampule.	____	____	____	____________
(5) Hold ampule upside down, or set it on a flat surface. Insert filter needle into center of ampule opening. Do not allow needle tip or shaft to touch rim of ampule.	____	____	____	____________
(6) Aspirate medication into syringe by gently pulling back on plunger.	____	____	____	____________

	S	U	NP	Comments
(7) Keep needle tip under surface of liquid. Tip ampule to bring all fluid within reach of the needle.	_____	_____	_____	_____
(8) If you aspirate air bubbles, do not expel air into ampule.	_____	_____	_____	_____
(9) To expel excess air bubbles, remove needle from ampule. Hold syringe with needle pointing up. Tap side of syringe to cause bubbles to rise toward needle. Draw back slightly on plunger, and then push plunger upward to eject air. Do not eject fluid.	_____	_____	_____	_____
(10) If syringe contains excess fluid, use sink for disposal. Hold syringe vertically with needle tip up and slanted slightly toward sink. Slowly eject excess fluid into sink. Recheck fluid level in syringe by holding it vertically.	_____	_____	_____	_____
(11) Cover needle with its safety sheath or cap. Replace filter needle with regular needle.	_____	_____	_____	_____
B. Vial Containing a Solution				
(1) Remove cap covering top of unused vial to expose sterile rubber seal. If a multidose vial has been used before, cap is removed already. Firmly and briskly wipe surface of rubber seal with alcohol swab, and allow it to dry.	_____	_____	_____	_____
(2) Pick up syringe and remove needle cap. Pull back on plunger to draw amount of air into syringe equivalent to volume of medication to be aspirated from vial.	_____	_____	_____	_____
(3) With vial on flat surface, insert tip of needle through center of rubber seal. Apply pressure to tip of needle during insertion.	_____	_____	_____	_____
(4) Inject air into the vial's air space, holding on to plunger. Hold plunger with firm pressure; plunger may be forced backward by air pressure within the vial.	_____	_____	_____	_____

	S	U	NP	Comments
(5) Invert vial while keeping firm hold on syringe and plunger. Hold vial between thumb and middle fingers of nondominant hand. Grasp end of syringe barrel and plunger with thumb and forefinger of dominant hand to counteract pressure in vial.	_____	_____	_____	____________________
(6) Keep tip of needle below fluid level.	_____	_____	_____	____________________
(7) Allow air pressure from the vial to fill syringe gradually with medication. If necessary, pull back slightly on plunger to obtain correct amount of solution.	_____	_____	_____	____________________
(8) When you obtain desired volume, position needle into vial's air space; tap side of syringe barrel carefully to dislodge any air bubbles. Eject any air remaining at top of syringe into vial.	_____	_____	_____	____________________
(9) Remove needle from vial by pulling back on barrel of syringe.	_____	_____	_____	____________________
(10) Hold syringe at eye level, at 90-degree angle, to ensure correct volume and absence of air bubbles. Remove any remaining air by tapping barrel to dislodge any air bubbles. Draw back slightly on plunger, then push plunger upward to eject air. Do not eject fluid.	_____	_____	_____	____________________
(11) If you need to inject medication into patient's tissue, change needle to appropriate gauge and length according to route of medication.	_____	_____	_____	____________________
(12) For multidose vial, make label that includes date of opening vial and your initials.	_____	_____	_____	____________________

	S	U	NP	Comments
C. Vial Containing a Powder (Reconstituting Medications):				
(1) Remove cap covering vial of powdered medication and cap covering vial of proper diluent. Firmly swab both caps with alcohol swab, and allow to dry.	____	____	____	________________
(2) Draw up diluent into syringe.	____	____	____	________________
(3) Insert tip of needle through center of rubber seal of vial of powdered medication. Inject diluent into vial. Remove needle.	____	____	____	________________
(4) Mix medication thoroughly. Roll in palms. Do not shake.	____	____	____	________________
(5) Reconstituted medication in vial is ready to be drawn into new syringe. Read label carefully to determine dose after reconstitution.	____	____	____	________________
(6) Draw up reconstituted medication in syringe.	____	____	____	________________
3. Dispose of soiled supplies. Place broken ampule and/or used vials and used needle in puncture-proof and leak-proof container. Clean work area, and perform hand hygiene.	____	____	____	________________
Evaluation				
1. Compare dose in syringe with desired dose.	____	____	____	________________

Name ____________________ **Date** __________ **Instructor's Name** __________________________

Performance Checklist: Skill 14-5 Administering Injections

	S	U	NP	Comments
Assessment				
1. Check accuracy and completeness of each MAR or computer printout with prescriber's written medication order.	_____	_____	_____	__________________________
2. Assess patient's medical history.	_____	_____	_____	__________________________
3. Assess patient's history of allergies, and know substances patient is allergic to and normal allergic reaction.	_____	_____	_____	__________________________
4. Observe verbal and nonverbal responses toward receiving injection.	_____	_____	_____	__________________________
5. Assess for contraindications.	_____	_____	_____	__________________________
6. Assess patient's knowledge regarding medication to be received.	_____	_____	_____	__________________________
Planning				
1. Determine expected outcomes. Clarify order as necessary.	_____	_____	_____	__________________________
2. Recopy or re-print parts of MAR that are difficult to read.	_____	_____	_____	__________________________
Implementation				
1. Prepare medication.	_____	_____	_____	__________________________
2. Take medication to patient at the right time, and perform hand hygiene.	_____	_____	_____	__________________________
3. Close room curtain or door.	_____	_____	_____	__________________________
4. Verify patient's identity by using at least two patient identifiers.	_____	_____	_____	__________________________
5. Compare the label of the medicaton with the MAR at patient's bedside.	_____	_____	_____	__________________________
6. Explain steps of procedure, and tell patient injection will cause a slight burning or sting.	_____	_____	_____	__________________________
7. Apply clean disposable gloves.	_____	_____	_____	__________________________
8. Keep sheet or gown draped over body parts not requiring exposure.	_____	_____	_____	__________________________
9. Select appropriate injection site. Inspect skin surface over sites for bruises, inflammation, or edema.	_____	_____	_____	__________________________
a. *Sub-Q:* Palpate sites for masses or tenderness. Be sure needle is correct size by grasping skinfold at site with thumb and forefinger. Measure fold from top to bottom.	_____	_____	_____	__________________________

	S	U	NP	Comments
b. *IM:* Note integrity and size of muscle, and palpate for tenderness or hardness. Avoid these areas. If injections are given frequently, rotate sites.	_____	_____	_____	_____
c. *ID:* Note lesions or discolorations of skin. If possible, select site three or four fingerwidths below antecubital space and one handwidth above wrist. If forearm cannot be used, inspect the upper back.	_____	_____	_____	_____
10. Assist patient to comfortable position:	_____	_____	_____	_____
a. *Sub-Q:* Have patient relax arm, leg, or abdomen, depending on site chosen for injection.	_____	_____	_____	_____
b. *IM:* Position patient depending on site chosen.	_____	_____	_____	_____
c. *ID:* Have patient extend elbow and support it and forearm on flat surface.	_____	_____	_____	_____
d. Talk with patient about subject of interest.	_____	_____	_____	_____
11. Relocate site using anatomical landmarks.	_____	_____	_____	_____
12. Cleanse site with an antiseptic swab. Apply swab at center of the site, and rotate outward in a circular direction for about 5 cm (2 inches).	_____	_____	_____	_____
13. Hold swab or gauze between third and fourth fingers of nondominant hand.	_____	_____	_____	_____
14. Remove needle cap by pulling it straight off.	_____	_____	_____	_____
15. Hold syringe between thumb and forefinger of dominant hand.	_____	_____	_____	_____
a. *Sub-Q:* Hold as dart, palm down.	_____	_____	_____	_____
b. *IM:* Hold as dart, palm down.	_____	_____	_____	_____
c. *ID:* Hold bevel of needle pointing up.	_____	_____	_____	_____
16. Administer injection.				
A. Subcutaneous:				
(1) For average-size patient, spread skin tightly across injection site or pinch skin with nondominant hand.	_____	_____	_____	_____
(2) Inject needle quickly and firmly at 45- to 90-degree angle. Then release skin, if pinched.	_____	_____	_____	_____

	S	U	NP	Comments
(3) For obese patient, pinch skin at site and inject needle at 90-degree angle below tissue fold.	_____	_____	_____	_____
(4) Inject medication slowly.	_____	_____	_____	_____
B. Intramuscular:				
(1) Position nondominant hand just below site and pull skin approximately 2.5 to 3.5 cm down or laterally with ulnar side of hand to administer in a z-track. Hold position until medication is injected. With dominant hand, inject needle quickly at 90-degreee angle into muscle.	_____	_____	_____	_____
(2) *(Option)* If patient's muscle mass is small, grasp body of muscle between thumb and fingers.	_____	_____	_____	_____
(3) After needle pierces skin, grasp lower end of syringe barrel with nondominant hand to stabilize syringe. Continue to hold skin tightly with nondominant hand. Move dominant hand to end of plunger. Do not move syringe.	_____	_____	_____	_____
(4) Pull back on plunger 5 to 10 seconds. If no blood appears, inject medication slowly at a rate of 1 ml/10 sec.	_____	_____	_____	_____
(5) Wait 10 seconds, then smoothly and steadily withdraw needle and release skin.	_____	_____	_____	_____
C. Intradermal:				
(1) With nondominant hand, stretch skin over site with forefinger or thumb.	_____	_____	_____	_____
(2) With needle almost against patient's skin, insert it slowly at a 5- to 15-degree angle until resistance is felt. Then advance needle through epidermis to approximately 3 mm (1/8 inch) below skin surface. Needle tip can be seen through skin.	_____	_____	_____	_____

	S	U	NP	Comments
(3) Inject medication slowly. Normally, resistance is felt. If not, needle is too deep; remove and begin again.	_____	_____	_____	_____
(4) While injecting medication, note that small bleb (approximately 6 mm [1/2 inch]) resembling mosquito bite appears on skin surface.	_____	_____	_____	_____
17. After withdrawing needle, apply alcohol swab or gauze gently over site.	_____	_____	_____	_____
18. Apply gentle pressure. Do not massage site. Apply bandage if needed.	_____	_____	_____	_____
19. Assist patient to comfortable position.	_____	_____	_____	_____
20. Discard uncapped needle or needle enclosed in safety shield and attached syringe into puncture- and leak-proof receptacle.	_____	_____	_____	_____
21. Remove disposable gloves, and perform hand hygiene.	_____	_____	_____	_____
22. Stay with patient, and observe for any allergic reactions.	_____	_____	_____	_____
Evaluation				
1. Return to room, and ask if patient feels any acute pain, burning, numbness, or tingling at injection site.	_____	_____	_____	_____
2. Inspect site, noting any bruising or induration.	_____	_____	_____	_____
3. Observe patient's response to medication at times that correlate with the medication's onset, peak, and duration.	_____	_____	_____	_____
4. Ask patient to explain purpose and effects of medication.	_____	_____	_____	_____
5. *For ID injections,* use skin pencil and draw circle around perimeter of injection site. Read site within appropriate amount of time, designated by type of medication or skin test given.	_____	_____	_____	_____
6. Correctly record medication administration and patient's response.	_____	_____	_____	_____
7. Report any undesirable effects from medication to nurse in charge or physician.	_____	_____	_____	_____

Name ____________________ Date __________ Instructor's Name __________________________

Performance Checklist: Skill 14-6 Adding Medications to Intravenous Fluid Containers

	S	U	NP	Comments
Assessment				
1. Check accuracy and completeness of each MAR or computer printout with prescriber's written medication order.	_____	_____	_____	____________________
2. Assess patient's medical history.	_____	_____	_____	____________________
3. Collect information necessary to administer drug safely, including action, purpose, side effects, normal dose, time of peak onset, and nursing implications.	_____	_____	_____	____________________
4. When you add more than one medication to IV solution, assess for compatibility of medications.	_____	_____	_____	____________________
5. Assess patient's systemic fluid balance.	_____	_____	_____	____________________
6. Assess patient's history of drug allergies.	_____	_____	_____	____________________
7. Perform hand hygiene. Assess IV insertion site for signs of infiltration or phlebitis.	_____	_____	_____	____________________
8. Assess patient's understanding of purpose of drug therapy.	_____	_____	_____	____________________
Planning				
1. Determine expected outcomes. Clarify order as necessary.	_____	_____	_____	____________________
2. Assemble supplies in medication room.	_____	_____	_____	____________________
Implementation				
1. Prepare medication.				
2. Perform hand hygiene.	_____	_____	_____	____________________
3. Compare medication labels and IV fluid with MAR.	_____	_____	_____	____________________
4. Add medication to new container (usually done in medication room or at medication cart).	_____	_____	_____	____________________
a. *Solutions in a bag:* Locate medication injection port on plastic IV solution bag.	_____	_____	_____	____________________
b. *Solutions in bottles:* Locate injection site on IV solution bottle.	_____	_____	_____	____________________
c. Wipe off port or injection site with alcohol or antiseptic swab.	_____	_____	_____	____________________

	S	U	NP	Comments
d. Remove needle cap or sheath from syringe, and insert needle of syringe through center of injection port or site; inject medication.	_____	_____	_____	__________
e. Withdraw syringe from bag or bottle.	_____	_____	_____	__________
f. Mix medication and IV solution by holding bag or bottle and turning it gently end to end.	_____	_____	_____	__________
g. Complete medication label with name and dose of medication, date, time, and your initials. Stick it on bottle or bag. *Optional (check institution's policy): Apply a flow strip that identifies the time the solution was hung and intervals indicating fluid levels.*	_____	_____	_____	__________
h. If new tubing is required, spike bag or bottle with IV tubing, prime IV tubing.	_____	_____	_____	__________
5. Bring assembled items to patient's bedside, and perform hand hygiene.	_____	_____	_____	__________
6. Verify patient's identity by using at least two patient identifiers.	_____	_____	_____	__________
7. Compare label on IV bag with MAR a final time.	_____	_____	_____	__________
8. Prepare patient by explaining that you will give medication through existing IV line or that you will start a new IV line. Explain that no discomfort should be felt during drug infusion. Encourage patient to report symptoms of discomfort.	_____	_____	_____	__________
9. Connect new infusion tubing or spike container with existing tubing. Regulate infusion at ordered rate.	_____	_____	_____	__________
10. Add medication to existing container:				
a. Check volume of solution remaining in bottle or bag.	_____	_____	_____	__________
b. Close off IV infusion clamp.	_____	_____	_____	__________
c. Wipe off medication injection port with an alcohol or antiseptic swab.	_____	_____	_____	__________
d. Remove needle cap or sheath from syringe, insert syringe needle through injection port, and inject medication.	_____	_____	_____	__________
e. Withdraw syringe from bag or bottle.	_____	_____	_____	__________
f. Lower bag or bottle from IV pole, and gently mix. Rehang bag.	_____	_____	_____	__________

	S	U	NP	Comments
g. Complete medication label, and stick it to bag or bottle.	____	____	____	____________
h. Regulate infusion to desired rate.	____	____	____	____________
11. Properly dispose of equipment and supplies. Do not cap needle of syringe. Specially sheathed needles are discarded as a unit with needle covered.	____	____	____	____________
12. Perform hand hygiene.	____	____	____	____________
Evaluation				
1. Observe patient for signs or symptoms of drug reaction.	____	____	____	____________
2. Observe for signs and symptoms of fluid volume excess.	____	____	____	____________
3. Periodically return to patient's room to assess IV insertion site and rate of infusion.	____	____	____	____________
4. Observe for signs or symptoms of IV infiltration.	____	____	____	____________
5. Record solution and medication added to parenteral fluid on appropriate form.	____	____	____	____________
6. Report any side effects to nurse in charge or physician.	____	____	____	____________

Name ____________________ Date __________ Instructor's Name ____________________

Performance Checklist: Skill 14-7 Administering Medications by Intravenous Bolus

	S	U	NP	Comments
Assessment				
1. Check accuracy and completeness of each MAR or computer printout with prescriber's written medication order.	____	____	____	____________
2. Collect drug reference information necessary to administer drug safely.	____	____	____	____________
3. If you will give drug through existing IV line, determine compatibility of medication with IV fluids and any additives within IV solution.	____	____	____	____________
4. Perform hand hygiene. Assess condition of IV needle insertion site for signs of infiltration or phlebitis.	____	____	____	____________
5. Check patient's medical history and drug allergies.	____	____	____	____________
6. Check date of expiration for medication vial or ampule.	____	____	____	____________
7. Assess patient's understanding of purpose of drug therapy.	____	____	____	____________
Planning				
1. Determine expected outcomes. Clarify order as necessary.	____	____	____	____________
Implementation				
1. Prepare medication.	____	____	____	____________
2. Take medication to patient at the right time, and perform hand hygiene.	____	____	____	____________
3. Verify patient's identity by using at least two patient identifiers.	____	____	____	____________
4. Compare the label of the medication with the MAR one more time at the patient's bedside.	____	____	____	____________
5. Explain procedure to patient. Encourage patient to report symptoms of discomfort at IV site.	____	____	____	____________
6. Put on disposable gloves.	____	____	____	____________
7. **Intravenous push (existing line):**				
a. Select injection port of IV tubing closest to patient.	____	____	____	____________
b. Clean port with antiseptic swab.	____	____	____	____________
c. Connect syringe to IV line: Insert needleless tip of syring or small-gauge needle containing drug through center of port.	____	____	____	____________

	S	U	NP	Comments
d. Occlude IV line by pinching tubing just above injection port. Pull back gently on syringe's plunger to aspirate for blood return.	____	____	____	____________
e. Release tubing and inject medication within amount of time recommended. Allow IV fluids to infuse when not pushing medication.	____	____	____	____________
f. Withdraw syringe and recheck fluid infusion rate after injecting medication.	____	____	____	____________
8. **Intravenous push (IV lock):**				
a. Prepare flush solutions according to hospital policy:	____	____	____	____________
(1) *Saline flush method (preferred):*	____	____	____	____________
(a) Prepare two syringes filled with 2 to 3 ml of normal saline.	____	____	____	____________
(2) *Heparin flush method (traditional):*	____	____	____	____________
(a) Prepare one syringe with ordered amount of heparin flush solution.	____	____	____	____________
(b) Prepare two syringes with 2 to 3 ml of normal saline (0.9%).	____	____	____	____________
b. Administer medication:				
(1) Clean lock's injection port with antiseptic swab.	____	____	____	____________
(2) Insert syringe with normal saline (0.9%) through injection port of IV lock.	____	____	____	____________
(3) Pull back gently on syringe plunger and check for blood return.	____	____	____	____________
(4) Flush IV site with normal saline by pushing slowly on plunger.	____	____	____	____________
(5) Remove saline-filled syringe.	____	____	____	____________
(6) Clean lock's injection port with antiseptic swab.	____	____	____	____________
(7) Insert syringe containing prepared medicaiton through injection port of IV lock.	____	____	____	____________
(8) Inject medication within amount of time recommended.	____	____	____	____________
(9) After administering bolus, withdraw syringe.	____	____	____	____________

	S	U	NP	Comments
(10) Clean lock's injection site with antiseptic swab.	_____	_____	_____	_____
(11) Flush injection port.				
(a) Attach syringe with normal saline, and inject normal saline flush at the same rate the medication was given.	_____	_____	_____	_____
(b) *Heparin flush option:* After instilling saline, attach syringe containing heparin flush, inject slowly, and remove syringe.	_____	_____	_____	_____
9. Dispose of uncapped needles and syringes in puncture-proof and leakproof container.	_____	_____	_____	_____
10. Remove gloves, and perform hand hygiene.	_____	_____	_____	_____
Evaluation				
1. Observe patient closely for adverse reactions during administration and for several minutes thereafter.	_____	_____	_____	_____
2. Observe IV site during injection for sudden swelling.	_____	_____	_____	_____
3. Assess patient's status after giving medication to evaluate its effectiveness.	_____	_____	_____	_____
4. Ask patient to explain the drug's purpose and side effects.	_____	_____	_____	_____
5. Record medication administration, including drug name, dose, route, and time of administration.	_____	_____	_____	_____
6. Report and record any adverse reactions.	_____	_____	_____	_____

Name ____________ Date ________ Instructor's Name ____________

Performance Checklist: Skill 14-8 Administering Intravenous Medications by Piggyback, Intermittent Intravenous Infusion Sets, and Mini-Infusion Pumps

	S	U	NP	Comments
Assessment				
1. Check accuracy and completeness of each MAR or computer printout with prescriber's written medication order.	____	____	____	____________
2. Determine patient's medical history.	____	____	____	____________
3. Collect information necessary to administer drug safely, including action, purpose, side effects, normal dose, time of peak onset, and nursing implications.	____	____	____	____________
4. Assess compatibility of drug with existing IV solution.	____	____	____	____________
5. Assess patency of patient's existing IV infusion line.	____	____	____	____________
6. Perform hand hygiene. Assess IV insertion site for signs of infiltration or phlebitis: redness, pallor, swelling, or tenderness on palpation.	____	____	____	____________
7. Assess patient's history of drug allergies.	____	____	____	____________
8. Assess patient's understanding of purpose of drug therapy.	____	____	____	____________
Planning				
1. Determine expected outcomes. Clarify order as necessary.	____	____	____	____________
2. Assemble supplies at bedside. Prepare patient by informing patient that medication will be given through IV equipment.	____	____	____	____________
Implementation				
1. Assemble medications and supplies at bedside.	____	____	____	____________
2. Compare the lable of the medication with the MAR at least two times while preparing supplies.	____	____	____	____________
3. Give medication to patient at the right time, and perform hand hygiene.	____	____	____	____________
4. Verify patient's identity by using at least two patient identifiers.	____	____	____	____________

	S	U	NP	Comments
5. Explain purpose of medication and side effects to patient, and explain that medication is to be given through existing IV line. Encourage patient to report symptoms of discomfort at site.	_____	_____	_____	_____
6. Compare the label of the medication with the MAR one more time.	_____	_____	_____	_____
7. Administer infusion:				
A. Piggyback Infusion				
(1) Connect infusion tubing to medication bag. Allow solution to fill tubing by opening regulator flow clamp. Once tubing is full, close clamp and cap end of tubing.	_____	_____	_____	_____
(2) Hang piggyback medication bag above level of primary fluid bag. (Use hook to lower main bag.)	_____	_____	_____	_____
(3) Connect tubing of piggyback infusion to appropriate connector on primary infusion line.	_____	_____	_____	_____
(a) *Needleless system:* Wipe off needleless port of IV line, and insert tip of piggyback infusion tubing.	_____	_____	_____	_____
(b) *Stopcock:* Wipe off stopcock port with alcohol swab, and connect tubing. Turn stopcock to open position.	_____	_____	_____	_____
(c) *Needle system:* Connect sterile needle to end of piggyback infusion tubing, remove cap, cleanse injection port on main IV line, and insert needle through center of port. Secure by taping connection.	_____	_____	_____	_____
(4) Regulate flow rate of medication solution by adjusting regulator clamp.	_____	_____	_____	_____
(5) After medication has infused, check flow regulator on primary infusion.	_____	_____	_____	_____
(6) Regulate main infusion line to desired rate if necessary.	_____	_____	_____	_____

	S	U	NP	Comments
(7) Leave IV piggyback bag and tubing in place for future drug administration or discard in appropriate containers.	_____	_____	_____	_____
B. Mini-infusion Administration				
(1) Connect prefilled syringe to mini-infusion tubing.	_____	_____	_____	_____
(2) Carefully apply pressure to syringe plunger, allowing tubing to fill with medication.	_____	_____	_____	_____
(3) Place syringe into mini-infusion pump (follow product directions). Be sure syringe is secure.	_____	_____	_____	_____
(4) Connect mini-infusion tubing to main IV line.	_____	_____	_____	_____
(a) *Needleless system:* Wipe off needleless port of IV tubing, and insert tip of the mini-infusion tubing.	_____	_____	_____	_____
(b) *Stopcock:* Wipe off stopcock port with alcohol swab, and connect tubing. Turn stopcock to open position.	_____	_____	_____	_____
(c) *Needle system:* Connect sterile needle to mini-infusion tubing, remove cap, cleanse injection port on main IV line or saline lock, and insert needle through center of port. Consider placing tape where IV tubing enters port to keep connection secured.	_____	_____	_____	_____
(5) Hang infusion pump with syringe on IV pole alongside main IV bag. Set pump to deliver medication within time recommended. Press button on pump to begin infusion.	_____	_____	_____	_____
(6) After medication has infused, check flow regulator on primary infusion. Regulate main infusion line to desired rate as needed.	_____	_____	_____	_____

	S	U	NP	Comments
C. Volume Control Set				
(1) Fill Volutrol with desired amount of fluid (50 to 100 ml) by opening clamp between Volutrol and main IV bag.	____	____	____	____
(2) Close clamp, and check to be sure clamp on air vent of volume control set chamber is open.	____	____	____	____
(3) Clean injection port on top of Volutrol with antiseptic swab.	____	____	____	____
(4) Remove needle cap or sheath, and insert syringe needle through port; then inject medication. Gently rotate Volutrol between hands.	____	____	____	____
(5) Regulate IV infusion rate to allow medication to infuse in time recommended.	____	____	____	____
(6) Label Volutrol with name of drug, dosage, total volume including diluent, and time of administration.	____	____	____	____
(7) Dispose of uncapped needle or needle enclosed in safety shield and syringe in appropriate container.	____	____	____	____
Evaluation				
1. Observe patient for signs of adverse reactions.	____	____	____	____
2. During infusion, periodically check infusion rate and condition of IV site.	____	____	____	____
3. Ask patient to explain purpose and side effects of medication.	____	____	____	____
4. Record drug, dose, route, and time administered.	____	____	____	____
5. Record volume of fluid in medication bag or volume control set.	____	____	____	____
6. Report any adverse reactions to nurse in charge or physician.	____	____	____	____

Name ____________________ Date __________ Instructor's Name ________________________

Procedural Guidelines 14-1 Giving Medications through a Nasogastric Tube, G-Tube, J-Tube, or Small-Bore Feeding Tube

	S	U	NP	Comments
1. Check accuracy and completeness of each MAR or computer printout with prescriber's written mediation order.	____	____	____	____________
2. Investigate and use alternative routes of medication administration if possible.	____	____	____	____________
3. Avoid complicated medication regimens that frequently interrupt enteral feedings.	____	____	____	____________
4. Prepare medication. Check label of medication with MAR two times.	____	____	____	____________
5. Be sure the medication is compatible with the enteral feeding before administering medications. If the medication is incompatible with the feeding, stop the feeding 1 to 2 hours before giving the medication, and restart the feeding 1 to 2 hours after giving the medication. Never add medications directly to the tube feeding.	____	____	____	____________
6. Administer medications in a liquid form when possible to prevent obstruction of the tube.	____	____	____	____________
7. Before crushing medications, be sure they should be crushed. Do not crush buccal, sublingual, enteric-coated, or sustained-release medications.	____	____	____	____________
8. Take medications to patient at correct time, and perform hand hygiene.	____	____	____	____________
9. Verify patient's identity by using at least two patient identifiers.	____	____	____	____________
10. Compare label of medications against MAR one more time at patient's bedside.	____	____	____	____________
11. Explain procedure to patient, and educate patient about medications.	____	____	____	____________
12. Dissolve crushed tablets, gelatin capsules, and powders in 15 to 30 ml of warm water.	____	____	____	____________
13. Do not give whole or undissolved medications through the feeding tube.	____	____	____	____________
14. Put on clean, disposabel gloves.	____	____	____	____________

	S	U	NP	Comments
15. Verify placement of any tube that enters the mouth or nose using pH testing.	_____	_____	_____	_____
16. Assess gastric residual.	_____	_____	_____	_____
17. Flush tube with 30 ml warm water.	_____	_____	_____	_____
18. Draw up each medication in syringe. Do **not** mix medications together.	_____	_____	_____	_____
19. Connect syringe with medication to nasogastric tube, G-tube, J-tube, or small-bore feeding tube.	_____	_____	_____	_____
20. Administer medication by either pushing the medication through the tube with the syringe or by allowing medication to flow into body freely by using gravity. Administer each medication separately.	_____	_____	_____	_____
21. Flush tube once more with 30 ml of warm water once all medications are given.	_____	_____	_____	_____
22. Once you have give all medications, flush tube once more with 30 ml warm water.	_____	_____	_____	_____
23. Clean area, and put supplies away.	_____	_____	_____	_____
24. Remove gloves, and perform hand hygiene.				
25. Document administration of medications on MAR.	_____	_____	_____	_____
26. Continually evaluate the patient's response to medication therapy. If the patient does not achieve the desired effect, a different medication or route of administration may be indicated because of problems with drug bioavailability when given by the enteral route.	_____	_____	_____	_____

Name ____________________ Date __________ Instructor's Name ____________________________

Procedural Guidelines 14-2 Administering Nasal Instillations

	S	U	NP	Comments
1. Check accuracy and completeness of each MAR or computer printout with prescriber's original medication order.	_____	_____	_____	______________________
2. Determine which sinus is affected by referring to medical record.	_____	_____	_____	______________________
3. Assess patient's history of hypertension, heart disease, diabetes mellitus, and hyperthyroidism.	_____	_____	_____	______________________
4. Using a penlight, inspect condition of nose and sinuses. Palpate sinuses for tenderness.	_____	_____	_____	______________________
5. Assess patient's knowledge regarding use of nasal instillations and technique for instillation and willingness to learn self-administration.	_____	_____	_____	______________________
6. Prepare medication.	_____	_____	_____	______________________
7. Take medications to patient at correct time, and perform hand hygiene.	_____	_____	_____	______________________
8. Verify patient's identity by using at least two patient identifiers.	_____	_____	_____	______________________
9. Compare MAR with medication labels at bedside.	_____	_____	_____	______________________
10. Explain procedure to patient regarding positioning and sensations to expect.	_____	_____	_____	______________________
11. Arrange supplies and medications at bedside. Apply gloves if patient has nasal drainage.	_____	_____	_____	______________________
12. Gently roll or shake container.	_____	_____	_____	______________________
13. Instruct patient to clear or blow nose gently unless contraindicated.	_____	_____	_____	______________________
14. Administer nasal drops:				
a. Assist patient to supine position and position head properly.	_____	_____	_____	______________________
(1) For access to posterior pharynx, tilt patient's head backward.	_____	_____	_____	______________________
(2) For access to ethmoid or sphenoid sinus, tilt head back over edge of bed or place small pillow under patient's shoulders and tilt head back.	_____	_____	_____	______________________

	S	U	NP	Comments
(3) For access to frontal or maxillary sinus, tilt head back over edge of bed or pillow with head turned toward side to be treated.	____	____	____	____________
b. Support patient's head with nondominant hand.	____	____	____	____________
c. Instruct patient to breathe through mouth.	____	____	____	____________
d. Hold dropper 1 cm ($^1/_2$ inch) above nares, and instill prescribed number of drops toward midline of ethmoid bone.	____	____	____	____________
e. Have patient remain in supine position 5 minutes.	____	____	____	____________
f. Offer facial tissue to blot runny nose, but caution patient against blowing nose for several minutes.	____	____	____	____________
15. Assist patient to a comfortable position after drug is absorbed.	____	____	____	____________
16. Dispose of soiled supplies in proper container, and perform hand hygiene.	____	____	____	____________
17. Document administration of medications on MAR.	____	____	____	____________
18. Observe patient for onset of side effects 15 to 30 minutes after administration. Ask if patient is able to breathe through nose after decongestant administration. May be necessary to have patient occlude one nostril at a time and breathe deeply.	____	____	____	____________
19. Evaluate patient's response to medication at times that correlate with the medication's onset, peak, and duration. Evaluate patient for both desired effect and adverse effacts.	____	____	____	____________

Name ____________________ Date __________ Instructor's Name __________________________

Procedural Guidelines 14-3 Administering Ear Medications

	S	U	NP	Comments
1. Check accuracy and completeness of each MAR or computer printout with prescriber's written mediation order. Check patient's name, drug name and dosage, route of administration, and time for administration.	_____	_____	_____	__________
2. Prepare medication. Be sure to compare the label of the medication with the MAR at least two times during medication preparation.	_____	_____	_____	__________
3. Take medication to patient at correct time, and perform hand hygiene.	_____	_____	_____	__________
4. Verify patient's identity by using at least two patient identifiers.	_____	_____	_____	__________
5. Compare the label of the medication with the MAR one more time at the patient's bedside.	_____	_____	_____	__________
6. Explain procedure to patient regarding postioning and sensations to expect.	_____	_____	_____	__________
7. Teach patient about medication.	_____	_____	_____	__________
8. *Administer ear drops:*				
a. Place patient in side-lying position if not contraindicated by patient's condition, with ear to be treated facing up. The patient may also sit in a chair or at the bedside.	_____	_____	_____	__________
b. Straighten ear canal by pulling auricle down and back for children or upward and outward for adults.	_____	_____	_____	__________
c. Instill prescribed drops holding dropper 1 cm ($^1/_2$ inch) above ear canal.	_____	_____	_____	__________
d. Ask patient to remain in side-lying position for 2 to 3 minutes. Apply gentle massage or pressure to tragus of ear with finger.	_____	_____	_____	__________
e. If you place a cotton ball into the outermost part of the ear canal, do not press cotton ball into the canal. Remove cotton after 15 minutes.	_____	_____	_____	__________

	S	U	NP	Comments
9. *Administer ear irrigations:*				
a. Assesss the tympanic membrane, or review medical record for history of eardrum perforation, which contraindicates ear irrigation.	____	____	____	____
b. Assist patient into sitting or lying position with head tilted or turned toward affected ear. Place towel under patient's head and shoulder, and have patient hold basin under affected ear.	____	____	____	____
c. Fill irrigation syringe with solution (approximately 50 ml) at room temperature.	____	____	____	____
d. Gently grasp auricle, and straighten ear by pulling it down and back for children or upward and outward for adults.	____	____	____	____
e. Slowly instill irrigating solution by holding tip of syringe 1 cm (1/2 inch) above opening of ear canal. Allow fluid to drain out during instillation. Continue until you cleanse the canal or use all solution.	____	____	____	____
10. Clean area, and put supplies away.	____	____	____	____
11. Remove gloves, and perform hand hygiene.	____	____	____	____
12. Document medication administration on MAR.	____	____	____	____
13. Evaluate patient's response to the medication.	____	____	____	____

Name ____________________ Date __________ Instructor's Name ________________________

Procedural Guidelines 14-4 Administering Vaginal Medications

	S	U	NP	Comments
1. Check accuracy and completeness of each MAR or computer printout with prescriber's written medication order.	____	____	____	____________
2. Prepare medication.	____	____	____	____________
3. Take medication to patient at the correct time, and perform hand hygiene.	____	____	____	____________
4. Verify patient's identity by using at least two patient identifiers.	____	____	____	____________
5. Compare label of medication against the MAR one more time at the patient's bedside.	____	____	____	____________
6. Explain procedure to patient regarding positioning and sensationsto expect. Be sure patient understands the procedure if she plans to self-administer medication. Teach patient about the medication.	____	____	____	____________
7. Close room door or pull curtain to provide privacy.	____	____	____	____________
8. Put on clean gloves.	____	____	____	____________
9. Be sure there is adequate lighting to visualize vaginal opening. Assess vaginal area, noting the appearance of any discharge and the condition of the external genitalia. Cleanse area with towel or washcloth if needed.	____	____	____	____________
10. *Administer vaginal suppository:*				
a. Remove suppository from wrapper and apply liberal amount of sterile water-based lubricating jelly to smooth or rounded end. Lubricate gloved index finger of dominant hand.	____	____	____	____________
b. With nondominant gloved hand, gently separate and hold labial folds.	____	____	____	____________
c. With dominant gloved hand, gently insert rounded end of suppository along posterior wall of vaginal canal entire length of finger (7.5 to 10 cm or 3 to 4 inches).	____	____	____	____________
d. Withdraw finger and wipe away remaining lubricant from around vaginal opening and labia.	____	____	____	____________

	S	U	NP	Comments
11. *Administer cream or foam:*				
a. Fill cream or foam applicator following package directions.	____	____	____	____
b. With nondominant gloved hand, gently separate and hold labial folds.	____	____	____	____
c. With dominant gloved hand, gently insert applicator about 5 to 7.5 cm (2 to 3 inches). Push applicator plunger to deposit medication into vagina.	____	____	____	____
d. Withdraw applicator and place on paper towel. Wipe off residual cream from labia or vaginal opening.	____	____	____	____
12. Dispose of supplies, remove gloves, and perform hand hygiene.	____	____	____	____
13. Instruct patient to remain on back for at least 10 minutes.	____	____	____	____
14. Document medication administration on MAR.	____	____	____	____
15. If applicator is used, wearing gloves, wash with soap and warm water, rinse, and store for future use.	____	____	____	____
16. Offer perineal pad to patient when she begins to ambulate.	____	____	____	____
17. Evaluate patient's response to medication.	____	____	____	____

Name ____________________ Date __________ Instructor's Name ________________________

Procedural Guidelines 14-5 Administering Rectal Suppositories

	S	U	NP	Comments
1. Check accuracy and completeness of each MAR or computer printout with prescriber's written medication order.	_____	_____	_____	____________________
2. Prepare medication.	_____	_____	_____	____________________
3. Take medication to patient at the correct time, and perform hand hygiene.	_____	_____	_____	____________________
4. Verify patient's identity by using at least two patient identifiers.	_____	_____	_____	____________________
5. Compare the label of the medication with the MAR one more time at the patient's bedside.	_____	_____	_____	____________________
6. Explain procedure to patient regarding positioning and sensations to expect. Be sure patient understands the procedure if he or she plans to self-administer medication. Teach patient about the medication.	_____	_____	_____	____________________
7. Close room door or pull curtain to provide privacy.	_____	_____	_____	____________________
8. Put on clean gloves.	_____	_____	_____	____________________
9. Assist patient to the Sims' position. Keep patient draped with only anal area exposed.	_____	_____	_____	____________________
10. Be sure there is adequate lighting to visualize anus. Assess external condition of anus and palpate rectal walls as needed. Dispose of gloves in proper receptacle if soiled.	_____	_____	_____	____________________
11. Apply disposable gloves if gloves were thrown away in previous step.	_____	_____	_____	____________________
12. Remove suppository from wrapper and lubricate rounded end with sterile water-soluble lubricating jelly. Lubricate index finger of dominant hand with water-soluble jelly.	_____	_____	_____	____________________
13. Ask patient to take slow deep breath through mouth and relax anal sphincter.	_____	_____	_____	____________________
14. Retract buttocks with nondominant hand. Using dominant hand, insert suppository gently through anus, past internal sphincter and against rectal wall, 10 cm (4 inches) in adults, or 5 cm (2 inches) in children and infants. You may need to apply gentle pressure to hold buttocks together momentarily.	_____	_____	_____	____________________

	S	U	NP	Comments
15. Withdraw finger and wipe anal area with tissue.	_____	_____	_____	_____
16. Dispose of supplies, remove gloves, and perform hand hygiene.	_____	_____	_____	_____
17. Instruct patient to remain on side for at least 5 minutes.	_____	_____	_____	_____
18. If suppository is a laxative or stool softener, place call light within reach of the patient.	_____	_____	_____	_____
19. Document medication administration on MAR.	_____	_____	_____	_____
20. Evaluate patient's response to medication.	_____	_____	_____	_____

Name ____________________ Date __________ Instructor's Name ____________________________

Procedural Guidelines 14-6 Mixing Two Kinds of Insulin in One Syringe

	S	U	NP	Comments
1. Check accuracy and completeness of each MAR or computer printout with prescriber's written medication order.	____	____	____	____________
2. Verify insulin labels carefully against the MAR before preparing the dose to ensure that you give the correct type of insulin.	____	____	____	____________
3. Perform hand hygiene.	____	____	____	____________
4. If patient takes insulin that is cloudy, roll the bottle of insulin between the hands to resuspend the insulin preparation.	____	____	____	____________
5. Wipe off tops of both insulin vials with alcohol swab.	____	____	____	____________
6. Verify insulin dosages against MAR a second time.	____	____	____	____________
7. If mixing rapid- or short-acting insulin with intermediate- or long-acting insulin, take insulin syringe and aspirate volume of air equivalent to dose to be withdrawn from intermediate- or long-acting insulin first. If two intermediate- or long-acting insulins are mixed, it makes no difference which vial you prepare first.	____	____	____	____________
8. Insert needle and inject air into vial of intermediate- or long-acting insulin. Do not let the tip of the needle touch the insulin.	____	____	____	____________
9. Remove the syringe from the vial of insulin without aspirating medication.	____	____	____	____________
10. With the same syringe, inject air, equal to the dose of rapid- or short-acting insulin, into the vial and withdraw the correct dose into the syringe.	____	____	____	____________
11. Remove the syringe from the rapid- or short-acting insulin, and get rid of air bubbles to ensure accurate dosing.	____	____	____	____________

	S	U	NP	Comments
12. After verifying insulin dosages with MAR a third time, determine which point on the syringe scale combined units of insulin measure by adding the number of units of both insulins together.	____	____	____	____________
13. Place the needle of the syringe back into the vial of intermediate- or long-acting insulin. Be careful not to push plunger and inject insulin in syringe into the vial.	____	____	____	____________
1. Invert the vial, and carefully withdraw the desired amount of insulin into syringe.	____	____	____	____________
2. Withdraw needle, and check fluid level in syringe. Keep needle of prepared syringe sheathed or capped until ready to administer medication.	____	____	____	____________
3. Dispose of soiled supplies in proper receptacle and perform hand hygiene.	____	____	____	____________

15 Fluid, Electrolyte, and Acid-Base Balances

Case Studies

1. The patient is taking Digoxin and Lasix.
   a. What patient teaching is indicated in relation to possible fluid and electrolyte imbalances?
2. You are working with two patients today. One of the patients is unconscious, and is experiencing a period of prolonged immobility. The other patient has a long history of alcoholism. You are alert to possible alterations in fluid and electrolyte imbalance.
   a. What specific signs and symptoms may these patients exhibit as a result of their present conditions?
3. An adult male patient has come to the outpatient clinic for an examination. During the initial interview, the patient tells you that he has smoked $2^1/2$ packs of cigarettes each day for the last 25 years.
   a. What physical signs do you anticipate finding because of the patient's history?
   b. What acid-base imbalance is this patient most likely to experience?

Chapter Review

Match the description/definition in Column A with the correct term in Column B.

	Column A	Column B
_______	1. Positively charged electrolytes	a. Anions
_______	2. Having the same osmotic pressure	b. Diffusion
_______	3. Movement of water across a semipermeable membrane	c. Filtration
_______	4. Ability of a solution to create osmotic pressure	d. Active transport
_______	5. Movement of molecules from an area of higher concentration to an area of lower concentration	e. Cations
		f. Isotonic
_______	6. Negatively charged electrolytes	g. Osmolality
_______	7. Movement of solutes out of a solution with greater hydrostatic pressure	h. Hypotonic
		i. Osmosis
_______	8. Number of molecules in a liter of solution	j. Osmolarity
_______	9. Having a lower osmotic pressure	k. Hypertonic
_______	10. Movement of molecules to an area of higher concentration	

Complete the following:

11. Identify the following terms:
    a. All fluids outside of the cell:
    b. Fluid between the cells and outside the blood vessels:
    c. All fluids within the cell:
12. Identify if the following electrolytes are cations or anions and whether they are primarily extracellular or intracellular:
    a. Sodium

b. Potassium

c. Calcium

d. Magnesium

e. Chloride

f. Bicarbonate

13. Acid-base balance in the body is regulated by:

14. What two age-groups are most susceptible to fluid and acid-base imbalances?

15. Identify whether the following solutions are isotonic, hypertonic, or hypotonic:
    a. Dextrose 5% in water (D_5W)

    b. 0.45% sodium chloride (0.45% NS)

    c. 0.9% sodium chloride (0.9% NS)

    d. Lactated Ringer's (LR)

    e. Dextrose 5% in 0.45% sodium chloride ($D_5\frac{1}{2}$ NS)

16. Identify three types of medications that may cause fluid, electrolyte, or acid-base imbalances.

17. Specify two possible nursing diagnoses for patients experiencing fluid, electrolyte, or acid-base imbalances.

18. Identify the sites for an IV infusion.

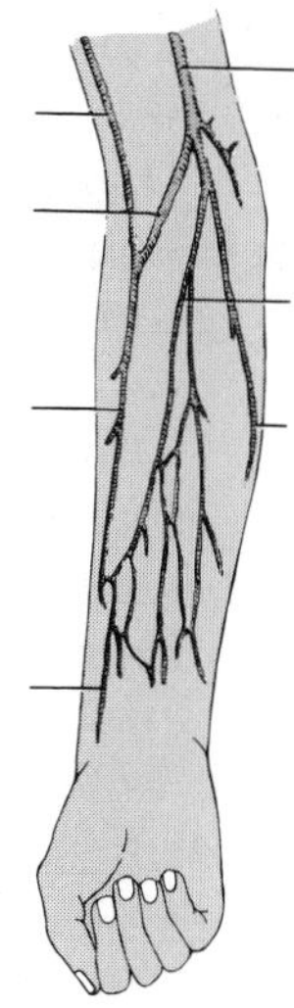

19. A patient who is NPO and receiving intravenous fluids needs to have ____________________ added to the solution.

20. A patient with a peripherally inserted central catheter (PICC) line develops a fever and increased white blood cell (WBC) count. The nurse anticipates that the health care provider will order:

21. A priority assessment before the administration of a blood transfusion is to:

22. Transfusion of a patient's own blood is termed:

23. Identify the electrolyte imbalance that is associated with each of the following test results:
    a. Serum sodium level—125 mEq/L

    b. Serum potassium level—5.8 mEq/L

    c. Serum calcium level—3.7 mEq/L

d. Serum magnesium level—1.2 mEq/L

24. Calculate the following IV infusion rates:
   a. IV 500 ml of D_5W to infuse in 5 hours; administration set = 15 gtt/ml
   How many gtt/min should infuse?

   b. IV 1000 ml of NS to infuse in 8 hours; administration set = 10 gtt/ml
   How many gtt/min should infuse?

   c. IV 200 ml of NS to infuse in 4 hours; administration set = 60 gtt/ml
   How many gtt/min should infuse?

   d. IV 2 L of D_5W to infuse in 18 hours
   How many ml/hour should be set on the infusion pump?

25. Identify the following hormones that control fluid balance:
   a. Pituitary

   b. Adrenal

26. If a hypotonic solution is given intravenously to a patient, the fluid will move into the cells.
   True _____ False _____
27. Arterial pH is an indirect measurement of:

28. Oxygen moves into the lungs via the process of:

29. An average adult's daily intake of fluid is approximately ____________________ ml.

Select the best answer for each of the following questions:

30. The patient has hypernatremia with a fluid deficit. The nurse anticipates finding:
   1. Dry, sticky mucous membranes
   2. Orthostatic hypotension
   3. Abdominal cramping
   4. Diarrhea
31. The patient who is experiencing a gastrointestinal problem has had periods of prolonged vomiting. The nurse is observing the patient for signs of:
   1. Metabolic acidosis
   2. Metabolic alkalosis
   3. Respiratory acidosis
   4. Respiratory alkalosis
32. The nurse is working with a patient who has had emphysema for many years. The nurse believes that the patient has uncompensated respiratory acidosis. This belief is a result of an analysis of the patient's blood gas values that reveals:
   1. pH = 7.35, $Paco_2$ = 40 mm Hg, HCO_3^- concentration = 22 mEq/L
   2. pH = 7.40, $Paco_2$ = 45 mm Hg, HCO_3^- concentration = 28 mEq/L
   3. pH = 7.30, $Paco_2$ = 50 mm Hg, HCO_3^- concentration = 24 mEq/L
   4. pH = 7.45, $Paco_2$ = 55 mm Hg, HCO_3^- concentration = 18 mEq/L
33. The patient has been admitted to the medical center for stabilization of congestive heart failure. The physician has prescribed Lasix (a diuretic) for the patient. This patient should be observed for:
   1. Diarrhea
   2. Edema
   3. Dysrhythmia
   4. Hyperactive reflexes
34. The patient has a potassium level above the normal value. The nurse anticipates that treatment for this patient with hyperkalemia will include:
   1. Fluid restrictions
   2. Foods high in potassium
   3. Administration of diuretics
   4. IV infusion of calcium

35. The patient has lost a large amount of body fluid. In assessment of this patient with hypovolemia (fluid volume deficit, FVD), the nurse expects to find:
    1. Oliguria
    2. Hypertension
    3. Periorbital edema
    4. Neck vein distention
36. The nurse is determining the care that is to be provided to the patients on the medical unit. There are a number of patients who have the potential for a fluid and electrolyte imbalance. A nurse-initiated (independent) intervention for these patients is:
    1. Administration of IV fluids
    2. Monitoring of intake and output
    3. Performance of diagnostic tests
    4. Dietary replacement of necessary fluids/electrolytes
37. For a patient who is experiencing a fluid volume excess, the nurse plans to determine the fluid status. The best way to determine the fluid balance for the patient is to:
    1. Obtain diagnostic test results
    2. Monitor IV fluid intake
    3. Weigh the patient daily
    4. Assess vital signs
38. The patient is admitted to the trauma unit following an accident while using power tools at home. The patient experienced significant blood loss and required a large infusion of citrated blood. The nurse assesses this patient for the development of:
    1. Urinary retention
    2. Poor skin turgor
    3. Increased blood pressure reading
    4. Positive Trousseau's sign
39. The patient is experiencing a severe anxiety reaction and the respiratory rate has increased significantly. Nursing intervention for this patient who may develop respiratory alkalosis is:
    1. Placing the patient in a sitting position
    2. Providing the patient with nasal oxygen
    3. Having the patient breathe into a paper bag
    4. Having the patient cough and deep breathe
40. A patient with normal renal function is to be maintained NPO. An IV of 1000 ml of D_5W is ordered to infuse over 8 hours. The nurse should:
    1. Infuse the IV at a faster rate
    2. Add multivitamins to the solution
    3. Provide oral fluids as a supplement
    4. Question the prescriber about adding potassium to the IV
41. A patient with an IV infusion may develop phlebitis. The nurse recognizes this condition by the presence at the IV infusion site of:
    1. Pallor
    2. Swelling
    3. Redness
    4. Cyanosis
42. The patient has had an IV line inserted. Upon observation of the IV site, the nurse notes that there is evidence of an infiltration. The nurse should first:
    1. Slow the infusion
    2. Discontinue the infusion
    3. Change the IV bag and tubing
    4. Contact the prescriber immediately
43. The nurse is reviewing the hospital policy for maintenance of IV infusions. The current guidelines for changing IV tubing (non–blood administration sets) are based on the IV tubing remaining sterile for:
    1. 24 hours
    2. 36 hours
    3. 48 hours
    4. 72 hours
44. The patient has just started to receive the blood transfusion. The nurse is performing the patient assessment and notes the patient has chills and flank pain. The nurse stops the infusion and then:
    1. Calls the physician
    2. Administers epinephrine
    3. Collects a urine specimen
    4. Sets up a piggyback IV infusion with 0.9% saline
45. A patient who has been admitted with a renal dysfunction is demonstrating signs and symptoms of a fluid volume excess (hypervolemia). Upon completing the

patient assessment, the nurse anticipates finding:
1. Poor skin turgor
2. Decreased blood pressure
3. Neck vein distention
4. Increased urine specific gravity

46. The nurse is assisting the patient with a fluid volume deficit to select an optimum replacement fluid. The nurse suggests that the patient drink:
1. Tea
2. Milk
3. Coffee
4. Fruit juice

47. A patient with congestive heart failure and fluid retention is placed on a fluid restriction of 1000 ml/24 hours. On the basis of guidelines for patients with restrictions, for the time period from 7:00 AM to 3:30 PM the nurse plans to provide the patient:
1. 250 ml
2. 400 ml
3. 500 ml
4. 750 ml

48. The patient has come to the orthopedist's office for treatment of osteoporosis. The nurse is explaining to the patient some of the possible complications from this disorder that may affect fluid and electrolyte balance. The nurse informs the patient to report:
1. Low back pain
2. Tingling in the fingers
3. Muscle twitching
4. Positive Trousseau's sign

49. The patient has a history of alcoholism and is admitted to the medical center in a malnourished state. The nurse specifically checks the lab values for:
1. Hypercalcemia
2. Hyponatremia
3. Hyperkalemia
4. Hypomagnesemia

50. The patient who is most prone to respiratory acidosis is the individual who is experiencing:
1. A narcotic overdose
2. An anxiety reaction
3. Renal failure
4. Asthma

51. Older adults have a greater risk of fluid imbalance as a result of:
1. Increased thirst response
2. Decreased glomerular filtration
3. Increased body fluid percentage
4. Increased basal metabolic rate

52. An example of a type of medication that can lead to metabolic alkalosis is a:
1. Narcotic
2. Diuretic
3. Potassium supplement
4. Nonsteroidal anti-inflammatory drug

53. A moderate to severe fluid volume excess is indicated with a weight change of:
1. 1% to 2%
2. 3% to 4%
3. 5% to 8%
4. 9% to 12%

54. An appropriate technique when initiating an intravenous infusion is to:
1. Use hard, stiff veins
2. Shave the arm hair with a razor
3. Use the proximal site in the dominant arm
4. Apply the tourniquet 4 to 6 inches above the selected site

55. A unit of packed cells or whole blood usually transfuses over:
1. 1/2 hour
2. 1 hour
3. 2 hours
4. 5 hours

56. An individual with type O blood is able to receive:
1. Type A or type B
2. Type AB
3. Type O
4. All types

57. A specific technique for initiating intravenous therapy for an older adult is to:
1. Select sites in the hands
2. Use the largest possible IV cannula gauge
3. Insert at a decreased angle of 5 to 15 degrees
4. Set the IV flow rate at 150 to 200 ml/hour

Study Group Questions

- How are body fluids distributed in the body?
- What is the composition of body fluids?
- How do fluids move throughout the body?
- How is the intake of body fluids regulated?
- What are the major electrolytes, and what is their function in the body?
- How is acid-base balance maintained?
- What are the major fluid, electrolyte, and acid-base imbalances and their causes?
- What signs and symptoms will the patient exhibit in the presence of a fluid, electrolyte, or acid-base imbalance?
- What diagnostic tests are used to determine the presence of imbalances?
- What information is critical to obtain in a patient assessment in order to determine the presence of a fluid, electrolyte, or acid-base imbalance?
- What health deviations increase a patient's susceptibility to an imbalance?
- What nursing interventions should be implemented for patients with various fluid, electrolyte, and acid-base imbalances?
- What information should be included in patient/family teaching for prevention of imbalances, or restoration of fluid, electrolyte, or acid-base balance?
- What are the nursing responsibilities associated with the initiation and maintenance of IV therapy?
- What are the responsibilities of the nurse with regard to blood transfusions?

Study Charts

Create study charts to compare:

a. Electrolyte Imbalances and Patient Responses, *including etiology, diagnostic test results, patient assessment, and nursing interventions for sodium, potassium, calcium, and magnesium imbalances*

b. Acid-Base Imbalances and Patient Responses, *including etiology, diagnostic test results, patient assessment, and nursing interventions both for metabolic acidosis and alkalosis and for respiratory acidosis and alkalosis*

Name ____________________ Date __________ Instructor's Name ________________________

Performance Checklist: Skill 15-1 Initiating a Peripheral Intravenous Infusion

	S	U	NP	Comments
Assessment				
1. Review physician's health care provider's order for type and amount of IV fluid and rate of administration.	____	____	____	____________
2. Assess for clinical factors/conditions that will respond to or be affected by IV fluid administration.	____	____	____	____________
3. Assess patient's previous or perceived experience with IV therapy and arm placement preference.	____	____	____	____________
4. Obtain information from drug reference books or pharmacist about composition of IV fluids, purposes of administration, potential incompatibilities, and possible side effects for which to monitor.	____	____	____	____________
5. Determine if patient is to undergo any planned surgeries or is to receive blood infusion later.	____	____	____	____________
6. Assess for risk factors.	____	____	____	____________
7. Assess laboratory data and patient's history of allergies.	____	____	____	____________
Planning				
1. Collect and organize equipment.	____	____	____	____________
2. Check patient's identity using at least two patient identifiers.	____	____	____	____________
3. Prepare patient and family by explaining the procedure, its purpose, and what is expected of patient. Also explain sensations patient will experiernce.	____	____	____	____________
4. Assist patient to comfortable sitting or supine position. Position yourself at same level as the patient.	____	____	____	____________
Implementation				
1. Perform hand hygiene.	____	____	____	____________
2. Organize equipment on clean, clutter-free area.	____	____	____	____________
3. Change patient's gown to the more easily removed gown with snaps at the shoulder, if available.	____	____	____	____________
4. Open sterile packages using sterile aseptic technique.	____	____	____	____________

	S	U	NP	Comments
5. Prepare IV infusion tubing and solution.	_____	_____	_____	____________________
a. Check IV solution, using six rights of medication administration. Make sure prescribed additives, such as potassium and vitamins, have been added. Check solution for color, clarity, and expiration date. Check bag for leaks, preferably before reaching the bedside.	_____	_____	_____	____________________
b. Open infusion set, maintaining sterility of both ends of tubing. Many sets allow for priming of tubing without removal of end cap.	_____	_____	_____	____________________
c. Place roller clamp about 2 to 5 cm (1 to 2 inches) below drip chamber, and move roller clamp to "off" position.	_____	_____	_____	____________________
d. Remove protective covering from IV tubing port on plastic IV solution bag.	_____	_____	_____	____________________
e. Insert infusion set into fluid container. Remove protector cap from tubing insertion spike, not touching spike, and insert spike into opening of IV bag. Cleanse rubber stopper on bottled solution with antiseptic, and insert spike into black rubber stopper of IV bottle.	_____	_____	_____	____________________
f. Prime infusion tubing by filling with IV solution:	_____	_____	_____	____________________
(1) Compress drip chamber and release.	_____	_____	_____	____________________
(2) Allow it to fill one-third to one-half full.	_____	_____	_____	____________________
g. Remove protector cap on end of tubing (some tubing can be primed without removal), and slowly release roller clamp to allow fluid to travel from drip chamber through tubing to needle adapter. Return roller clamp to "off" position after tubing is primed (filled with IV fluid).	_____	_____	_____	____________________

	S	U	NP	Comments
h. Be certain tubing is clear of air and air bubbles. To remove small air bubbles, firmly tap IV tubing where air bubbles are located. Check entire length of tubing to ensure that all air bubbles are removed. If you use a multiple port tubing, turn ports upside down and tap to fill and remove air.				
i. Replace cap protector on end of infusion tubing.				
6. *Option:* Prepare heparin or normal saline lock for infusion.				
a. If a loop or short extension tubing is needed because of an awkward VAD site placement, use sterile technique to connect the IV plug to the loop of short extension tubing. Inject 1 to 3 ml of normal saline through the plug and through the loop or short extension tubing.				
7. Identify accessible vein for placement of VAD. Apply tourniquet around arm above antecubital fossa or 4 to 6 inches (10 to 15 cm) above proposed insertion site. Do not apply tourniquet too tightly to avoid injury or bruising to skin. Check for presence of radial pulse. Tourniquet may be applied on top of a thin layer of clothing such as a gown sleeve. *Optional:* Apply BP cuff.				
8. Select the vein for VAD insertion.				
a. Use the most distal site in the nondominant arm, if possible.				
b. Avoid areas that are painful to palpation.				
c. Select a vein large enough for VAD.				
d. Choose a site that will not interfere with patient's activities of daily living (ADLs) or planned procedures.				
e. Using your index finger, palpate the vein by pressing downward and noting the resilient, soft, bouncy feeling as you release pressure.				
f. If possible, place extremity in dependent position from the heart.				

	S	U	NP	Comments
g. Select well-dilated vein. Methods to foster venous distention include:	____	____	____	____
(1) Stroking the extremity from distal to proximal below the proposed venipuncture site.	____	____	____	____
(2) Applying warmth to the extremity for several minutes, for example, with a warm washcloth.	____	____	____	____
h. Avoid sites distal to previous venipuncture site, veins in antecubital fossa or inner wrist, sclerosed or hardened veins, infiltrate site or phlebotic vessels, bruised areas, and areas of venous valves.	____	____	____	____
i. Avoid fragile dorsal veins in older adult patients and vessels in an extremity with compromised circulation.	____	____	____	____
9. Release tourniquet temporarily and carefully.	____	____	____	____
10. Apply disposable gloves. Wear eye protection if splash or spray of blood is possible.				
11. Place VAD adapter end of infusion set nearby on sterile gauze or sterile towel.	____	____	____	____
12. If area of insertion appears to need cleansing, use soap and water first. Use antiseptic swab to cleanse insertion site; allow the agent to dry.	____	____	____	____
13. Reapply tourniquet 10 to 12 cm (4 to 5 inches) above anticipated insertion site. Check presence of distal pulse.	____	____	____	____
14. Perform venipuncture. Anchor vein below site by placing thumb over vein and by stretching the skin against the direction of insertion 2 to 3 inches (5 to 7.5 cm) distal to the site. Warn patient of a sharp, quick stick.	____	____	____	____
a. *Over-the-needle catheter (ONC):* Insert with bevel up at 20- to 30-degree angle slightly distal to actual site of venipuncture in the direction of the vein.	____	____	____	____
b. *IV catheter with safety device:* Insert using same position as for ONC.	____	____	____	____

	S	U	NP	Comments
c. *Winged cannula:* Hold needle at 20- to 30-degree angle with bevel up slightly distal to actual site of venipuncture.	____	____	____	____
15. Observe for blood return through flashback cannula indicating that VAD has entered vein. Lower catheter until almost flush with skin. Advance catheter another 1/4 inch into vein and then loosen stylet. Continue to hold skin taut and advance catheter into vein until hub rests at venipuncture site. *Do not reinsert the stylet once it is loosened.* (If available, advance the safety device by using push-off tab to thread the catheter.) Advance butterfly needle until hub rests at venipuncture site.	____	____	____	____
16. Stabilize cannula with one hand, and release tourniquet with other. Apply gentle but firm pressure with index finger of nondominant hand 1 1/4 inches (3 cm) above the insertion site. Keep cannula stable. For a safety device, slide the catheter off the stylet while gliding the protective guard over the stylet. A click indicates the device is locked over the stylet. Remove the stylet of ONC. Do not recap the stylet. (NOTE: Techniques will vary with each IV device.)	____	____	____	____
17. Quickly connect end of the prepared saline lock or the infusion tubing set to end of catheter. Do not touch point of entry of connection. Secure connection.	____	____	____	____
18. *Intermittent infusion:* Hold the sterile heparin/saline lock firmly with nondominant hand. Insert prefilled syringe containing flush solution into injection cap. Flush slowly with flush solution. Withdraw the syringe while still flushing.	____	____	____	____
19. *Continuous infusion:* Begin infusion by slowly opening the slide clamp or adjusting the roller clamp of the IV tubing.	____	____	____	____

	S	U	NP	Comments
20. Secure cannula (follow agency policy).	___	___	___	___
a. *Transparent dressing:* Secure catheter with nondominant hand while preparing to apply dressing.	___	___	___	___
b. *Sterile gauze dressing:* Place narrow piece (1/2 inch) of sterile tape under catheter hub with sticky side up and cross tape over catheter hub. Place tape only on the catheter, never over the insertion site. Secure site to allow easy visual inspection. Avoid applying tape around the arm.	___	___	___	___
21. Apply sterile dressing over site.				
A. Transparent Dressing:				
(1) Carefully remove adherent backing. Apply one edge of dressing, and then gently smooth remaining dressing over IV site, leaving connection between IV tubing and catheter hub uncovered. Remove outer covering, and smooth dressing gently over site. (2) Take 1-inch piece of tape, and place it down from end of hub of catheter to insertion site, placing it over transparent dressing. (3) Apply chevron, and place over tape.	___	___	___	___
B. Sterile Gauze Dressing:				
(1) Fold a 2 × 2 gauze in half and cover with a 1-inch–wide tape extending about 1 inch from each side. Place under the tubing/catheter hub junction. Curl a loop of tubing alongside the arm, and place a second piece of tape directly over the tubing and padded 2 × 2, securing tubing in two places.	___	___	___	___
(2) Place 2 × 2 gauze pad over insertion site and catheter hub. Secure all edges with tape. Do not cover connection between IV tubing and catheter hub.	___	___	___	___

	S	U	NP	Comments
22. Loop tubing alongside the arm and place a second piece of tape over the tape covering the transparent dressing.	____	____	____	____________
23. For IV fluid administration, recheck flow rate to correct drops per minute.	____	____	____	____________
24. Label dressing agency per policy.	____	____	____	____________
25. Dispose of sheathed stylet or other sharps in appropriate sharps container. Discard supplies. Remove gloves and wash hands.	____	____	____	____________
26. Instruct patient how to change position in and out of bed without dislodging VAD.	____	____	____	____________
Evaluation				
1. Observe peripheral IV access. Peripheral IV access should be changed every 72 to 96 hours or per physician orders, or more frequently if complications occur.	____	____	____	____________
2. Observe patient every 1 to 2 hours.				
a. Check if correct amount of IV solution has infused by looking at time tape on IV bag or by checking infusion pump record.	____	____	____	____________
b. Count drip rate (if gravity drip) or check rate on infusion pump.	____	____	____	____________
c. Check patency of VAD.	____	____	____	____________
d. Observe patient during compression of vessel for signs of discomfort.	____	____	____	____________
e. Inspect insertion site, and note color. Inspect for presence of swelling. Palpate temperature of skin above dressing.	____	____	____	____________
3. Observe patient every 1 to 2 hours to determine response to therapy.	____	____	____	____________
4. Record IV insertion, type of fluid, insertion site by vessel, flow rate, size, and type of catheter or needle, and when infusion was begun.	____	____	____	____________
5. Record IV infusion and patient's response.	____	____	____	____________
6. Report type of fluid, flow rate, status of venipuncture site, amount of fluid remaining in present solution, expected time to hang next IV bag or bottle, and any side effects.	____	____	____	____________

Name ____________________ Date __________ Instructor's Name __________________________

Performance Checklist: Skill 15-2 Regulating Intravenous Flow Rate

	S	U	NP	Comments
Assessment				
1. Check patient's medical record for correct solution and additives. Follow six rights of medication administration.	____	____	____	____________
2. Perform hand hygiene. Observe for patency of VAD and IV tubing.	____	____	____	____________
3. Assess patients knowledge of how positioning of IV site affects flow rate.	____	____	____	____________
4. Inspect IV site, and verify with patient how venipuncture site feels.	____	____	____	____________
Planning				
1. Collect and organize equipment.	____	____	____	____________
2. Check patient's identification using two identifiers. Explain procedure.	____	____	____	____________
3. Have paper and pencil available to calculate flow rate.	____	____	____	____________
4. Acquire calibration (drop factor) in drops per milliliter (gtt/ml) of infusion set.	____	____	____	____________
5. A formula to calculate flow rate after determining ml/hr.	____	____	____	____________
Implementation				
1. Read physician's or health care provider's orders, and follow six rights for correct solution and proper additives.	____	____	____	____________
2. Obtain IV fluid/medication and tubing.	____	____	____	____________
3. Confirm hourly rate by dividing volume by hours, for example, and place marked adhesive tape or commercial fluid indicator tape on IV bottle or bag next to volume markings.	____	____	____	____________
4. *For gravity transfusion:* Confirm hourly rate and minute rate calculated in planning.	____	____	____	____________
5. Determine flow rate by counting drops in drip chamber for 1 minute by watch; then adjust roller clamp to increase or decrease rate of infusion.	____	____	____	____________
6. *For infusion using EID:* Follow manufacturer's guidelines for setup of EID:				
a. Place electronic eye on drip chamber. If gravity controller is used, ensure that IV container is 36 inches above IV site.	____	____	____	____________

	S	U	NP	Comments
b. Insert tubing into chamber of control mechanism, according to manufacturer's directions.	____	____	____	____________
c. Required drops per minute or volume per hour are selected, door to control chamber is closed, power button is turned on, and start button is pressed.	____	____	____	____________
d. Open regulator clamp completely while EID is in use.	____	____	____	____________
e. Monitor infusion rates and IV site for complications according to agency policy. Use watch to check rate of infusion, even when using EID.	____	____	____	____________
f. Assess patency of system when alarm sounds.	____	____	____	____________
7. For a volume-control device:				
a. Place volume-metric device between IV bag and insertion spike of infusion set.	____	____	____	____________
b. Place 2-hours' allotment of fluid into device.	____	____	____	____________
c. Assess system at least hourly; add fluid to volume-control device. Regulate flow rate.	____	____	____	____________
Evaluation				
1. Monitor IV infusion at least every hour, noting volume of IV fluid infused and rate.	____	____	____	____________
2. Observe patient for signs of overhydration or dehydration to determine response to therapy and restoration of fluid and electrolyte balance.	____	____	____	____________
3. Evaluate for signs of complications with IV flow rate: inflammation at site, clot in catheter, or kink or knot in infusion tubing.	____	____	____	____________
4. Record solution and rate of infusion every 4 hours or according to agency policy.	____	____	____	____________
5. Immediately record any new IV fluid rates.	____	____	____	____________
6. Document use of any electronic infusion device or controlling device and lot number on that device.	____	____	____	____________
7. Report rate of infusion to nurse in charge or next nurse assigned to care for patient.	____	____	____	____________

Name ____________________ Date __________ Instructor's Name ____________________

Performance Checklist: Skill 15-3 Changing Intravenous Solution and Infusion Tubing

	S	U	NP	Comments
Assessment				
1. Check physician's or health care provider's orders for type of fluid and infusion rate.	____	____	____	____________
2. Note date and time when IV tubing and solution were last changed.	____	____	____	____________
3. Determine the compatibility of all IV fluids and additives by consulting appropriate literature or the pharmacy.	____	____	____	____________
4. Determine patient's understanding of need for continued IV therapy.	____	____	____	____________
5. Assess patency of current IV access site.	____	____	____	____________
Planning				
1. Collect appropriate equipment. Have next solution prepared at least 1 hour before needed. If solution is prepared in pharmacy, be sure it has been delivered to the patient's hospital unit. Check that solution is correct and properly labeled. Check solution expiration date.	____	____	____	____________
2. Check patient's identification by using at least two patient identifiers.	____	____	____	____________
3. Prepare to change solution when about 50 ml of fluid remains in ottle or bag.	____	____	____	____________
4. Coordinate tubing changes with bag changes whenever possible.	____	____	____	____________
5. Prepare patient and family by explaining the procedure, its purpose, and what you expect of the patient.	____	____	____	____________
Changing IV solution				
Implementation				
1. Perform hand hygiene.	____	____	____	____________
2. *To change IV tubing without new tubings:*				
a. Prepare new solution for changing. If using plastic bag, remove protective cover from IV tubing port. If using glass bottle, remove metal cap and metal and rubber disks.	____	____	____	____________

	S	U	NP	Comments
b. Position roller clamp to stop flow rate.	_____	_____	_____	_____
c. Remove old IV fluid container from IV pole.	_____	_____	_____	_____
d. Quickly remove spike from old solution bag or bottle and, without touching tip, insert spike into new bag or bottle.	_____	_____	_____	_____
e. Hang new bag or bottle of solution.	_____	_____	_____	_____
f. Check for air in tubing. If bubbles form, they can be removed by closing the roller clamp, stretching the tubing downward, and tapping the tubing with the finger. For a larger amount of air, insert syringe into a port below the air and aspirate the air into the syringe. Swab port with alcohol and allow to dry before inserting syringe into port. Reduce air in tubing by priming slowly instead of allowing a wide-open flow.	_____	_____	_____	_____
g. Make sure drip chamber is one-third to one-half full. If the drip chamber is too full, pinch off tubing below the drip chamber, invert the container, squeeze the drip chamber, hang up the bottle, and release the tubing.	_____	_____	_____	_____
3. To change IV tubing without new solution:				
a. Open new infusion set and connect filter and/or extension tubing, keeping protective coverings over infusion spike and end of tubing.	_____	_____	_____	_____
b. Apply clean, disposable gloves.	_____	_____	_____	_____
c. If VAD is not visible, remove dressing. Hold VAD securely with nondominant hand. Do not remove tape securing VAD to skin.	_____	_____	_____	_____
d. For IV without injection cap:				
(1) Move roller clamp on new IV tubing to "off" position.	_____	_____	_____	_____
(2) Slow rate of infusion by regulating drip rate on old tubing. Be sure rate is at KVO.	_____	_____	_____	_____
(3) With old tubing in place, compress drip chamber and fill chamber.	_____	_____	_____	_____

	S	U	NP	Comments
(4) Remove old tubing from solution and hang or tape the drip chamber on IV pole 36 inches above IV pole.	_____	_____	_____	_____
(5) Place insertion spike of new tubing into old solution bag opening and hang solution bag on IV pole.	_____	_____	_____	_____
(6) Compress and release drip chamber on new tubing; slowly fill drip chamber one-third to one-half full.	_____	_____	_____	_____
(7) Slowly open roller clamp, remove protective cap from needle adapter (if necessary), and flush tubing with solution. Replace cap.	_____	_____	_____	_____
(8) Turn roller clamp on old tubing to "off" position.	_____	_____	_____	_____
(9) Stabilize hub of catheter or needle, and apply pressure over vein just above insertion site. Gently disconnect old tubing. Maintain stability of hub and quickly insert adapter of new tubing or saline lock into hub.	_____	_____	_____	_____
e. For saline/heparin lock or injection cap:				
(1) If you need to replace the loop or short extension tubing swab injection cap with alcohol. Insert syringe with 1 to 3 ml of saline, and inject through the injection cap into the loop or tubing.	_____	_____	_____	_____
(2) Position roller clamp of existingtubing to "off" position and disconnect tubing from injection cap.	_____	_____	_____	_____
(3) Take existing IV solution bag off IV pole.	_____	_____	_____	_____
(4) Prime tubing by spiking IV solution bag.	_____	_____	_____	_____
(5) Swab injection port of IV with alcohol and allow to dry.	_____	_____	_____	_____
4. Open roller clamp on new tubing. Allow solution to run rapidly for 30 to 60 seconds.	_____	_____	_____	_____
5. Regulate IV drip rate according to physician's orders, and monitor rate hourly.	_____	_____	_____	_____

	S	U	NP	Comments
6. If necessary, apply new dressing. Secure tubing to extremity with tape.	____	____	____	________________
7. Discard old tubing in proper container.	____	____	____	________________
8. Remove and dispose of gloves. Perform hand hygiene.	____	____	____	________________
Evaluation				
1. Evaluate flow rate and observe connection site for leakage.	____	____	____	________________
2. Observe patient for signs of overhydration or dehydration.	____	____	____	________________
3. Check IV system for patency and development.	____	____	____	________________
4. Record changing of tubing and solution on patient's record.	____	____	____	________________
5. Place a piece of tape or preprinted label with the date and time of tubing change and attach to tubing below the level of drip chamber.	____	____	____	________________

Name ____________________ Date __________ Instructor's Name ____________________________

Performance Checklist: Skill 15-4 Changing a Peripheral Intravenous Dressing

	S	U	NP	Comments
Assessment				
1. Determine when dressing was last changed.	_____	_____	_____	______________
2. Observe present dressing for moisture and intactness.	_____	_____	_____	______________
3. Observe IV system for proper functioning or complications: current flow rate, presence of kinks in infusion tubing or VAD. Palpate the VAD through the intact dressing for subjective complaints of pain or burning.	_____	_____	_____	______________
4. Inspect exposed VAD site for inflammation and swelling.	_____	_____	_____	______________
5. Monitor body temperature.	_____	_____	_____	______________
6. Assess patient's understanding of the need for continued IV infusion.	_____	_____	_____	______________
Planning				
1. Explain procedure and purpose to patient and family. Explain that affected extremity must be held still and describe length of procedure.	_____	_____	_____	______________
2. Collect equipment.	_____	_____	_____	______________
Implementation				
1. Perform hand hygiene. Apply disposable gloves and mask.	_____	_____	_____	______________
2. Remove tape, gauze, and/or transparent dressing from old dressing one layer at a time by pulling toward the insertion site, leaving tape that secures VAD intact. Be cautious if catheter tubing becomes tangled between two layers of dressing. When removing transparent dressing, hold catheter hub and tubing with nondominant hand.	_____	_____	_____	______________
3. Observe insertion site for signs and/or symptoms of infection, namely, redness, swelling, and presence of exudate.	_____	_____	_____	______________
4. If complication exists or if ordered by physician, discontinue infusion.	_____	_____	_____	______________
5. If IV is infusing properly, gently remove tape securing VAD. Use adhesive remover to cleanse skin and remove adhesive residue, if needed.	_____	_____	_____	______________

	S	U	NP	Comments
6. Clean insertion site with antiseptic swab using circular friction motion.	____	____	____	____________
7. Apply skin protectant and allow to dry.	____	____	____	____________
8. *Apply dressing.*				
a. *Applying gauze dressing:* Place a narrow piece (1/2 inch) of tape under hub of catheter with adhesive side up, and cross tape over hub. Place tape only on the catheter, never over the insertion site.	____	____	____	____________
b. *Applying transparent dressing:* Secure catheter with nondominant hand while preparing to apply dressing.	____	____	____	____________
9. Apply sterile dressing over site.				
a. Sterile gauze dressing				
(1) Fold a 2 × 2 gauze in half and cover with a 1-inch–wide piece of tape extending about 1 inch from each side. Place gauze under the tubing/catheter hub junction. Curl a loop of tubing alongside the arm and place a second piece of tape directly over the padded 2 × 2, securing tubing in two places.	____	____	____	____________
(2) Place another 2 × 2 gauze pad over the venipuncture site and catheter hub. Secure all edges with tape. Do not cover connection between IV tubing and catheter hub.	____	____	____	____________
b. Transparent dressing				
(1) Carefully remove adherent backing. Apply one edge of dressing, and then gently smooth remaining dressing over IV site, leaving end of catheter hub uncovered.	____	____	____	____________
(2) Place 1 inch of tape from end of catheter insertion site over dressing. Apply chevron.	____	____	____	____________
10. Remove and discard gloves.	____	____	____	____________
11. Label dressing per agency policy.	____	____	____	____________
12. Apply securement device.	____	____	____	____________
13. Discard equipment, and perform hand hygiene.	____	____	____	____________

	S	U	NP	Comments
Evaluation				
1. Observe IV flow rate, and compare with rate at time dressing change began.	_____	_____	_____	_____
2. Inspect condition of site.	_____	_____	_____	_____
3. Monitor patient's body temperature.	_____	_____	_____	_____
4. Record and report dressing change and observation of IV system.	_____	_____	_____	_____

16 Caring in Nursing Practice

Case Study

1. The daughter of a patient in an extended care facility has traveled from another state to visit. When she arrives with her husband and teenage son, she finds that her mother has deteriorated dramatically from the last time she spoke with her. The patient, in the terminal stages of liver disease, is now only minimally responsive, with episodes of agitation and disorientation. The family, especially the daughter, is emotionally distraught.
   a. What can be done to demonstrate caring for this patient's family?

Chapter Review

Complete the following:

1. Match the theorist with the theoretical concept:
   Patricia Benner and Judith Wrubel
   Jean Watson
   Madeleine Leininger
   Kristen Swanson
   a. Five processes and subdimensions
   b. Transpersonal caring
   c. Caring is primary
   d. Transcultural caring
2. For the following nursing behaviors, identify an example of a clinical intervention:
   a. Providing presence
   b. Comforting
   c. Listening
   d. Knowing the patient
3. A patient is to have an intravenous (IV) line inserted. The nurse demonstrates caring behaviors by:

Select the best answer for each of the following questions:

4. The nurse is discussing with her peers how much a patient matters to her. She states that she does not want the patient to suffer. The nurse is implementing the theory described by:
   1. Patricia Benner
   2. Jean Watson
   3. Kristen Swanson
   4. Madeleine Leininger
5. The patient was admitted to the hospital to have diagnostic tests to rule out a cancerous lesion in the lungs. The nurse is sitting with the patient in the room awaiting the results of the tests. The nurse is demonstrating the caring behavior of:
   1. Knowing
   2. Comforting
   3. Providing presence
   4. Maintaining belief

6. The nurse manager would like to promote more opportunities for the staff on the busy unit to demonstrate caring behaviors. The manager elects to implement:
   1. More time off for the staff
   2. A strict schedule for patient treatments
   3. Staff selection of patient assignments
   4. Staff appointment to hospital committees
7. The new graduate is looking at theories of caring. He selects Leininger's theory because it is most agreeable with his belief system. Leininger defines caring as a(n):
   1. New consciousness and moral idea
   2. Nurturing way of relating to a valued other
   3. Central, unifying domain necessary for health and survival
   4. Improvement in the human condition, using a transcultural perspective
8. The nurse is working with a patient who has been admitted to the oncology unit for treatment of a cancerous growth. This nurse is applying Swanson's theory of caring and demonstrating the concept of maintaining belief when:
   1. Performing the patient's dressing changes
   2. Providing explanations about the medications
   3. Keeping the patient draped during the physical exam
   4. Discussing how the radiation therapy will assist in decreasing the tumor's size
9. The new graduate is assigned to the surgical unit, where there are a large number of procedures to be performed during each shift. This nurse demonstrates a caring behavior in this situation by:
   1. Avoiding situations that may be uncomfortable or difficult
   2. Attempting to do all of the treatments independently and quickly
   3. Seeking assistance before performing new or difficult skills
   4. Telling the patients that he or she is a new graduate and unfamiliar with all of the procedures
10. A subdimension of Swanson's process of caring, "doing for others as he/she would do for self," involves:
    1. Being there
    2. Performing skillfully
    3. Generating alternatives
    4. Offering realistic optimism
11. Additional teaching is required if the nurse observes a nursing assistant working with an older adult patient and:
    1. Having the patient select the clothes to wear
    2. Addressing the patient as "Honey"
    3. Carefully organizing the patient's personal items
    4. Combing and styling the patient's hair

Study Group Questions

- What is "caring" in the nursing profession?
- What are the major theories of caring and the key concepts in each one?
- How is caring perceived by patients?
- What are caring behaviors?
- How can the nurse demonstrate caring to patients and families?

17 Cultural Diversity

Case Study

1. For the following situations, identify how the nurse should approach the patient and significant others in order to recognize cultural concerns and health care needs:
   a. The male patient comes from a culture with a matriarchal organization.
   b. Large numbers of family members surround the patient on the acute care unit.
   c. Dietary practices of the patient prohibit the eating of meat or meat products.
   d. A traditional healer makes calls to the patient's home in between the patient's visits to the physician.
   e. The patient and her family speak another language.

Chapter Review

Match the description/definition in Column A with the correct term in Column B.

	Column A	*Column B*
_______	1. Process of adapting to and adopting a new culture	a. Culture
_______	2. Shared identity related to social and cultural heritage	b. Race
_______	3. Tendency to categorize people into particular patterns without further assessment	c. Ethnicity
		d. Ethnocentrism
_______	4. Attitudes associating negative characteristics to people perceived to be different from oneself	e. Acculturation
		f. Assimilation
_______	5. Integrated patterns of human behavior, including language, customs, and beliefs	g. Prejudices
		h. Worldview
_______	6. Common biological characteristics shared by a group of people	i. Transcultural nursing
		j. Stereotypes
_______	7. Cognitive stance or perspective about phenomena characteristic of a particular cultural group	k. Subculture
_______	8. Giving up ethnic identity in favor of the dominant culture	
_______	9. Holding one's own way of life as superior to others	
_______	10. Distinct discipline focused on the comparative study of cultures to understand similarities	

Complete the following:

11. Currently in the United States, the largest minority group is _______________, and the largest growth rate is occurring for:

12. Subcultures have the same life patterns, values, and norms as the dominant culture.
    True _____ False _____

13. Select all of the following ways that a variant culture is more likely to approach illness causation and treatment:
    a. Causation is magic-religious based. _______
    b. Treatment is organ specific. _______
    c. Practitioners are sought who have uniform qualifications and follow universalistic standards. _______

d. Approach to illness is group reliability and interdependence. _______

14. Identify two possible nursing diagnoses that may be related to a patient's cultural needs.

15. It is predicted that by the year 2020 the percentage of people of European origin in North America will increase to 85%.
True _____ False _____

16. The nurse anticipates that a patient who has a present time orientation will arrive at the clinic for his/her appointment:

17. Select all of the following that are correct statements concerning cultural beliefs of pregnancy and childbirth:
   a. Hindu women are encouraged to eat "hot" foods when pregnant. _______
   b. Arab women seek out male practitioners. _______
   c. Hispanic women tend to avoid early baby showers. _______
   d. Filipino and South Asian women tend to endure labor without complaining or asking for medication. _______
   e. Orthodox Jewish fathers play an active role in the delivery room. _______

18. The nurse may anticipate that decision making for African or Asian patients near death will be made by family members.
True _____ False _____

Select the best answer for each of the following questions:

19. The nurse is seeing patients in the outpatient clinic who are Asian-American. A patient from this cultural group who demonstrates traditional health practices may use a(n):
   1. Herbalist
   2. *Curandero*
   3. Root worker
   4. Medicine man

20. The nurse recognizes that physiological characteristics of cultural groups may affect overall health, and that there may be an increased prevalence of particular disease processes within certain groups. In working with Native American Indians, the nurse is alert to the signs and symptoms that may indicate:
   1. Cancer of the esophagus
   2. Diabetes mellitus
   3. Parasites
   4. Sickle cell anemia

21. The community center where the nurse volunteers has a very culturally diverse population. The nurse wants to promote communication with all of the patients from different cultures. A beneficial technique for the nurse is to:
   1. Explain nursing terms that are used
   2. Use direct and consistent eye contact with all patients
   3. Call patients by their first names to establish rapport
   4. Wait for responses to all questions that are asked

22. The patient expresses to the nurse that traditional Western or American practices are used in the home for health promotion. The nurse expects that the patient will use:
   1. Acupuncture
   2. Guided imagery
   3. Aromatic therapy
   4. Over-the-counter medications

23. When working with an interpreter for a patient who speaks another language, the nurse should:
   1. Direct questions to the interpreter
   2. Expect word for word translation
   3. Ensure that the interpreter speaks the patient's dialect
   4. Ask the interpreter to evaluate the patient's nonverbal behaviors

24. When asking a patient specifically about his or her social organization, the nurse will focus on the patient's:
   1. Position in the family hierarchy
   2. Preferred manner of communication
   3. Age at the time of immigration
   4. Dietary practices

25. The nurse is working with a patient who is Muslim. There are foods that are prohibited (*Haram*), and the

nurse recognizes that this will include:
1. Pork
2. Fish
3. Fresh fruit
4. Vegetables

26. An Orthodox Jewish patient has just died. The nurse anticipates:
 1. A request for an autopsy
 2. Preparation for cremation
 3. Refusal to move the body
 4. Scheduling for immediate burial

27. When working with patients of other cultures, the nurse anticipates that a curandero may be sought for a patient who is:
 1. Hispanic
 2. Chinese
 3. African
 4. Korean

Study Group Questions

- What is culture?
- What are the major ethnocultural groups in the country/community, their health and illness beliefs and practices, and their traditional remedies?
- How can the nurse promote communication with individuals who are from other cultures and/or individuals that speak different languages?
- How can the nurse identify and respond to the patient's cultural needs?
- What information may be obtained from a cultural assessment?
- What nursing approaches may be successful in assisting multicultural patients in health care settings?
- What resources are available to assist the nurse in learning about and working with patients from other cultures?

Spiritual Health 18

Case Study

1. You are working with a patient in an acute care facility who practices Buddhism.
   a. What information should be obtained in relation to the patient's spiritual practices?
   b. What adaptations may need to be made by the nurse, the other members of the health care team, and the acute care facility to meet the patient's spiritual needs?

Chapter Review

Match the description/definition in Column A with the correct term in Column B.

	Column A	Column B
______	1. Does not believe in the existence of God	a. Faith
______	2. Cultural or institutional religion	b. Hope
______	3. Awareness of one's inner self and a sense of connection to a higher being	c. Connectedness d. Atheist
______	4. Multidimensional concept that gives comfort while a person endures hardship and challenges	e. Spirituality f. Self-transcendence
______	5. Awareness of that which cannot be seen or known in ordinary ways	g. Agnostic h. Religion
______	6. Believes that ultimate reality is unknown or unknowable	
______	7. Having close spiritual relationships with oneself, others, and God or other spiritual being	

Complete the following:

8. Four themes of spirituality are:

9. An example of a nursing intervention for a patient who has had a near death experience is:

10. Identify two possible nursing diagnoses relating to spirituality or spiritual health.

11. Identify what each letter in the BELIEF assessment tool acronym designates:
    B:
    E:
    L:
    I:
    E:
    F:

12. Formulate a question that may be asked to determine the patient's spiritual belief system.

Select the best answer for each of the following questions:

13. A patient is admitted to the medical center for surgery to repair a fractured hip. Upon reviewing the patient's admission history, the nurse finds that the patient attends religious services fairly routinely. The nurse supports the patient's spiritual needs by stating:
    1. "Do you really go to services often?"
    2. "Don't worry. God will take care of you."

3. "I'll call your minister and have him stop by to see you."
4. "Is there any way that I may be able to help you with your spiritual needs?"

14. A patient who is of the Jewish faith is admitted to the long-term care facility. The nurse seeks to provide support of the usual health practices that are part of this religion. The nurse discovers that one component of usual Jewish tradition states:
   1. No euthanasia should be used
   2. A faith healer should be used
   3. Modern medical treatment should be refused
   4. Physical exams should be performed only by individuals of the same gender
15. While caring for a patient in the intensive care unit, the patient has a cardiac arrest. The patient is successfully resuscitated. Following this near death experience, the patient is progressing physically, but appears withdrawn and concerned. The nurse assists the patient by stating:
   1. "The experience that you had is easy to explain and understand."
   2. "That was a very close call. It must be very frightening for you."
   3. "Other people have had similar experiences and worked through their feelings."
   4. "If you would like to talk about your experience, I will stay with you."
16. For the patient with a diagnosis of a chronic disease, the nurse wishes to support feelings of hope. The nurse recognizes that hope provides:
   1. A meaning and purpose for the patient
   2. An organized approach to dealing with the disease process
   3. A connection to the cultural background of the patient
   4. A binding relationship with the divine being of the patient's religion
17. The nurse is reviewing the plan of care for a 66-year-old home care patient who is experiencing the beginning stages of Alzheimer's disease. Several nursing diagnoses have been identified from the initial home visit and assessment. The nurse believes that the patient may need to be assessed for spiritual needs based on the diagnosis of:
   1. *Impaired memory*
   2. *Altered health maintenance*
   3. *Ineffective individual coping*
   4. *Altered thought process*
18. According to Erikson's stages of psychosocial development, with regard to spiritual beliefs it is expected that a 6-year-old child will:
   1. Begin to ask about God or a supreme being
   2. Have spiritual well-being provided by the parents
   3. Interpret meanings literally
   4. Begin to learn the difference between right and wrong
19. The nurse recognizes that a group whose members may *reject* modern medicine based on religious beliefs is:
   1. Hindu
   2. Islamic
   3. Catholic
   4. Navajo
20. According to Erikson's stages of psychosocial development, with regard to spiritual beliefs it is expected that a middle-age person will begin to:
   1. Reflect on inconsistencies in religious stories
   2. Form independent beliefs and attitudes
   3. Review value systems during a crisis
   4. Sort fantasy from fact

Study Group Questions

- What is spirituality and how does it relate to an individual's health status?
- What are the concepts of spirituality/spiritual health?
- What spiritual or religious problems may arise during patient care?
- How can the nurse assess a patient's spirituality/spiritual health?

- What is the role of the nurse in promoting spiritual health?
- How can the nurse avoid imposing his or her own beliefs on the patient?
- What are the differences and similarities in spiritual practices and health beliefs between the major religious sects?
- How is hope related to spirituality?

19 Growth and Development

Case Studies

1. You are a student nurse on an inpatient pediatric unit in a medical center. You have two patients—an infant and a 5-year-old child.
   a. How will you promote growth and developmental needs for these two patients in the acute care environment?
2. Your patient in the extended care facility is an 86-year-old woman who is occasionally disoriented to time, place, and person.
   a. How will you approach this patient to assist her in meeting her developmental needs?
3. You are working as a summer camp nurse with children 8 to 10 years old. It is your turn to select diversional activities for your group.
   a. What types of games or activities are appropriate for this age-group?
4. You are teaching the parents of adolescents the signs that may indicate a potential suicidal tendency in their children.
   a. What signs/behaviors will you identify for these parents?

Chapter Review

Match the description in Column A with the correct theorist in Column B.

	Column A	Column B
________	1. Development of cognition	a. Freud
________	2. Psychosexual focus	b. Erikson
________	3. Based on human needs	c. Maslow
________	4. Male and female personality development	d. Piaget
________	5. Moral development	e. Kohlberg
________	6. Psychosocial development	f. Gillian

Complete the following:

7. An example of a teratogen is:

8. The leading cause of death in the toddler and preschool age-groups is:

9. Select the age-group *(Infant, Toddler, Preschool Age, School Age, Adolescent, Young Adult, Middle Adult, or Older Adult)* in which each of the following behaviors is evident or usually begins:
   a. Toilet training
   b. Tripling of birth weight
   c. Use of script handwriting
   d. Separation anxiety
   e. Moving away from the family
   f. Parallel play
   g. Search for personal identity

h. Menopause

i. Speaking in short sentences

j. More graceful running and jumping

k. Development of fears

l. Presbycusis

m. Loss of primary teeth

n. Development of primary and secondary sexual characteristics

o. Low risk of chronic illness

p. Diminished skin turgor and appearance of wrinkles

q. Socioeconomic stability

10. To promote awareness of time, place, and person in an extended care environment, the nurse implements:

11. Prescriptive use or administration of more medication than indicated clinically is termed:

12. Identify safety concerns in the home environment for the following age-groups:
    a. Toddler:

    b. Older adult:

Select the best answer for each of the following questions:

13. You are assigned to prepare a teaching plan for a group of preschool age children. For individuals of this age-group, the nurse includes:
    1. Appropriate use of medications
    2. Cooking safety, including use of the stove
    3. Information on prevention of obesity and hypertension
    4. Guidelines for crossing the street or actions to take during a fire
14. Children who are admitted to a hospital may experience a great deal of fear regarding the hospitalization. To reduce the fear of school-age children in an acute care environment, the nurse:
    1. Restrains them for all assessments and procedures
    2. Shows them the equipment that is to be used for procedures
    3. Provides in-depth information on how procedures are done
    4. Tells them that everything will be all right and the procedures will not hurt
15. During a clinical rotation the student nurse is observing children in a day care center. The student is asked to assist with the activities for the preschool age children. Children in this age-group are usually able to:
    1. Make detailed drawings
    2. Skip, throw, and catch balls
    3. Easily hold a pencil and print letters
    4. Use a vocabulary of more than 8000 words
16. A parent of an infant asks the nurse what the infant should be able to do at the end of the first year. You identify that the infant will be able to:
    1. Participate in simple games, like peek-a-boo
    2. Use symbols to represent objects or persons
    3. Differentiate strangers from family members
    4. Recognize his or her own name
17. The parents of a 6-month-old infant are asking about the usual activities that can be expected of a child this age. The nurse informs the parents that a major

milestone in gross motor development for a 6-month-old infant is:
1. Banging hand-held blocks together
2. Pulling self to a standing position
3. Sitting up independently
4. Crawling on the abdomen

18. The nurse is working with a group of young adults at the community center. There are many discussions about life and health issues. The nurse is aware that a health-related concern for young adults is that:
1. Attachment needs must be enhanced
2. "Labeling" may alter their self-perceptions
3. Adaptation to chronic disease is developing
4. Fast-paced lifestyles may place them at risk for illnesses or disabilities

19. As part of the assignment in the home health agency, the nurse visits a local senior citizen housing development on a weekly basis. During the visit, the nurse provides information on issues that affect older adults, including how:
1. Cognitive development is limited
2. Depression and stress-related illnesses are common
3. Health maintenance programs are important to promote well-being
4. Accidents and injuries are the major cause of death in this age-group

20. The nurse is seeking to evaluate the effectiveness of teaching provided to the parents of an infant. The nurse determines that the teaching has been successful when the parents:
1. Place small pillows in the infant's crib
2. Position the infant on the stomach for sleeping
3. Purchase a crib with slats that are less than 2 inches apart
4. Prop a bottle up for the infant to suck on while falling asleep

21. When presenting a program for a group of individuals in their middle-adult years, the nurse informs the members to expect the following physical change:
1. A decrease in skin turgor
2. An increased breast size
3. Palpable lateral thyroid lobes
4. A visual acuity that is greater than 20/50

22. Parents of a 3½-year-old boy are concerned when, following hospitalization, the boy begins to suck his thumb again. The boy had not sucked his thumb for over a year. The nurse informs the parents that:
1. Their physician must be informed about this behavior
2. The child was probably not ready to stop this behavior previously
3. The child is feeling neglected by his parents and they should spend more time with him
4. The behavior should be ignored as it is common for the child to regress when anxious

23. An adolescent female has come to the family planning center for information about birth control. The patient asks the nurse what she should use to avoid getting pregnant. The nurse responds:
1. "Are your parents aware of your sexual activity?"
2. "You've been using some kind of protection before, right?"
3. "What are your friends doing to protect themselves?"
4. "What can you tell me about your past sexual experiences?"

24. A patient has come to the outpatient obstetric clinic for a routine checkup. The patient asks the nurse what is happening with the baby now that she is in her second trimester. The nurse informs the patient that:
1. The heartbeat can be heard
2. The fingers and toes are well-developed
3. The organ systems are just beginning to develop
4. The brain undergoes a tremendous growth spurt

25. The patient in the nursing center has pneumonia. The nurse suspects the potentially reversible cognitive impairment of:
1. Delirium
2. Dementia

3. Depression
4. Disengagement

Study Group Questions

- What are the principles of growth and development?
- How can growth and development be influenced both internally and externally?
- What are the differences and similarities of the major developmental theorists?
- How can the nurse apply the different developmental theories to patient situations?
- What are the major physical, psychosocial, and cognitive changes that occur throughout the life span?
- What are the specific health needs for each developmental stage?
- How does the approach of the nurse differ for individuals in each developmental stage in order to meet their developmental needs?
- What are the different teaching/learning needs of each developmental stage?

Study Chart

Create a study chart to compare Growth and Development across the Life Span, *identifying the physical abilities, psychosocial/cognitive activities, and health promotion behaviors and strategies for each age-group from infancy to older adulthood.*

20 Self-Concept and Sexuality

Case Studies

1. A 17-year-old male patient is admitted to the rehabilitation facility. He was seriously injured during a school football game, and now is paraplegic. Although medically stable, it appears that he is having difficulty dealing with his physical limitations. The patient speaks frequently about his involvement in athletics, as well as other school-related activities.
   a. What self-concept and sexuality issues are involved in this situation?
   b. Formulate a plan of care for this patient.
2. A patient that you suspect is the victim of sexual abuse arrives at the clinic.
   a. What behaviors may the patient exhibit that would lead to this assessment?
   b. What questions should you ask to get more information from the patient about the possible abuse?

Chapter Review

Match the description/definition in Column A with the correct term in Column B.

Column A

_____ 1. Set of conscious and unconscious feelings and beliefs about oneself

_____ 2. Set of behaviors that have been approved by the family, community, and culture as appropriate in particular situations

_____ 3. Clear, persistent preference for persons of one sex

_____ 4. Emotional evaluation of self-worth

_____ 5. Involves experiences and attitudes related to appearance and physical abilities

_____ 6. Sense of femaleness or maleness

_____ 7. Irrational fear of homosexuality

_____ 8. Persistent individuality and sameness of a person over time and in various circumstances

Column B

a. Sexuality
b. Self-concept
c. Homophobia
d. Self-esteem
e. Sexual orientation
f. Role
g. Identity
h. Body image

Complete the following:

9. Identify two examples of general positive influences on and stressors to self-concept:

10. Select the behaviors that may indicate an altered self-concept:
    a. Eye contact maintained _______
    b. Straight posture _______
    c. Hesitant speech _______
    d. Overly angry response _______
    e. Independence _______
    f. Passive attitude _______
    g. Able to make decisions _______
    h. Unkempt appearance _______

11. For the following patients, identify the potential concerns related to self-concept and sexuality:
    a. A woman who has had a mastectomy

b. A woman who is undergoing chemotherapy for cancer and who has a young child at home

c. A 7-year-old child who has been severely burned

d. A middle-adult man who has had a heart attack

12. A way in which the nurse may promote self-concept in an acute care setting is by:

13. An example of an alteration in sexual health is:

14. Specify an area for patient teaching to promote sexual functioning:

15. For the nursing diagnosis *Situational low self-esteem,* related to being unable to successfully pass a required college course, identify a patient goal/outcome and nursing interventions.

16. The capacity for sexuality diminishes significantly in older adults.
    True _____ False _____
17. Cultural background does not directly influence self-concept.
    True _____ False _____
18. An example of an intervention that the nurse may implement to promote self-concept for an older adult is:

Select the best answer for each of the following questions:

19. The nurse recognizes that which of the following age-groups are most vulnerable to identity stressors?
    1. Infancy
    2. Preschool
    3. Adolescence
    4. Middle adulthood
20. An adolescent patient has come to the nurse's office in the school to discuss some personal issues. The nurse wishes to determine the sexual health of this adolescent. The nurse begins by asking:
    1. "Do you use contraception?"
    2. "Have you already had sexual relations?"
    3. "Are your parents aware of your sexual activity?"
    4. "Do you have any concerns about sex or your body's development?"
21. During an interview and physical assessment of a female patient in the clinic, the nurse finds that the individual has multiple lacerations and bruises, and that she has experienced headaches and difficulty sleeping. The nurse suspects:
    1. Sexual dysfunction
    2. Emotional conflict
    3. Sexually transmitted disease
    4. Physical and/or sexual abuse
22. The patient has come to the family planning center for assistance in selecting a birth control method. She asks the nurse about contraception that requires a prescription. The nurse responds by discussing:
    1. Condoms
    2. Abstinence
    3. Spermicides
    4. Birth control pills
23. The patient is admitted to the coronary care unit following an acute myocardial infarction. He tells the nurse, "I won't be able to do what I used to at the hardware store." The nurse recognizes that the patient is experiencing a problem with the self-concept component of:
    1. Role
    2. Identity

3. Self-esteem
4. Body image

24. An adolescent patient has just been diagnosed with scoliosis and will need to wear a corrective brace. She tells the nurse angrily, "I don't know why I have to have this stupid problem!" The nurse responds most appropriately by saying:
    1. "Tell me what you do when you get angry and upset."
    2. "Don't be angry. You'll be getting the best care available."
    3. "You'll heal quickly and the brace can come off pretty soon."
    4. "It's okay to be angry around your friends, but try not to be upset around your parents."

25. During an initial assessment at the outpatient clinic, the nurse wants to determine the patient's perception of identity. The nurse asks the patient:
    1. "What is your usual day like?"
    2. "How would you describe yourself?"
    3. "What activities do you enjoy doing at home?"
    4. "What changes would you make in your personal appearance?"

26. The patient has been in the rehabilitation facility for several weeks following a cerebral vascular accident (CVA/stroke). During the hospitalization the nurse has identified that the patient has become progressively more depressed about his physical condition. Although the patient is able to, he will not participate in personal grooming, and now is refusing any visitors. At this point, the nurse intervenes by:
    1. Telling the patient to think more positively about the future
    2. Helping the patient to get washed and dressed every day
    3. Leaving the patient to complete activities of daily living independently
    4. Contacting a representative of a support group and investigating a psychological consultation with the physician

27. The nurse is working with a patient who has had a colostomy. The patient asks about resuming a sexual relationship with a partner. The nurse begins by determining:
    1. The patient's knowledge about sexual activity
    2. How the patient has dealt with other life changes in the past
    3. The partner's feelings about the colostomy
    4. How comfortable the patient and the partner are in communicating with each other

28. The nurse who is using Erikson's theory expects that a 5-year-old boy will begin to:
    1. Accept body changes and maturation
    2. Incorporate feedback from peers into his personality
    3. Distinguish himself from the environment around him
    4. Identify with a specific gender group

29. The patient asks the nurse about a prescription for Cialis (tadalafil). The nurse recognizes, however, that this drug is definitely contraindicated for the patient who is taking:
    1. Antibiotics
    2. Beta blockers
    3. Antihistamines
    4. Nonsteroidal anti-inflammatory agents

30. The nurse is aware that which of the following strategies is appropriate to teach a patient for promotion of a positive sexual experience?
    1. Encouraging the use of only one position for intercourse
    2. Instructing couples to work harder at the beginning of intercourse
    3. Discussing side effects of medications that may alter responsiveness
    4. Emphasizing a shorter period of foreplay

31. Correction is required if the new nurse in the women's clinic is observed:
    1. Closing the door during an examination
    2. Determining the patient's cultural beliefs
    3. Identifying physiological changes for the patient
    4. Discussing findings with the patient in the examination room

32. Which of the following is anticipated as a sexual change related to the aging process?
    1. Increased vaginal secretions
    2. Decreased time for ejaculation to be achieved
    3. Decreased time for maintenance of an erection
    4. Increased orgasmic contractions
33. During an initial assessment at the outpatient clinic, the nurse wants to determine the patient's self-esteem. The nurse asks the patient:
    1. "What is your usual day like?"
    2. "How do you feel about yourself?"
    3. "What hobbies do you enjoy doing at home?"
    4. "What changes would you make in your personal appearance?"

Study Group Questions

- What are the components of self-concept?
- What stressors may influence an individual's self-concept?
- How may the nurse promote an individual's self-concept in different health care settings?
- What is sexuality and how does it develop throughout the life span?
- How can sexual health be defined?
- What are some of the current issues related to sexuality and sexual health?
- How may sexual health be altered?
- What health-related factors may influence sexual function?
- How are self-concept and sexuality related?
- How can the nurse determine an individual's self-concept and sexual health?
- What adaptations may be made by the nurse in approaching different age-groups for the assessment and promotion of self-concept and sexual health?
- How can the nurse apply critical thinking and nursing processes to the areas of self-concept and sexuality?
- What resources are available to assist individuals to promote optimum self-concept and sexual health?
- How can the nurse make the patient feel more at ease when completing an assessment of sexual health?

Study Chart

Create a study chart on Stressors Affecting Self-Concept, *identifying how the components of self-concept may be influenced and nursing interventions that may be implemented to promote the patient's self-concept.*

21 Family Context in Nursing

Case Study

1. A 65-year-old male has been admitted to the coronary care unit in the medical center. The patient experienced a myocardial infarction (heart attack) while working late in his store. His wife, who accompanied him to the medical center, not only has been the "homemaker" for the family for over 25 years but also has assisted in the family business run by her husband. They have two children who live on their own. Their son lives with a male roommate in a homosexual relationship, while their younger daughter is married and has two children of her own. The patient and his wife speak readily about the younger daughter, but avoid talking about her older brother.
   a. What factors related to family roles and function are involved in this situation?
   b. What stage of the family life cycle is this family in currently?
   c. What strategies may the nurse use to promote communication in this family?
   d. How may the role of the patient and his wife influence the health education plan?
   e. Identify a family-oriented nursing diagnosis for this situation.

Chapter Review

Match the family stages in Column A with the key principle identified for that stage in Column B.

Column A (Family Stages)

_____ 1. Unattached young adult
_____ 2. Newly married couple
_____ 3. Family with adolescents
_____ 4. Launching children and moving on
_____ 5. Family in later life

Column B (Key Principles)

a. Increasing flexibility of family's boundaries to include children's independence
b. Accepting parent-offspring separation
c. Accepting shifting of generational roles
d. Committing to a new system
e. Accepting a multitude of exits from and entries into the family system

---

Complete the following:

6. Identify a nursing diagnosis for a family coping with the difficult care of an older adult parent in the home:

7. Select all of the following that are correct statements regarding today's society:
   a. Families are larger. _______
   b. Divorce rates have tripled since the 1950s. _______
   c. Less people are living alone. _______
   d. From the 1970s to the 1990s, the number of single-parent families has doubled. _______
   e. Less than one third of gay male couples live together. _______
   f. Father-only families have increased. _______
   g. The fastest growing age-group is 65 years and older. _______

8. Identify an effect that inadequate functioning may have on a family. _______

Select the best answer for each of the following questions:

9. The nurse is working with a family where the parents, both previously divorced, have brought a total of three unrelated children together. This type of family structure is classified as:
   1. Nuclear
   2. Extended
   3. Blended
   4. Multi-adult
10. The community health nurse has been assigned to work with a patient who is being discharged from a psychiatric facility. The nurse recognizes when dealing with families that:
    1. All family members do not need to understand and agree to the plan of care
    2. Health behaviors of the family do not influence the health of individual family members
    3. The nurse needs to change the structure of the family to meet the needs of the patient
    4. Health promotion behaviors need to be tied to the developmental stage of the family
11. Preparation for working with families includes the understanding of the life cycle stage that the patient is experiencing. The nurse is working with a family that is in the "launching children and moving on" stage. It is expected that a family in this stage may also need to deal with:
    1. A review of life events
    2. Determining career goals
    3. The death of an older parent
    4. Development of intimate peer relationships
12. The nurse is working with a family that has been taking care of a parent with Alzheimer's disease for several years in their home. A nursing diagnosis of *Risk for caregiver role strain* is identified. The nurse initially plans for:
    1. Respite care
    2. More medication for the parent
    3. Placement in a long-term care facility
    4. Consultation with a family therapist
13. Following an initial assessment, the nurse determines that this is a healthy family. This assessment is based on the finding that:
    1. The family responds passively to stressors
    2. Change is viewed negatively and strongly resisted
    3. The family structure is flexible enough to adapt to crises
    4. Minimum influence is exerted by the members upon their environment
14. A patient who has had surgery is going to be discharged tomorrow. The patient has a visual deficit and will need dressing changes twice a day. To meet this specific need, the nurse first:
    1. Refers the patient to an adult day care center
    2. Arranges for a private duty nurse to take care of the patient 24 hours a day
    3. Informs the patient that the dressing changes will have to be managed independently
    4. Investigates the availability of a family member or neighbor to perform the dressing changes
15. While working in the community health center, the nurse employs principles of family care. The nurse is concerned with:
    1. Caring for the expectant family
    2. Strengthening the family unit
    3. Providing care outside of the hospital for the family members
    4. Promoting the health of the family as a unit and the health of the individual members
16. The concept of the family being able to transcend divorce and remarriage is termed:
    1. Family resiliency
    2. Family diversity
    3. Family durability
    4. Family functioning
17. To determine the family form and membership, the nurse asks the patient:
    1. "How are financial decisions made?"
    2. "Who drives the children to school?"
    3. "Where do you go on vacation?"
    4. "Who do you consider your family?"

18. Members of which one of the following groups have been found less likely to live in an extended family situation?
    1. Caucasian
    2. Asian
    3. Hispanic
    4. African American

Study Group Questions

- What are the attributes of a family?
- What are the different family forms?
- What are the current issues/trends influencing the family of today?
- How do the structure and function of the family influence family relationships?
- How does communication affect family relationships?
- How are the nursing approaches to the family as patient and the family as context similar/different?
- How may critical thinking and nursing processes be applied to family nursing?
- What specific assessments should the nurse make in relation to the family?
- How does the nurse plan for the educational needs of the patient within a family?
- What does the nurse need to consider to meet the health needs of patients within families?
- How are psychosocial/cultural factors involved in family processes and the nursing approach to families?
- What resources are available within the health care setting and community to assist and support family functioning?

Stress and Coping 22

Case Study

1. A young adult female patient is preparing to be married in a few months. She has also received a recent job promotion that requires many additional hours to be spent at work. She is seen in the nurse practitioner's office for vague symptoms.
   a. What possible signs and symptoms may be demonstrated if this patient is experiencing a stress reaction?
   b. Identify a possible nursing diagnosis for this patient.
   c. What relaxation techniques may be presented to this patient?

Chapter Review

Complete the following:

1. Evaluating an event for its personal meaning is called:

2. Select all of the following that are correct statements about stress:
   a. Increased self-confidence results in decreased tension. _______
   b. The emotional concern of others can increase negative effects. _______
   c. Shorter, less intense stressors increase the stress response. _______
   d. The same event can cause different stress levels in different people. _______
   e. The greater the perceived magnitude of the stressor, the greater the stress response. _______
   f. Stress is decreased if a person is unable to anticipate the occurrence of an event. _______

3. A priority nursing intervention for safety for a patient under extreme stress is to determine: _______

4. Depression in later adulthood is a common problem.
   True _______ False _______

5. An example of a positive benefit of exercise for stress reduction is:

6. For the following, select the type of factor that may produce stress: *Situational, Maturational, Sociocultural, Posttraumatic stress disorder*
   a. Divorce _______________
   b. Poverty _______________
   c. Rape _______________
   d. Immigration status _______________
   e. Job change _______________
   f. Adolescent identity crisis _______________
   g. Hypertension _______________
   h. Children moving away from home _______________
   i. September 11th _______________
   j. Homelessness _______________

7. Identify an indicator of stress for each of the following areas:
   Cognitive

   Cardiovascular

   Gastrointestinal

Behavioral

Neuroendocrine

Select the best answer for each of the following questions:

8. The patient has been hospitalized with a serious systemic infection. If the patient is in the resistance stage of the general adaptation syndrome and moving toward recovery, the nurse expects that the patient will demonstrate a:
   1. Stabilization of hormone levels
   2. Greater degree of tissue damage
   3. Reduction in cardiac output
   4. Greater involvement of the sympathetic nervous system
9. While working in the psychiatric emergency department, the nurse is alert to patients who are having severe difficulty in coping. A priority for the nurse is the safety of the patient and others; therefore the nurse asks patients:
   1. "How can we help you?"
   2. "Are you thinking of harming yourself?"
   3. "What physical symptoms are you having?"
   4. "What happened that is different in your life?"
10. As a result of the patient's health problem, the family is experiencing an economic difficulty and demonstrating signs of crisis. As part of crisis intervention, the nurse:
    1. Refers the patient for financial assistance
    2. Recommends inpatient psychiatric therapy
    3. Plans to teach the family about long term health needs
    4. Has the patient avoid discussions about personal feelings and emotions
11. A nurse working on the surgical unit notes that the patient has been exhibiting nervous behavior the evening before the surgical procedure. To assess the degree of stress that the patient is experiencing, the nurse asks:
    1. "Would you like me to call your family for you?"
    2. "How dangerous do you think the surgery will be?"
    3. "You seem anxious. Would you like to talk about the surgery?"
    4. "How would you like to speak with another patient who has had the procedure already?"
12. The nurse determines that the patient is experiencing a stress reaction. To determine how the patient may cope with the event, the nurse should ask:
    1. "Are you taking any hypnotics?"
    2. "What do you think caused your stress?"
    3. "How long have you felt this way?"
    4. "Have you dealt with this reaction before?"
13. An 80-year-old patient was admitted to the hospital with a diagnosis of pneumonia. The patient is very lethargic and not communicating, and the patient's respirations are extremely labored. The nurse assesses that the patient is experiencing the general adaptation stage of:
    1. Alarm
    2. Resistance
    3. Exhaustion
    4. Reflex response
14. The patient has come to the employee support center with complaints of fatigue and general uneasiness. The patient believes that the symptoms may be related to the increased amount of work that is expected in the job. The nurse recommends initially that the patient attempt to reduce or control the stress by:
    1. Leaving the job immediately
    2. Enrolling in a self-awareness course
    3. Seeking the assistance of a psychiatrist
    4. Employing relaxation techniques, such as deep breathing
15. According to the general adaptation syndrome (GAS), the nurse expects which one of the following signs of an alarm reaction?
    1. Pupil dilation
    2. Decreased blood glucose levels
    3. Decreased heart rate
    4. Stabilized hormone levels
16. The nurse identifies that the patient is under stress. To determine the patient's

perception of the stress, the nurse should ask:

1. "Are you sure you are not taking drugs or alcohol?"
2. "What does the situation mean to you?"
3. "How did you handle this in the past?"
4. "Why aren't you seeing a counselor?"

Study Group Questions

- What is stress?
- What theories are associated with stress and the stress response?
- How does the general adaptation syndrome (GAS) work?
- How do nursing theorists explain stress and the stress response?
- What factors influence the response to stress?
- What assessment data may indicate the presence of a stress reaction?
- How does stress relate to illness?
- What are coping/defense mechanisms and how may they be used by individuals to deal with stress?
- What is the role of the nurse in reducing or eliminating stress for patients in health promotion, acute care, and restorative care settings?
- What is involved in crisis intervention?
- What are possible relaxation/stress reduction techniques?

23 Loss and Grief

Case Study

1. Mrs. R.'s husband committed suicide and she is devastated by the event. In anticipation of potential difficulties, the nurse should be alert to the possibility of a complicated bereavement.
   a. What assessment data may indicate that Mrs. R. is experiencing a complicated period of bereavement?
   b. Identify a possible nursing diagnosis, goals, and nursing interventions for an individual who is experiencing a complicated bereavement.

Chapter Review

Match the nursing intervention in Column A with the related dimension of hope in Column B.

	Column A	*Column B*
_____	1. Promoting the patient's experience of time and development of short-term goals	a. Contextual
_____	2. Offering information about the illness and treatment	b. Affective
_____	3. Reminiscing	c. Cognitive
_____	4. Showing an empathetic understanding of the patient's strengths	d. Behavioral
_____	5. Strengthening or fostering relationships with others	e. Affiliative
_____	6. Assisting the patient to use personal resources	f. Temporal

Complete the following:

7. Grief resolution may be affected by:

8. Unexpected unemployment may be perceived as a loss.
   True _____ False _____

9. Provide an intervention that the nurse should implement for a family dealing with a patient's diagnosis of a terminal illness.

10. Select all of the appropriate interventions for a terminally ill patient with constipation:
    a. Maintenance of complete bed rest _______
    b. Increased intake of coffee _______
    c. Consumption of fresh vegetables _______
    d. Consumption of whole grain products _______

Select the best answer for each of the following questions:

11. The nurse is working with a patient who has been diagnosed with a terminal disease. The patient, who is moving into Kübler-Ross's bargaining stage of grieving, may respond:
    1. "I understand what the diagnosis means, and I know that I may die."
    2. "I would like to be able to make it to my son's wedding in June."
    3. "I think that the diagnostic tests are wrong, and they should be re-done."

4. "I don't think that I can stand to have any more treatments. I just want to feel better."

12. While working with young children in the day care center, the nurse responds to instances that occur in their lives. Toddlers at the center generally experience loss and grief associated with:
    1. Anticipation of loss
    2. Separation from the parents
    3. Changes in physical abilities
    4. Development of their identities
13. In the senior citizen center, the nurse is talking with a group of older adults. The recurrent theme associated with loss for this age-group is a:
    1. Confusion of fact and fantasy
    2. Perceived threat to their identity
    3. Change in status, role, and lifestyle
    4. Determination to reexamine life goals
14. A nurse who has recently graduated from nursing school is employed on an oncology unit. There are a number of patients who will not improve and will need assistance with dying. The nurse prepares for this experience by:
    1. Completing a detailed course on legal aspects of end of life issues
    2. Controlling his or her emotions about dying patients
    3. Experiencing the death of a close family member
    4. Identifying his or her own feelings about death and dying
15. The patient has had a long illness and is now approaching the end stages of his life. To assist this patient to meet his need for self-worth and support during this time, the nurse:
    1. Arranges for a grief counselor to visit
    2. Leaves the patient alone to deal with his life issues
    3. Asks the patient's family to take over his care
    4. Plans to visit the patient regularly throughout the day
16. The spouse of a patient who has just died is having more frequent episodes of headaches and generalized joint pain. The initial nursing intervention for this individual is to:
    1. Complete a thorough pain assessment
    2. Encourage more frequent use of analgesics
    3. Sit with the patient and encourage discussion of feelings
    4. Refer the patient immediately to a psychologist or grief counselor
17. The patient is experiencing a very serious illness that may not be curable. The nurse promotes hope for this patient in the affiliative dimension when:
    1. Reinforcing realistic goal setting
    2. Encouraging the development of supportive relationships
    3. Offering information about the illness and its treatment
    4. Demonstrating an understanding of the patient's strengths
18. A patient in the long-term care facility is to receive palliative care measures only during the end stages of a terminal illness. The nurse anticipates that this will include:
    1. Pain relief measures
    2. Emergency surgery
    3. Pulmonary resuscitation
    4. Transfer to intensive care if necessary
19. The patient arrives for outpatient chemotherapy. During this visit the patient tells the nurse that she is experiencing periods of nausea. The nurse promotes patient comfort by providing:
    1. Milk
    2. Coffee
    3. Ginger ale
    4. Orange juice
20. The loss of a known environment is associated with:
    1. Being hospitalized for several days
    2. The death of a pet
    3. Amputation of the right leg
    4. A recent burglary in the home
21. Of the following situations, a situational loss occurs when a:
    1. Traumatic automobile accident occurs
    2. Family friend dies
    3. Child goes off to college
    4. Job demotion and pay reduction occur

22. An individual in Bowlby's second phase of mourning, *yearning and searching,* may be expected to:
    1. Not be able to believe the loss
    2. Endlessly examine how the loss occurred
    3. Acquire new skills and build new relationships
    4. Experience emotional outbursts and sobbing
23. The nurse recognizes exaggerated grief in the person who:
    1. Has an active period of mourning that does not decrease and continues over time
    2. Postpones or holds back grieving and responds much later to the event
    3. Cannot function and is overwhelmed, with resulting substance abuse or phobias
    4. Is not aware that behaviors are interfering with daily activities, such as sleeping and eating
24. The nurse manager observes the new staff nurse performing care of the body after death. Which one of the following interventions requires correction and further instruction?
    1. The patient's remaining personal items are discarded.
    2. The family is allowed time alone with the deceased.
    3. Dentures are left in the patient's mouth.
    4. The patient's eyes are closed.

Study Group Questions

- What are loss and grief?
- What are the different types of loss, and possible reactions to these losses?
- What are the differences and similarities between the theories of grief and loss?
- What is anticipatory grief?
- How may the grieving process be influenced by special circumstances?
- How are hope, spirituality, and self-concept related to loss and grieving?
- What behaviors are associated with loss and grieving?
- What resources are available for the patient, family, and nurse to assist in the grieving process?
- What principles facilitate mourning?
- How may the nurse apply critical thinking and nursing processes to the patient/family experiencing loss and grieving?
- How are religious and cultural beliefs associated with loss, grief, death, and dying?
- How may the nurse intervene to assist the patient/family with loss and the grieving process?
- What is involved in care of the body after death?

Study Chart

Create a study chart on Theories of Loss and Grief, *comparing the components of the theories of Kübler-Ross, Bowlby, and Worden, and identifying how the patient may behave in the different stages.*

Managing Patient Care 24

Case Studies

1. You are a nurse working on a busy surgical unit. This evening you have eight postoperative patients assigned to you.
   a. What types of activities could be delegated to an unlicensed nursing assistant?
   b. What determination do you need to make before safely delegating activities to the nursing assistant?
2. As a nurse on the surgical unit, you will be involved in identifying quality improvement (QI) projects.
   a. What possible areas could be important to the nurses and patients on this unit?
3. A friend tells you that she is interested in becoming a nurse practitioner. She has just started to take general courses at a 4-year university that has a nursing program.
   a. What information can you provide to this individual about the preparation for this career role?

Chapter Review

Complete the following:

1. Upon completion of an RN or LPN/LVN program, the graduate nurse must pass the:

2. A person who is reasonably independent and self-governing in decision making and practice is demonstrating:

3. The most important aspect of delegation is:

4. Provide the correct term for the following definitions:
   a. Duties and activities an individual is employed to perform:
   b. Official power to act:
   c. Being accountable for one's actions:

Select the best answer for each of the following questions:

5. In the course of a day, the nurse is responsible for and carries out all of the following interventions. The caring aspect of nursing is specifically evident when the nurse:
   1. Documents care accurately
   2. Inserts a urinary catheter using sterile technique
   3. Coordinates care with other members of the health care team
   4. Acquires an order for the liquid version of the medication when the patient has difficulty swallowing pills
6. The student nurse is working with a patient who has begun to have respiratory difficulty. It is the student nurse's initial responsibility to:
   1. Call the pharmacy
   2. Alert the primary nurse
   3. Contact the attending physician
   4. Administer the prescribed medication
7. The nurses on a medical unit are discussing plans to change the focus of the unit to the primary nursing care model. With this model, the assignment for nurse A is:
   1. Mrs. J., Mrs. R., and Mrs. T. for the length of their stays

2. To receive reports from the nursing assistant on the care of Mrs. J., Mrs. R., and Mrs. T.
3. Side 1 of the unit in cooperation with nurse B and the nursing assistant
4. Medication administration for all of the patients on the unit, while nurse B does the physical care with the nursing assistant

8. The nurse in the long-term care facility is delegating care to the nursing assistant. It is appropriate for the nurse to delegate the care of the patient who requires:
   1. Catheter care
   2. An admission history
   3. Administration of oral medications
   4. Vital sign measurements following episodes of arrhythmias
9. The student nurse is assigned to care for a patient in the hospital. While taking the patient's vital signs, the student cannot obtain the blood pressure reading after two attempts. The student should:
   1. Keep trying to get the blood pressure measurement
   2. Use the closest measurement to the last reading
   3. Ask another nurse to obtain the blood pressure measurement
   4. Inform the instructor about the difficulty and request assistance
10. A nurse is working with a patient who has just returned from surgery. The nurse has no experience working with the patient's postoperative surgical dressing. During an assessment, the nurse notices that the dressing has come loose and has fallen away from the surgical wound. The patient tells the nurse, "Oh, you can fix it." The nurse:
   1. Asks the patient to help replace the dressing
   2. Replaces the loosened dressing as best as possible
   3. Asks the surgeon to replace the dressing
   4. Covers the wound with a sterile dry dressing until assistance is obtained
11. The nurse has been assigned to work on a very busy medical unit in the hospital. It is important for the nurse to employ time management skills. The nurse implements a plan to:
   1. Have all of the patients' major needs met in the morning hours
   2. Anticipate possible interruptions by therapists and visitors
   3. Complete assessments and treatments for each patient at different times each day
   4. Leave each day totally unstructured in order to allow for changes in treatments and patient assignments
12. The nurses in the medical center have been working together on quality improvement (QI) projects. A threshold of 90% has been identified as an outcome indicator. Further review is indicated for the finding that:
   1. Waiting time in the clinic is decreased by 96%
   2. Renal dialysis patients express a 95% satisfaction with care
   3. 93% of patients express a reduction in postoperative discomfort
   4. Infections are evident in 92% of patients following urinary catheter insertion
13. When designing a quality improvement program, the indicators that evaluate the way in which nursing care is delivered to patients are identified as:
   1. Team indicators
   2. Patient indicators
   3. Process indicators
   4. Structure indicators
14. Nurses working on a surgical unit will be part of a work redesign effort. This is evidenced by the staff:
   1. Determining the best work day and vacation schedules
   2. Investigating personnel who should be reassigned or laid off
   3. Shifting the decision making from the unit to the supervisors
   4. Delegating non-nursing activities and tasks to unlicensed personnel
15. One specific measurement criterion for the standard of "quality of practice" is:
   1. Using creativity to improve nursing care delivery
   2. Discussing concerns with fellow staff members

3. Attending workshops on new technologies
4. Speaking on behalf of the patient's family and their concerns

16. The medical unit in the acute care facility is experiencing a staffing shortage. The staff members, working with the unit manager, decide that nurse A will administer all of the medications, nurse B will complete all of the treatments, and nurse C will perform vital sign measurements and patient teaching. This is an example of:
    1. Functional nursing
    2. Primary nursing
    3. Total patient care
    4. Team nursing
17. One specific measurement criterion for the standard of practice of "collegiality" is:
    1. Seeking experiences to maintain clinical skills
    2. Contributing to a healthy work environment
    3. Assigning tasks based on patient needs
    4. Serving as a patient advocate
18. The student nurse has a multiple patient assignment. In reviewing the report obtained from the primary nurse, the student should decide to see which patient first? The patient who is:
    1. Experiencing nausea
    2. Asking for the bedpan
    3. Having a severe anxiety attack
    4. Thirsty and wants another drink for breakfast

Study Group Questions

- What are the applications of theoretical models in nursing?
- What are the standards of practice and standards of care?
- How do nurse practice acts influence nursing, including entry into practice, licensure, and role?
- What are the different types of nursing education programs and the preparation required of their graduates?
- To whom may the nurse delegate care responsibilities? What types of responsibilities may be delegated legally and safely?
- What does an advanced practice nurse require in education and experience?
- How does the nurse manager function within the health care team?
- How do the different types of nursing care delivery models differ from one another?
- What is quality improvement (QI) and what does it mean to nurses?
- How are the QI processes and results communicated to other members of the health care team?
- What are some of the challenges for nurses and nursing in the future?

25 Exercise and Activity

Case Study

1. You are assigned to work with Mrs. T., an 80-year-old woman residing in a nursing home. There is conflicting information in the chart about Mrs. T.'s ability to move around independently. You are concerned about meeting Mrs. T.'s needs for proper body mechanics, as well as safety.
   a. What important assessment information is needed to plan meeting Mrs. T.'s needs?
   b. If Mrs. T. is unable to ambulate independently, what nursing interventions should be planned?

Chapter Review

Match the description/definition in Column A with the correct term in Column B.

	Column A	Column B
______	1. Awareness of the position of the body and its parts	a. Body mechanics
______	2. Resistance that moving body meets from the surface on which it moves	b. Prone
		c. Range of motion
______	3. Manner or style of walking	d. Posture
______	4. Lying face up	e. Circumduction
______	5. Movement of the joint in a full circle	f. Dorsal flexion
______	6. Lying face down	g. Supine
______	7. Movement of the foot where the toes point upward	h. Friction
______	8. Maintenance of optimal body position	i. Gait
______	9. Actions of walking, turning, lifting, or carrying	j. Proprioception
______	10. Mobility of the joint	

Complete the following:

11. The three components to assess for a patient's mobility are:

12. From the following, select all of the correct principles of body mechanics:
    a. Maintain a narrow base of support.
    b. Face the direction of movement.
    c. Maintain a higher center of gravity.
    d. Divide balanced activity between the arms and legs.
    e. Increase friction between the object and surface.
    f. Alternate periods of rest and activity.

13. The best way to determine a patient's level of pain is to observe for redness or swelling of the joints.
    True _____ False _____

14. Before ambulating a patient who has been in bed, the nurse should prepare the patient by:

15. Range of motion can be determined by observing the patient's gait and ability to perform activities of daily living.
    True _____ False _____

16. An example of a physiological factor that may influence activity tolerance is:

17. Identify a nursing diagnosis associated with a change in a patient's ability to maintain physical activity.

18. For the patient who has severe arthritis and is unable to perform activities of daily living because of discomfort on movement, the priority is to:

19. A patient with a respiratory condition should be positioned in:

20. The nurse's priority during patient transfers is:

21. Identify the following patient positions:

a. ______________________________

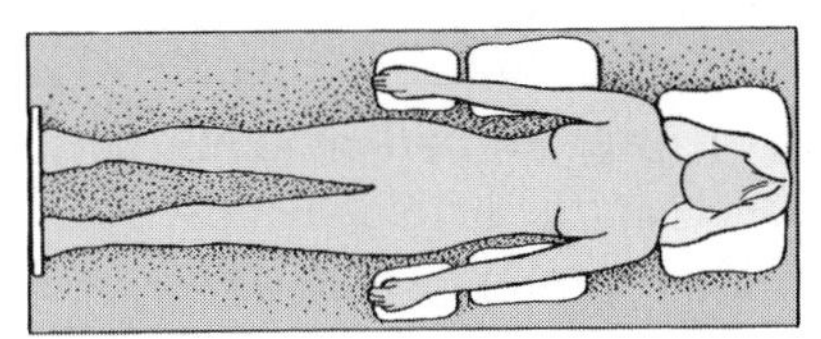

b. ______________________________

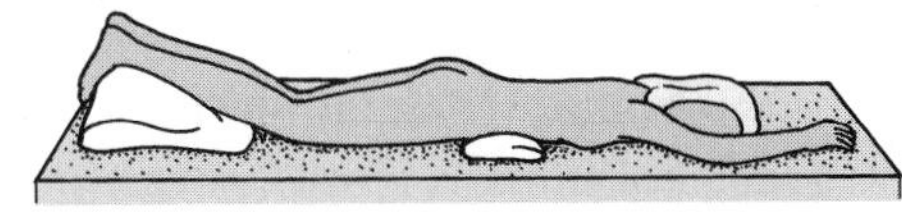

c. ______________________________

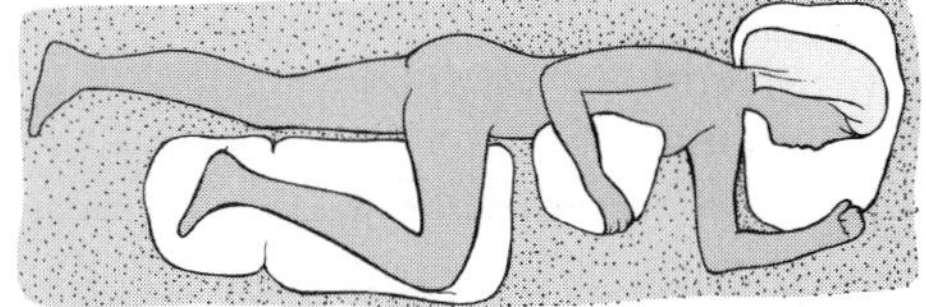

22. Select all of the expected findings for assessment of the patient while standing:
   a. Head is erect and midline. _______
   b. Body parts are asymmetrical. _______
   c. The spine has a lateral curve. _______
   d. The abdomen protrudes. _______
   e. The knees are in a straight line between the hips and ankles. _______
   f. The feet are pointed at an angle and close together. _______
   g. The arms hang comfortably at the sides. _______
23. For the patient who is observed using crutches, select all of the appropriate findings and/or techniques:
   a. The patient leans on the crutches to support his or her weight. _______
   b. The rubber tips are cracked and worn. _______
   c. Crutches are placed 1 foot to the front and side of the feet. _______
   d. The patient has a non–weight-bearing left leg and is using a three-point gait. _______
   e. The unaffected leg is advanced first when the patient goes up the stairs. _______

Select the best answer for each of the following questions:

24. The patient is able to bear weight on one foot. The crutch walking gait that the nurse teaches this patient is the:
   1. Two-point gait
   2. Swing-through gait
   3. Three-point alternating gait
   4. Four-point alternating gait
25. The nurse is working with a patient who is only able to minimally assist the nurse in moving from the bed to the chair. The nurse needs to help the patient up. The correct technique for lifting the patient to stand and pivot to the chair is to:
   1. Keep the legs straight
   2. Maintain a wide base with the feet
   3. Keep the stomach muscles loose
   4. Support the patient away from the body

26. The nurse is assisting a patient who has been prescribed total bed rest to perform range-of-motion exercises. The nurse performs the exercises by:
    1. Hyperextending the joints
    2. Working from proximal to distal joints
    3. Flexing the joints beyond where slight resistance is felt
    4. Providing support for joints distal to the joint being exercised
27. A patient has experienced an injury to his lower extremity. The orthopedist has prescribed the use of crutches and a four-point gait. The nurse instructs the patient using this gait to:
    1. Move the right foot forward first
    2. Move both crutches forward together
    3. Move the right foot and the left crutch together
    4. Move the right foot and the right crutch together
28. The patient has had a CVA (cerebral vascular accident/stroke) with resultant left hemiparesis. The nurse is instructing the patient on the use of a cane for support during ambulation. The nurse instructs the patient to:
    1. Use the cane on the right side
    2. Use the cane on the left side
    3. Move the left foot forward first
    4. Move the right foot forward first
29. A patient is admitted to the rehabilitation facility for physical therapy following an automobile accident. To conduct an assessment of the patient's body alignment, the nurse should begin by:
    1. Observing the patient's gait
    2. Putting the patient at ease
    3. Determining the level of activity tolerance
    4. Evaluating the full extent of joint range of motion
30. An average-size female patient who resides in the extended care facility requires assistance to ambulate down the hall. The nurse has noticed that the patient has some weakness to her right side. The nurse assists this patient to ambulate by:
    1. Standing at her left side and holding the patient's arm
    2. Standing at her right side and holding the patient's arm
    3. Standing at her left side and encircling one arm around the patient's waist
    4. Standing at her right side and encircling one arm around the patient's waist
31. The patient has a cast on the right foot and is being discharged home. Crutches will be used for ambulation, and the patient has stairs to manage to enter the house and to get to the bedroom and bathroom. The nurse evaluates the patient's correct technique in using the crutches on the stairs when the patient:
    1. Advances the crutches first to ascend the stairs
    2. Uses one crutch for support while going up and down
    3. Uses the banister or wall for support when descending the stairs
    4. Advances the affected leg after moving the crutches when descending the stairs
32. The patient has had a surgical procedure and is getting up to ambulate for the first time. While ambulating in the hallway, the patient complains of severe dizziness. The nurse should first:
    1. Call for help
    2. Lower the patient gently to the floor
    3. Lean the patient against the wall until the episode passes
    4. Support the patient and move quickly back to the room
33. During an assessment of the patient's range of motion, the nurse notes that there are significant limitations. This limited range of motion is associated with:
    1. Fluid in the joints
    2. Connective tissue disorders
    3. Ligament tears
    4. Joint fractures
34. One of the expected benefits of exercise is:
    1. Decreased diaphragmatic excursion
    2. Decreased cardiac output
    3. Increased fatigue
    4. Decreased resting heart rate

35. The nurse selects which of the following for maintaining dorsiflexion of the patient?
    1. Pillows
    2. Foot boots
    3. Bed boards
    4. Trochanter rolls
36. The nurse recognizes that the position that is contraindicated for a patient who is at risk for aspiration is:
    1. Fowler's
    2. Lateral
    3. Sims'
    4. Supine
37. The patient has had total hip replacement surgery and requires careful postoperative positioning to maintain the legs in abduction. The nurse will obtain a:
    1. Foot boot
    2. Trapeze bar
    3. Bed board
    4. Wedge pillow

Study Group Questions

- What are body mechanics?
- How is body movement regulated by the musculoskeletal and nervous systems?
- What general changes occur in the body's appearance and function throughout growth and development?
- How may body mechanics be influenced by pathological conditions?
- What patient assessment data should be obtained regarding body mechanics?
- What is activity tolerance?
- How may proper body mechanics be promoted for patients in different health care settings?
- What safety measures should be implemented before patient transfers and ambulation?
- What are the proper procedures for range-of-motion exercises, transfers, positioning, and ambulation?
- How should the patient be instructed to use assistive devices, such as canes, walkers, and crutches?

Study Chart

Create a study chart to describe how to Safely Use Assistive Devices for Ambulation, *identifying the nursing actions and patient instruction required to reduce possible hazards for the following devices: gait belt, cane, walker, crutches.*

Name ____________________ Date __________ Instructor's Name __________________________

Performance Checklist: Skill 25-1 Moving and Positioning Patients in Bed

	S	U	NP	Comments
Assessment				
1. Assess patient's body alignment and comfort level while patient is lying down.	_____	_____	_____	____________________
2. Assess for risk factors that may contribute to complications of immobility.	_____	_____	_____	____________________
3. Assess patient's physical ability to help with moving and positioning.	_____	_____	_____	____________________
4. Assess health care provider's orders. Clarify whether conditions are contraindicated by any positions.	_____	_____	_____	____________________
5. Assess for tubes, incisions, and equipment.	_____	_____	_____	____________________
6. Assess ability and motivation of patient, family members, and primary caregiver to participate in moving and positioning patient in bed in anticipation of discharge to home.	_____	_____	_____	____________________
Planning				
1. Collect appropriate equipment.	_____	_____	_____	____________________
2. Perform hand hygiene.	_____	_____	_____	____________________
3. Correctly identify patient, and explain procedure.	_____	_____	_____	____________________
4. Position patient flat in bed if tolerated.	_____	_____	_____	____________________
5. Keep patient aligned.	_____	_____	_____	____________________
Implementation				
1. Position patient in bed.				
A. Assist Patient in Moving Up in Bed (Two Nurses)				
(1) Remove pillow from under head and shoulders, and place pillow at head of bed.	_____	_____	_____	____________________
(2) Face head of bed.	_____	_____	_____	____________________
(3) Each nurse should have one arm under patient's shoulders and one arm under patient's thighs.	_____	_____	_____	____________________

	S	U	NP	Comments
(4) Alternative position: position one nurse at patient's upper body. Nurse's arm nearest head of bed should be under patient's head and opposite shoulder; other arm should be under patient's closest arm and shoulder. Position other nurse at patient's lower torso. The nurse's arms should be under patient's lower back and torso.	____	____	____	____
(5) Place feet apart, with foot nearest head of bed behind other foot (forward-backward stance).	____	____	____	____
(6) When possible, ask patient to flex knees with feet flat on bed.	____	____	____	____
(7) Instruct patient to flex neck, tilting chin toward chest.	____	____	____	____
(8) Instruct patient to assist moving by pushing with feet on bed surface.	____	____	____	____
(9) Flex knees and hips, bringing forearms closer to level of bed.	____	____	____	____
(10) Instruct patient to push with heels and elevate trunk while breathing out, thus moving toward head of bed on count of three.	____	____	____	____
(11) On count of three, rock and shift weight from front to back leg. At the same time patient pushes with heels and elevates trunk.	____	____	____	____
B. Move Immobile Patient Up in Bed With Drawsheet (Two Nurses)	____	____	____	____
(1) Place drawsheet under patient by turning side to side. Extend sheet from shoulders to thighs. Return patient to supine position.	____	____	____	____
(2) Position one nurse at each side of patient's hips.	____	____	____	____
(3) Grasp drawsheet firmly near the patient.	____	____	____	____

	S	U	NP	Comments
(4) Place feet apart with forward-backward stance. Flex knees and hips. Shift weight from front to back leg, and move patient and drawsheet to desired position in bed.	____	____	____	____
(5) Realign patient in correct body alignment.	____	____	____	____
C. Position Patient in Supported Fowler's Position	____	____	____	____
(1) Elevate head of bed 45 to 60 degrees.	____	____	____	____
(2) Rest head against mattress or on small pillow.	____	____	____	____
(3) Use pillows to support arms and hands if patient does not have voluntary control or use of hands and arms.	____	____	____	____
(4) Position pillow at lower back.	____	____	____	____
(5) Place small pillow or roll under thigh.	____	____	____	____
(6) Place small pillow or roll under ankles.	____	____	____	____
D. Position Hemiplegic Patient in Supported Fowler's Position	____	____	____	____
(1) Elevate head of bed 45 to 60 degrees.	____	____	____	____
(2) Position patient in sitting position as straight as possible.	____	____	____	____
(3) Position head on small pillow with chin slightly forward. If patient is totally unable to control head movement, hyperextension of the neck.	____	____	____	____
(4) Flex knees and hips by using pillow or folded blanket under knees.	____	____	____	____
(5) Support feet in dorsiflexion with firm pillow or footboard.	____	____	____	____
E. Position Patient in Supine Position				
(1) Be sure patient is comfortable on back with head of bed flat.	____	____	____	____
(2) Place small rolled towel under lumbar area of back.	____	____	____	____
(3) Place pillow under upper shoulders, neck, or head.	____	____	____	____

	S	U	NP	Comments
(4) Place trochanter rolls or sandbags parallel to lateral surface of patient's thighs.	_____	_____	_____	__________
(5) Place small pillow or roll under ankle to elevate heels.	_____	_____	_____	__________
(6) Place footboard or firm pillows against bottom of patient's feet.	_____	_____	_____	__________
(7) Place pillows under pronated forearms, keeping upper arms parallel to patient's body.	_____	_____	_____	__________
(8) Place hand rolls in patient's hands.	_____	_____	_____	__________
F. Position Hemiplegic Patient in Supine Position				
(1) Place head of bed flat.	_____	_____	_____	__________
(2) Place folded towel or small pillow under shoulder or affected side.	_____	_____	_____	__________
(3) Keep affected arm away from body with elbow extended and palm up. (Alternative is to place arm out to side, with elbow bent and hand toward head of bed.)	_____	_____	_____	__________
(4) Place folded towel under hip of involved side.	_____	_____	_____	__________
(5) Flex affected knee 30 degrees by supporting it on pillow or folded blanket.	_____	_____	_____	__________
(6) Support feet with soft pillows at right angle to leg.	_____	_____	_____	__________
G. Position Patient in Prone Position				
(1) With patient supine, roll patient over arm positioned close to body, with elbow straight and hand under hip. Position on abdomen in center of bed.	_____	_____	_____	__________
(2) Turn patient's head to one side and support head with small pillow.	_____	_____	_____	__________
(3) Place small pillow under patient's abdomen below level of diaphragm.	_____	_____	_____	__________

	S	U	NP	Comments
(4) Support arms in flexed position level at shoulders.	____	____	____	____
(5) Support lower legs with pillow to elevate toes.	____	____	____	____
H. Position Hemiplegic Patient in Prone Position				
(1) With patient lying supine, Move patient toward unaffected side.	____	____	____	____
(2) Roll patient onto side.	____	____	____	____
(3) Place pillow on patient's abdomen.	____	____	____	____
(4) Roll patient onto abdomen by positioning involved arm close to patient's body, with elbow straight and hand under hip. Roll patient carefully over arm.	____	____	____	____
(5) Turn head toward involved side.	____	____	____	____
(6) Position involved arm out to side, with elbow bent, hand toward head of bed, and fingers extended (if possible).	____	____	____	____
(7) Flex knees slightly by placing pillow under legs from knees to ankles.	____	____	____	____
(8) Keep feet at right angle to legs by using pillow high enough to keep toes off mattress.	____	____	____	____
I. Position Patient in Lateral (Side-Lying) Position				
(1) Lower head of bed completely or as low as patient can tolerate.	____	____	____	____
(2) Position patient to side of bed.	____	____	____	____
(3) Prepare to turn patient onto side. Flex patient's knee that will not be next to mattress. Place one hand on patient's hip and one hand on patient's shoulder.	____	____	____	____
(4) Roll patient onto side toward you.	____	____	____	____
(5) Place pillow under patient's head and neck.	____	____	____	____
(6) Bring shoulder blade forward.	____	____	____	____

	S	U	NP	Comments
(7) Position both arms in slightly flexed position. Upper arm is supported by pillow level with shoulder; other arm, or mattress supports other arm.	____	____	____	____
(8) Place tuck-back pillow behind patient's back. (Make by folding pillow lengthwise. Smooth area is slightly tucked under patient's back.)	____	____	____	____
(9) Place pillow under semiflexed upper leg level at hip from groin to foot.	____	____	____	____
(10) Place sandbag parallel to plantar surface of dependent foot.	____	____	____	____
J. Position Patient in Sims' (Semiprone) Position				
(1) Lower head of bed completely.	____	____	____	____
(2) Be sure patient is comfortable in supine position.	____	____	____	____
(3) Position patient to one side of bed, then roll over one arm positioned close to body. Roll patient to lateral position, lying partially on abdomen. Position dependent arm out from body.	____	____	____	____
(4) Place small pillow under patient's head.	____	____	____	____
(5) Place pillow under flexed upper arm, supporting arm level with shoulder.	____	____	____	____
(6) Place pillow under flexed upper legs, supporting leg level with hip.	____	____	____	____
(7) Place sandbags parallel to plantar surface of foot.	____	____	____	____
K. Logrolling the Patient (Three Nurses)				
(1) Place pillow between patient's knees.	____	____	____	____
(2) Cross patient's arms on chest.	____	____	____	____
(3) Position two nurses on side of bed to which the patient will be turned. Position third nurse on the other side of bed.	____	____	____	____
(4) Fanfold or roll the drawsheet.	____	____	____	____

	S	U	NP	Comments
(5) Move the patient as one unit in a smooth, continuous motion on the count of three.	____	____	____	____
(6) Nurse on the opposite side of the bed places pillows along the length of the patient.	____	____	____	____
(7) Gently lean the patient as a unit back toward the pillows for support.	____	____	____	____
2. Perform hand hygiene.	____	____	____	____
Evaluation				
1. Evaluate patient's body alignment, position, and comfort.	____	____	____	____
2. Measure range of motion.	____	____	____	____
3. Observe for areas of erythema or breakdown involving skin.	____	____	____	____
4. Record each position change, including frequency, amount of assistance needed, and patient's response and tolerance.	____	____	____	____
5. Record and report any signs of redness in areas such as over bony prominences.	____	____	____	____

Name ____________ Date ________ Instructor's Name ____________

Performance Checklist: Skill 25-2 Using Safe and Effective Transfer Techniques

	S	U	NP	Comments
Assessment				
1. Assess patient's muscle strength, joint range of motion and contracture formation, and paralysis or paresis.	___	___	___	________
2. Assess patient's sensory status.	___	___	___	________
3. Assess patient's cognitive status.	___	___	___	________
4. Assess patient's level of motivation.	___	___	___	________
5. Assess previous mode of transfer (if applicable).	___	___	___	________
6. Assess patient's specific risk of falling when transferred.	___	___	___	________
7. Assess special transfer equipment needed for home setting. Assess home environment for hazards.	___	___	___	________
Planning				
1. Gather appropriate equipment.	___	___	___	________
2. Perform hand hygiene.	___	___	___	________
3. Explain procedure to patient.	___	___	___	________
Implementation				
1. Transfer patient.				
A. Assist Patient to Sitting Position (Bed at Waist Level)	___	___	___	________
(1) Place patient in supine position.	___	___	___	________
(2) Face head of bed at a 45-degree angle, and remove pillows.	___	___	___	________
(3) Position feet apart with foot nearer bed behind other foot, continuing at a 45-degree angle to the head of the bed.	___	___	___	________
(4) Place hand farther from patient under shoulders, supporting patient's head and cervical vertebrae.	___	___	___	________
(5) Place other hand on bed surface.	___	___	___	________
(6) Raise patient to sitting position by shifting weight from front to back leg.	___	___	___	________
(7) Push against bed using arm that is placed on bed surface.	___	___	___	________

	S	U	NP	Comments
B. Assist Patient to Sitting Position on Side of Bed With Bed in Low Position				
(1) Turn patient to side, facing you on side of bed on which patient will be sitting.	_____	_____	_____	__________________
(2) With patient in supine position, raise head of bed 30 degrees.	_____	_____	_____	__________________
(3) Stand opposite patient's hips. Turn diagonally so you face patient and far corner of foot of bed.	_____	_____	_____	__________________
(4) Place feet apart with foot closer to head of bed in front of other foot.	_____	_____	_____	__________________
(5) Place arm nearer head of bed under patient's shoulders, supporting head and neck.	_____	_____	_____	__________________
(6) Place other arm over patient's thighs.	_____	_____	_____	__________________
(7) Move patient's lower legs and feet over side of bed. Pivot toward rear leg, allowing patient's upper legs to swing downward.	_____	_____	_____	__________________
(8) At same time, shift weight to rear leg and elevate patient.				
(9) Remain in front until patient regains balance, and continue to provide physical support to weak or cognitively impaired patient.	_____	_____	_____	__________________
C. Transferring Patient From Bed to Chair With Bed in Low Position				
(1) Assist patient to sitting position on side of bed. Have chair in position at 45-degree angle to bed.	_____	_____	_____	__________________
(2) Apply transfer belt or other transfer aids.	_____	_____	_____	__________________
(3) Ensure that patient has stable nonskid shoes. Place weight-bearing or strong leg is placed forward, with weak foot back.	_____	_____	_____	__________________
(4) Spread your feet apart.	_____	_____	_____	__________________
(5) Flex hips and knees, aligning knees with patient's knees.	_____	_____	_____	__________________

	S	U	NP	Comments
(6) Grasp transfer belt from underneath.	_____	_____	_____	_____
(7) Rock patient up to standing position on count of three while straightening hips and legs and keeping knees slightly flexed. Unless contraindicated, patient may be instructed to use hands to push up if applicable.	_____	_____	_____	_____
(8) Maintain stability of patient's weak or paralyzed leg with knee.	_____	_____	_____	_____
(9) Pivot on foot farther from chair.	_____	_____	_____	_____
(10) Instruct patient to use armrests on chair for support and ease into chair.	_____	_____	_____	_____
(11) Flex hips and knees while lowering patient into chair.	_____	_____	_____	_____
(12) Assess patient for proper alignment for sitting position. Provide support for paralyzed extremities. Lapboard or sling will support flaccid arm. Stabilize leg with bath blanket or pillow.	_____	_____	_____	_____
(13) Praise patient's progress, effort, or performance.	_____	_____	_____	_____
D. Perform Three-Person Carry From Bed to Stretcher (Bed at Stretcher Level)				
(1) Three nurses stand side by side facing side of patient's bed.	_____	_____	_____	_____
(2) Each person assumes responsibility for one of three areas: head and shoulders, hips and thighs, and ankles.	_____	_____	_____	_____
(3) Each person assumes wide base of support with foot closer to stretcher in front and knees slightly flexed.	_____	_____	_____	_____
(4) Arms of lifters are placed under patient's head and shoulders, hips and thighs, and ankles, with fingers securely around other side of patient's body.	_____	_____	_____	_____

	S	U	NP	Comments
(5) Lifters roll patient toward their chests. On count of three, patient is lifted and held against nurses' chests.	____	____	____	____________
(6) On second count of three, nurses step back and pivot toward stretcher, moving forward if needed.	____	____	____	____________
(7) Gently lower patient onto center of stretcher by flexing knees and hips until elbows are level with edge of stretcher.	____	____	____	____________
(8) Assess patient's body alignment, place safety straps across body, and raise side rails.	____	____	____	____________
E. Use Mechanical/Hydraulic Lift to Transfer Patient From Bed to Chair				
(1) Bring lift to bedside.	____	____	____	____________
(2) Position chair near bed, and allow adequate space to maneuver lift.	____	____	____	____________
(3) Raise bed to high position with mattress flat. Lower side rail.	____	____	____	____________
(4) Keep bed side rail up on side opposite you.	____	____	____	____________
(5) Roll patient away from you.	____	____	____	____________
(6) Place hammock or canvas strips under patient to form sling. With two canvas pieces, lower edge fits under patient's knees (wide piece), and upper edge fits under patient's shoulders (narrow piece).	____	____	____	____________
(7) Raise bed rail.	____	____	____	____________
(8) Go to opposite side of bed and lower side rail.	____	____	____	____________
(9) Roll patient to opposite side and pull hammock (strips) through.	____	____	____	____________
(10) Roll patient supine onto canvas seat.	____	____	____	____________
(11) Remove patient's glasses, if appropriate.	____	____	____	____________
(12) Place lift's horseshoe bar under side of bed (on side with chair).	____	____	____	____________

	S	U	NP	Comments
(13) Lower horizontal bar to sling level by releasing hydraulic valve. Lock valve.	____	____	____	____________
(14) Attach hooks on strap (chain) to holes in sling. Short chains or straps hook to top holes of sling; longer chains hook to bottom of sling.	____	____	____	____________
(15) Elevate head of bed.	____	____	____	____________
(16) Fold patient's arms over chest.	____	____	____	____________
(17) Pump hydraulic handle using long, slow, even strokes until patient is raised off bed.	____	____	____	____________
(18) Use steering handle to pull lift from bed and maneuver to chair.	____	____	____	____________
(19) Roll base around chair.	____	____	____	____________
(20) Release check valve slowly (turn to left) and lower patient into chair.	____	____	____	____________
(21) Close check valve as soon as patient is down and straps can be released.	____	____	____	____________
(22) Remove straps and mechanical/hydraulic lift.	____	____	____	____________
(23) Check patient's sitting alignment and correct if necessary.	____	____	____	____________
2. Perform hand hygiene.				
Evaluation				
1. Evaluate vital signs. Ask if patient feels fatigued.	____	____	____	____________
2. Observe for correct body alignment and presence of pressure points on skin.	____	____	____	____________
3. Ask if patient experienced pain.	____	____	____	____________
4. Record each transfer and position change and patient's response.	____	____	____	____________
5. Report patient progress and any unusual occurrence to nurse in charge.	____	____	____	____________

26 Safety

Case Studies

1. You will be accompanying the visiting nurse to the home of a family with two young children, ages 2 and 4 years.
   a. What general assessment information should be obtained regarding home safety during the visit?
   b. What specific safety observations should be made because there are two young children residing in the home?
2. A patient with diabetes mellitus is living at home and needs to take daily insulin injections.
   a. What are some of the precautions that this patient should take in relation to pathogen transmission and safety?

Chapter Review

Complete the following:

1. Identify an example of a problem that may be encountered if a basic human need of a safe environment is not met.

2. Identify an example of a possible physical hazard that may be found in the home.

3. Older adults are predisposed to accidents as a result of:

4. For each of the following, identify a nursing intervention that may be implemented to prevent the risk of injury and promote patient safety:
   a. Falls

   b. Patient-inherent accidents

   c. Procedure-related risks

   d. Equipment-related risks

5. The leading cause of unintentional death is:

6. Immunity that occurs as a result of injection of weakened or dead organisms and modified toxins is called:

7. For each of the following age-groups, identify an example of a potential hazard:
   a. Infant, toddler, preschool:

   b. School-age child:

   c. Adolescent:

   d. Adult:

   f. Older adult:

8. During an assessment, the nurse determines that a patient with a high risk for injury is an individual experiencing:

9. For each of the following potential bioterrorist methods, identify a possible agent that may be used:
   a. Biological:

   b. Chemical:

   c. Radiological:

10. The nurse determines that there is a greater risk for poisoning as a result of finding ______________________ ____________________ in the home of an older adult.
11. An example of safety instruction for a school-age child would be:

12. The primary goal when using restraints (safety reminder devices) is to:

13. When using restraints, nursing homes are required to:

14. Side rails may be used at any time to keep the patient in bed.
    True _____ False _____
15. An older adult patient who often forgets to take medication or does not remember if it was taken may benefit from a(n):

16. Identify an example of a medication safety strategy that is used in a health care agency:

17. For the following areas, identify a specific environmental adjustment that should be made to promote safety:
    a. Tactile deficit:

    b. Visual deficit:

18. Identify an example of an intervention that may be implemented as an alternative to patient restraint:

19. An example of a nursing diagnosis associated with patient safety concerns is:

Select the best answer for each of the following questions:

20. To prevent sudden infant death syndrome (SIDS), the nurse instructs the parents to:
    1. Use proper infant car seats
    2. Remove poisonous substances from the home
    3. Have the child immunized as recommended
    4. Place the infant on the back or side to sleep
21. An older adult patient is being discharged home. The patient will be taking Lasix (furosemide) on a daily basis. A specific consideration for this patient is:
    1. Exposure to the sun
    2. Food consumption when taking take the medication
    3. The location of the bathroom
    4. Financial considerations for long term care
22. While walking through the hallway in the extended care facility, the nurse notices smoke coming from the wastebasket in the patient's room. Upon closer investigation, the nurse identifies that there is a fire that is starting to flare up. The nurse should first:
    1. Extinguish the fire
    2. Remove the patient from the room
    3. Contain the fire by closing the door to the room
    4. Turn off all of the surrounding electrical equipment
23. The patient is newly admitted to the hospital and appears to be disoriented. There is a concern for the patient's immediate safety. The nurse is considering the use of restraints to prevent an injury.

The nurse recognizes that the use of restraints in a hospital requires:
1. A physician's order
2. The patient's consent
3. A family member's consent
4. Agreement among the nursing staff

24. The nurse is completing admission histories for the newly admitted patients on the unit. The nurse is alert that the patient with the greatest risk of injury:
 1. Is 84 years of age
 2. Uses corrective lenses
 3. Has a history of falls
 4. Has arthritis in the lower extremities

25. A child has ingested a poisonous substance. The parent is instructed by the nurse to:
 1. Bring the child to the hospital immediately
 2. Call the poison control center
 3. Take the child to the pediatrician
 4. Administer 30 ml of emetic

26. While practicing blood pressure measurement in the lab, the student nurse drops the sphygmomanometer. When it hits the floor, it breaks open and the mercury is spilled. The student should:
 1. Wipe the mercury up with a sponge
 2. Close all of the doors and windows
 3. Get the janitor to vacuum up the spill
 4. Evacuate the room

27. A restraint that may be used to prevent the adult patient from pulling on and removing tubes or an IV is a(n):
 1. Vest restraint
 2. Jacket restraint
 3. Extremity restraint
 4. Mummy restraint

28. An older adult patient in the extended care facility has been wandering outside of the room during the late evening hours. The patient has a history of falls. The nurse intervenes initially by:
 1. Placing an abdominal restraint on the patient during the night
 2. Keeping both the light and the television on in the patient's room all night
 3. Reassigning the patient to a room close to the nursing station
 4. Having the family members check on the patient during the night

29. A parent with three children has come to the outpatient clinic. The children range in age from 2½ to 15 years old. The nurse is discussing safety issues with the parent. The nurse evaluates that further teaching is required if the parent states:
 1. "I have spoken to my teenager about safe sex practices."
 2. "I make sure that my child wears a helmet when he rides his bicycle."
 3. "My 8-year-old is taking swimming classes at the local community center."
 4. "Now my 2½-year-old can finally sit in the front seat of the car with me."

30. A viral disease that is spread through contaminated food or water is:
 1. *Shigella*
 2. *E. coli*
 3. *Listeria*
 4. Hepatitis A

Study Group Questions

- What are the basic human needs regarding safety?
- What are some physical hazards and how can they be reduced or eliminated?
- What developmental changes and abilities predispose individuals to accidents/injury?
- What additional risk factors may affect an individual's level of safety?
- What risks exist in the health care agency, and how may they be prevented?
- What safety measures and patient teaching should be implemented in different health care settings?
- What are the procedures for the correct use of side rails and restraints?
- How can the nurse avoid the use of patient restraints?
- What assessment information should be obtained regarding patient/family safety?
- How can the nurse assist patients and families in reducing or eliminating safety hazards?

Name ____________________ Date __________ Instructor's Name ____________________________

Performance Checklist: Skill 26-1 Use of Restraints

	S	U	NP	Comments
Assessment				
1. Assess if the patient needs a restraint.	_____	_____	_____	____________________
2. Assess patient's behavior, such as confusion, disorientation, agitation, restlessness, combativeness, or inability to follow directions.	_____	_____	_____	____________________
3. Review agency policies regarding restraints. Check physician's order for purpose and type of restraint, location of restraint, and duration of restraint. Determine if signed consent for use of restraint is needed.	_____	_____	_____	____________________
Planning				
1. Review manufacturer's instructions for restraint application before entering patient's room.	_____	_____	_____	____________________
2. Perform hand hygiene and collect equipment.	_____	_____	_____	____________________
3. Correctly identify patient by checking armband and having patient state name if possible.	_____	_____	_____	____________________
4. Introduce self to patient and family and assess their feelings about restraint use. Explain that restraint is temporary and designed to protect patient from injury.	_____	_____	_____	____________________
5. Inspect area where restraint is to be placed. Assess condition of skin underlying area on which restraint is to be applied.	_____	_____	_____	____________________
6. Approach patient in a calm, confident manner. Explain what you plan to do.	_____	_____	_____	____________________
Planning				
1. Provide privacy. Position and drape patient as needed.	_____	_____	_____	____________________
2. Adjust bed to proper height and lower side rail on side of patient contact.	_____	_____	_____	____________________
3. Be sure patient is comfortable and in correct anatomical position.	_____	_____	_____	____________________
4. Pad skin and bony prominences (if necessary) that will be under the restraint.	_____	_____	_____	____________________

	S	U	NP	Comments
5. Apply proper-size selected restraint: **Always refer to manufacturer's directions.**	____	____	____	____
a. Jacket (vest or Posey) restraint: Apply jacket or vest over gown, pajamas, or clothes. Place patient's hands through armholes or sleeves. Vest restraints should have front and back of garment labeled as such. Secure vest according to manufacturer's directions. Adjust to patient's level of comfort.	____	____	____	____
b. Belt restraint: Have patient in a sitting position. Apply over clothes, gown, or pajamas. Remove wrinkles or creases from front and back of restraint while placing it around patient's waist. Bring ties through slots in belt. Help patient lie down if in bed. Avoid placing belt too tightly across patient's chest or abdomen.	____	____	____	____
c. Extremity (ankle or wrist) restraint: This restraint is designed to immobilize one or all extremities. Wrap limb restraint around wrist or ankle with soft part toward skin and secured snugly in place by Velcro straps.	____	____	____	____
d. Mitten restraint: Thumbless mitten device that restrains patient's hands. Place hand in mitten, being sure Velcro strap is around the wrist and not the forearm.	____	____	____	____
6. Attach restraint straps to portion of bed frame that moves when head of bed is raised or lowered. **Do not attach to side rails.** You can also attach restraint with patient in chair or wheelchair to chair frame.	____	____	____	____
7. When patient is in a wheelchair, secure jacket restraint by placing ties under armrests and securing at back of chair.	____	____	____	____

	S	U	NP	Comments
8. Secure restraints with a quick-release tie. Do not tie in a knot.	____	____	____	________
9. Insert two fingers under secured restraint.	____	____	____	________
10. Assess proper placement of restraint, skin integrity, pulses, temperature, color, and sensation of the restrained body part **at least every 2 hours** or more frequently as determined by agency policy.	____	____	____	________
11. Remove restraints at least every 2 hours (JCAHO, 2001). If patient is violent or noncompliant, remove one restraint at a time and/or have staff assistance while removing restraints.	____	____	____	________
12. Secure call light or intercom system within reach.	____	____	____	________
13. Leave bed or chair with wheels locked. Make sure bed is in the lowest position.	____	____	____	________
14. Perform hand hygiene.	____	____	____	________
Evaluation				
1. Inspect patient for any injury, including all hazards of immobility, while restraints are in use.	____	____	____	________
2. Observe IV lines, urinary catheters, and drainage tubes to determine that they are positioned correctly.	____	____	____	________
3. Reassess patient's need for continued use of restraint at least every 24 hours.	____	____	____	________
4. Provide appropriate sensory stimulation and reorient patient as needed.	____	____	____	________
5. Document patient's response and expected or unexpected outcomes after restraint is applied.	____	____	____	________

Name ____________________ Date __________ Instructor's Name ________________________

Procedural Guidelines 26-1 Intervening in Accidental Poisoning

	S	U	NP	Comments
1. Assess for signs or symptoms of accidental ingestion of harmful substances; symptoms may include nausea, vomiting, drooling, difficulty breathing, sweating, lethargy.	____	____	____	____________
2. Terminate the toxic exposure by emptying the mouth of pills, plant parts, or other material.	____	____	____	____________
3. If poisoning is due to skin or eye contact, irrigate the skin or eye with copious amounts of tap water for 15 to 20 minutes. In the case of an inhalation exposure, safely remove the victim from the potentially dangerous environment.	____	____	____	____________
4. Identify the type and amount of substance ingested to help determine the correct type and amount of antidote needed.	____	____	____	____________
5. If the victim is conscious and alert, call the local poison control center or the national toll-free poison control center number (1-800-222-1222) before attempting any intervention.	____	____	____	____________
6. If the victim has collapsed or stopped breathing, call 911 for emergency transportation to the hospital. Ambulance personnel will be able to provide emergency measures if needed. In addition, the parent or guardian is sometimes too upset to drive safely.	____	____	____	____________
7. Position victim with head turned to side to reduce risk of aspiration.	____	____	____	____________
8. Never induce vomiting with the following poisonous substances: lye, household cleaners, hair care products, grease or petroleum products, furniture polish, paint thinner, or kerosene.	____	____	____	____________
9. Never induce vomiting in an unconscious or convulsing victim because vomiting increases risk of aspiration.	____	____	____	____________

Hygiene 27

Case Studies

1. Your clinical experience is scheduled to be on a medical unit. It will be your responsibility to provide instruction to a patient who has just been diagnosed with diabetes mellitus.
   a. What specific information on hygienic care will be included for this patient's teaching session?
2. An older adult patient residing in an extended care facility requires assistance with hygienic care.
   a. What developmental changes are considered when assisting this patient to meet hygienic needs?

Chapter Review

Match the description/definition in Column A with the correct term in Column B.

	Column A	*Column B*
_______	1. Inflammation of the skin characterized by abrupt onset with erythema, pruritus, pain, and scaly oozing lesions	a. Abrasion
_______	2. Thickened portion of the epidermis, usually flat and painless, on the undersurface of the foot or hand	b. Callus
_______	3. Inflammation of the tissue surrounding the nail	c. Plantar wart
_______	4. Scraping or rubbing away of the epidermis, resulting in localized bleeding	d. Paronychia
_______	5. Keratosis caused by friction and pressure from shoes, mainly on toes	e. Contact dermatitis
_______	6. Fungating lesion that appears on the sole of the foot	f. Corn
_______	7. Loss of hair	g. Alopecia
		h. Ingrown nail

Complete the following:

8. Select all of the following techniques that are appropriate for diabetic foot care:
   a. Soaking the feet _______
   b. Rubbing the feet vigorously to dry them _______
   c. Walking barefoot to toughen the feet _______
   d. Applying bland powder if the feet perspire _______
   e. Applying lanolin for dryness _______
   f. Wearing clean, white cotton socks _______
   g. Using a heating pad to warm the feet _______
   h. Applying a mild antiseptic to small cuts _______
   i. Avoiding elastic stockings _______
9. A nurse-initiated treatment for a skin rash is:

10. When cleansing a patient's eyes, the nurse should use:

11. The patient's eyeglasses should be kept:

12. Ear irrigation is contraindicated in the presence of:

13. Asepsis is maintained during linen changes by the nurse when:

14. Provide an example of how the nurse prepares a comfortable environment for the patient in the health care facility:

15. The best type of light to use to assess a patient's skin is:

Select the best answer for each of the following questions:

16. The nurse is caring for an older adult patient in the extended care facility. The patient wears dentures and the nurse delegated their care to the nursing assistant. The nurse instructs the assistant that the patient's dentures should be:
    1. Cleaned in hot water
    2. Left in place during the night
    3. Brushed with a soft toothbrush
    4. Wrapped in a soft towel when not worn
17. The nurse determines, after completing the assessment, that an expected outcome for a patient with impaired skin integrity will be that the:
    1. Skin remains dry
    2. Skin has increased erythema
    3. Skin tingles in areas of pressure
    4. Skin demonstrates increased diaphoresis
18. A patient has been hospitalized following a traumatic injury. The nurse is now able to provide hair care for the patient. The nurse includes in this care:
    1. Using hot water to rinse the scalp
    2. Cutting away matted or tangled hair
    3. Using the nails to massage the patient's scalp
    4. Applying peroxide to dissolve blood in the hair and then rinsing with saline
19. While completing the patient's bath, the nurse notices a red, raised skin rash on the patient's chest. The next step for the nurse to take is to:
    1. Moisturize the skin with lotion
    2. Wash the area again with hot water and soap
    3. Discuss proper hygienic care with the patient
    4. Assess for any other areas of inflammation
20. The nurse is planning the patient assignment with the nursing assistant. In delegating the morning care for the patient, the nurse expects the assistant to:
    1. Cut the patient's nails with scissors
    2. Use soap to wash the patient's eyes
    3. Wash the patient's legs with long strokes from the ankle to the knee
    4. Place the unconscious patient in high-Fowler's position to provide oral hygiene
21. A patient is receiving chemotherapy and is experiencing stomatitis. To promote comfort for this patient, the nurse recommends that the patient use:
    1. A firm toothbrush
    2. Normal saline rinses
    3. A commercial mouthwash
    4. An alcohol and water mixture
22. For the patient with dry skin, the nurse should:
    1. Apply moisturizing lotion
    2. Use hot water for bathing
    3. Obtain a dehumidifier
    4. Wash the skin frequently
23. When integrating cultural considerations into hygienic care, the nurse recognizes that Hindu or Muslim patients:
    1. Consider the top part of the body cleaner
    2. Do not desire gender-congruent care
    3. Use the left hand for bathing
    4. Have no specific hygienic care practices

24. Use of an electric razor is specifically contraindicated for the patient who is being treated with:
    1. Diuretics
    2. Antibiotics
    3. Anticoagulants
    4. Narcotic analgesics

Study Group Questions

- What hygienic care measures are necessary for the integumentary system?
- What factors may influence a patient's hygienic care practices?
- How do growth and development influence hygienic care needs?
- What are the patient teaching needs for hygienic care across the life span?
- What assessments of the integumentary system are necessary to determine integumentary alterations and hygienic care needs?
- What are the correct procedures for providing hygienic care and a comfortable environment for patients?
- How does the patient's self-care ability influence the provision of hygienic care?
- How is physical assessment integrated into the provision of hygienic care?
- What actions should be taken if the patient refuses hygienic care?

Name ____________________ Date __________ Instructor's Name ________________________

Performance Checklist: Skill 27-1 Bathing and Perineal Care

	S	U	NP	Comments
Assessment				
1. Assess patient's tolerance for bathing.	____	____	____	____________
2. Assess patient's visual status, ability to sit without support, hand grasp, ROM of extremities.	____	____	____	____________
3. Assess for presence of equipment.	____	____	____	____________
4. Assess patient's bathing preferences.	____	____	____	____________
Planning				
1. Ask if patient has noticed any problems related to condition of skin and genitalia.	____	____	____	____________
2. Assess condition of patient's skin.	____	____	____	____________
3. Identify risks for skin impairment.	____	____	____	____________
4. Assess patient's knowledge of skin hygiene in terms of its importance, preventive measures to take, and common problems.	____	____	____	____________
5. Check physician's or health care provider's therapeutic bath order for type of solution, length of time for bath, and body part to be attended.	____	____	____	____________
6. Review orders for specific precautions concerning patient's movement or positioning.	____	____	____	____________
7. Explain procedure and ask patient for suggestions on how to prepare supplies. If partial bath, ask how much of bath patient wishes to complete.	____	____	____	____________
8. Adjust room temperature and ventilation, close room doors and windows, and draw room divider curtain.	____	____	____	____________
9. Prepare equipment and supplies.	____	____	____	____________
Implementation				
1. Complete or Partial Bed Bath				
a. Offer patient bedpan or urinal. Provide towel and washcloth.	____	____	____	____________
b. Perform hand hygiene.	____	____	____	____________

	S	U	NP	Comments
c. Place hospital be at comfortable working height. Lower side rail closest to you, and assist patient in assuming comfortable supine position, maintaining body alignment. Bring patient toward side closest to you.	_____	_____	_____	_____
d. Place bath blanket over patient, and then loosen and remove top covers without exposing patient. If possible, have patient hold top of bath blanket.	_____	_____	_____	_____
e. Remove patient's gown or pajamas. If an extremity is injured or has reduced mobility, begin removal from *unaffected* side. If patient has IV access, remove gown from arm *without* IV first. Then remove gown from arm with IV. Remove IV from pole, and slide IV tubing and bag through the arm of patient's gown. Rehang IV container and check flow rate.	_____	_____	_____	_____
f. Pull side rail up. Fill washbasin two-thirds full with warm water. Check water temperature, and also have patient place fingers in water to test temperature tolerance. Place plastic container of bath lotion in bathwater to warm if desired.	_____	_____	_____	_____
g. Lower side rail, remove pillow, and raise head of bed 30 to 45 degrees if allowed. Place bath towel under patient's head. Place second bath towel over patient's chest.	_____	_____	_____	_____
h. Wash face.				
(1) Ask if patient is wearing contact lenses. If so, perform correct eye care.	_____	_____	_____	_____
(2) Fold washcloth around fingers of your hand to form a mitt. Immerse mitt in water and wring thoroughly.	_____	_____	_____	_____

	S	U	NP	Comments
(3) Wash patient's eyes with plain warm water. Use different section of mitt for each eye. Move mitt from inner to outer canthus. Soak any crusts on eyelid for 2 to 3 minutes with damp cloth before attempting removal. Dry around eyes gently and thoroughly.	____	____	____	____
(4) Ask if patient prefers to use soap on face. Wash, rinse, and dry forehead, cheeks, nose, neck, and ears. (Men may wish to shave at this point or after bath.)	____	____	____	____
(5) Provide eye care for the unconscious patient.	____	____	____	____
i. Wash trunk and upper extremities.				
(1) Remove bath blanket from patient's arm closest to you. Place bath towel lengthwise under arm. Bathe with minimal soap and water using long, firm strokes from distal to proximal (fingers to axilla).	____	____	____	____
(2) Raise and support arm above head (if possible) to wash, rinse, and dry axilla thoroughly. Apply deodorant or powder to underarms if desired or needed.	____	____	____	____
(3) Move to other side of bed and repeat steps (1) and (2) with other arm.	____	____	____	____
(4) Cover patient's chest with bath towel and fold bath blanket down to umbilicus. Bathe chest using long, firm strokes. Take special care with skin under female's breasts, lifting breast upward, if necessary, using back of your hand. Rinse and dry well.	____	____	____	____

	S	U	NP	Comments
j. Wash hands and nails.				
(1) Fold bath towel in half and lay it on bed beside patient. Place basin on towel. Immerse patient's hand in water. Allow hand to soak for 2 to 3 minutes before washing hand and fingernails. Remove basin and dry hand well. Repeat for other hand.	_____	_____	_____	_____
k. Check temperature of bathwater and change if necessary.	_____	_____	_____	_____
l. Wash the abdomen.				
(1) Place bath towel lengthwise over chest and abdomen. (Two towels may be needed.) Fold bath blanket down to just above pubic region. Bathe, rinse, and dry abdomen with special attention to umbilicus and skinfolds of abdomen and groin. Keep abdomen covered between washing and rinsing. Dry well.	_____	_____	_____	_____
(2) Apply clean gown or pajama top.	_____	_____	_____	_____
m. Wash the lower extremities.				
(1) Cover chest and abdomen with top of bath blanket. Cover legs with bottom of blanket. Expose near leg by folding blanket toward midline. Be sure to drape perineum with blanket.	_____	_____	_____	_____
(2) Place bath towel under leg, supporting leg at knee and ankle. If appropriate, place patient's foot in the bath basin to soak while washing and rinsing. (Bend patient's leg at knee, and while grasping patient's heel, elevate leg from mattress slightly and place bath basin on towel.) If patient is unable to support leg, cleansing can simply be done by washing feet thoroughly with washcloth.	_____	_____	_____	_____

	S	U	NP	Comments
(3) Wash leg using long, firm strokes from ankle to knee, then knee to thigh. Do not rub or massage the back of the calf. Dry well. Wash between the toes of foot. Cleanse foot, making sure to bathe between toes. Clean and clip nails as needed. Dry toes and feet completely. Remove and discard towel.	____	____	____	____
(4) Raise side rail, move to opposite side of bed, lower side rail, and repeat steps (2) and (3) for other leg and foot.	____	____	____	____
n. Raise side rail for patient's safety, remove contaminated gloves, and change bathwater.	____	____	____	____
o. Provide perineal hygiene.				
(1) If patient is able to maneuver and handle washcloth, allow to cleanse perineum on own.	____	____	____	____
(2) Female patient				
(a) Apply new pair of disposable gloves. Lower side rail. Assist patient in assuming dorsal recumbent position. Note restrictions or limitations in patient's positioning. Be sure waterproof pad is positioned under patient's buttocks. Drape patient with bath blanket placed in the shape of a diamond. Lift lower edge of bath blanket to expose perineum.	____	____	____	____
(b) Fold lower corner of bath blanket up between patient's legs onto abdomen. Wash and dry patient's upper thighs.	____	____	____	____
(c) Wash labia majora. Use nondominant hand to gently retract labia from thigh: with dominant hand, wash carefully in skinfolds. Wipe in direction from perineum to rectum. Repeat on opposite side using separate section of washcloth. Rinse and dry area thoroughly.	____	____	____	____

	S	U	NP	Comments
(d) Gently separate labia with nondominant hand to expose urethral meatus and vaginal orifice. With dominant hand, wash downward from pubic area toward rectum in one smooth stroke the middle and both sides of the perineum. Use separate section of cloth for each stroke. Cleanse thoroughly around labia minora, clitoris, and vaginal orifice. Avoid placing tension on indwelling catheter if present, and clean area around it thoroughly.	_____	_____	_____	_____
(e) Provide catheter care as needed.	_____	_____	_____	_____
(f) Rinse area thoroughly. If patient uses bedpan, pour warm water over perineal area. Dry thoroughly, using front to back method.	_____	_____	_____	_____
(g) Fold lower corner of bath blanket back between patient's legs and over perineum. Ask patient to lower legs and assume comfortable position.	_____	_____	_____	_____
(3) Male patient				
(a) Lower side rail. Assist patient to supine position. Note any restriction in mobility.	_____	_____	_____	_____
(b) Fold lower half of bath blanket up to expose upper thighs. Wash and dry thighs.	_____	_____	_____	_____
(c) Cover thighs with bath towels. Raise bath blanket up to expose genitalia. Gently raise penis and place bath towel underneath. Gently grasp shaft of penis. If patient is uncircumcised, retract foreskin. If patient has an erection, defer procedure until later.	_____	_____	_____	_____

	S	U	NP	Comments
(d) Wash tip of penis at urethral meatus first. Using circular motion, cleanse from meatus outward. Discard washcloth and repeat with a clean cloth until penis is clean. Rinse and dry gently.	____	____	____	____________
(e) Return foreskin to its natural position. This is extremely important in patients with decreased sensation in their lower extremities.	____	____	____	____________
(f) Gently cleanse shaft of penis and scrotum by having patient abduct legs. Pay special attention to underlying surface of penis. Lift scrotum carefully, and wash underlying skinfolds. Rinse and dry thoroughly.	____	____	____	____________
(g) Avoid placing tension on indwelling catheter if.	____	____	____	____________
p. Dispose of bathwater and dispose of gloves.	____	____	____	____________
q. Wash back.				
(1) Reapply clean pair of gloves. Lower side rail. Assist patient in assuming prone or side-lying position (as applicable). Place towel lengthwise along patient's side, and keep patient covered with bath blanket.	____	____	____	____________
(2) If fecal material is present, enclose in a fold of underpad or toilet tissue, and remove with disposable wipes.	____	____	____	____________
(3) Keep patient draped by sliding bath blanket over shoulders and thighs during bathing. Wash, rinse, and dry back from neck to buttocks using long, firm strokes. Pay special attention to folds of buttocks and anus.	____	____	____	____________

	S	U	NP	Comments
(4) Cleanse buttocks and anus, washing front to back. Cleanse, rinse, and dry area thoroughly. If needed, place a clean absorbent pad under patient's buttocks. Remove contaminated gloves.	_____	_____	_____	_____
(5) Give a back rub.	_____	_____	_____	_____
r. Apply additional body lotion or oil as desired.	_____	_____	_____	_____
s. Remove soiled linen and place in dirty–linen bag. Clean and replace bathing equipment. Wash hands.	_____	_____	_____	_____
t. Assist patient in dressing. Comb patient's hair. Women may want to apply makeup.	_____	_____	_____	_____
u. Make patient's bed.	_____	_____	_____	_____
v. Check the function and position of external devices.	_____	_____	_____	_____
w. Place bed in lowest position.	_____	_____	_____	_____
2. Commercial Bag Bath or Cleansing Pack				
a. The cleansing pack contains 8 to 10 premoistened towels for cleansing. Warm the package contents in a microwave following package directions.	_____	_____	_____	_____
b. Use a single towel for each general body part cleansed. Follow the same order of cleansing as the total or partial bed bath.	_____	_____	_____	_____
c. Allow the skin to air-dry for 30 seconds. It is permissible to lightly cover patient with a bath towel to prevent chilling. NOTE: If there is excessive soiling (e.g., in the perineal region), use an extra Bag Bath or conventional washcloths, soap, water, and towels.	_____	_____	_____	_____
3. Tub Bath or Shower				
a. Consider patient's condition, and review orders for precautions concerning patient's movement or positioning.	_____	_____	_____	_____
b. Schedule use of shower or tub.	_____	_____	_____	_____
c. Check tub or shower for cleanliness. Use cleaning techniques outlined in agency policy. Place rubber mat on tub or shower bottom. Place disposable bath mat or towel on floor in front of tub or shower.	_____	_____	_____	_____

	S	U	NP	Comments
d. Collect all hygienic aids, toiletry items, and linens requested by patient. Place within easy reach of tub or shower.	____	____	____	____________
e. Assist patient to bathroom if necessary. Have patient wear robe and slippers to bathroom.	____	____	____	____________
f. Demonstrate how to use call signal for assistance.	____	____	____	____________
g. Place "occupied" sign on bathroom door.	____	____	____	____________
h. Fill bath tub halfway with warm water. Check temperature of bath water; then have patient test water and adjust temperature if water is too warm. Explain which faucet controls hot water. If patient is taking shower, turn shower on and adjust water temperature before patient enters shower stall. Use shower seat or tub chair if needed.	____	____	____	____________
i. Instruct patient to use safety bars when getting in and out of tub or shower. Caution patient against use of bath oil in tub water.	____	____	____	____________
j. Instruct patient not to remain in tub longer than 10 to 15 minutes. Check patient every 5 minutes.	____	____	____	____________
k. Return to bathroom when patient signals, and knock before entering.	____	____	____	____________
l. For patient who is unsteady, drain tub of water before patient attempts to get out of it. Place bath towel over patient's shoulders. Assist patient in getting out of tub as needed and assist with drying.	____	____	____	____________
m. Assist patient as needed with getting dressed in a clean gown or pajamas, slippers, and robe. (In home setting patient may put on regular clothing.)	____	____	____	____________
n. Assist patient to room and comfortable position in bed or chair.	____	____	____	____________

	S	U	NP	Comments
o. Clean tub or shower according to agency policy. Remove soiled linen and place in dirty linen bag. Discard disposable equipment in proper receptacle. Place "unoccupied" sign on bathroom door. Return supplies to storage area.	_____	_____	_____	_____
p. Perform hand hygiene.	_____	_____	_____	_____
Evaluation				
1. Observe skin, paying particular attention to areas that previously were soiled or reddened or showed early signs of breakdown.	_____	_____	_____	_____
2. Observe range of motion during bath.	_____	_____	_____	_____
3. Ask patient to rate level of comfort.	_____	_____	_____	_____
4. Record bath on flow sheet. Note level of assistance required.	_____	_____	_____	_____
5. Record condition of skin and any significant findings.	_____	_____	_____	_____
6. Report evidence of alterations in skin integrity to nurse in charge or physician.	_____	_____	_____	_____

Name ____________________ Date __________ Instructor's Name ____________________________

Performance Checklist: Skill 27-2 Performing Nail and Foot Care

	S	U	NP	Comments
Assessment				
1. Inspect all surfaces of fingers, toes, feet, and nails.	____	____	____	____________
2. Assess color and temperature of toes, feet, and fingers. Assess capillary refill of nails. Palpate radial and ulnar pulses of each hand and dorsalis pedis pulse of foot; note character of pulses.	____	____	____	____________
3. Observe patient's walking gait. Have patient walk down hall or walk straight line (if able).	____	____	____	____________
4. Ask female patients about whether they use nail polish and polish remover frequently.	____	____	____	____________
5. Assess type of footwear worn by patients.	____	____	____	____________
6. Obtain physician's order for cutting nails if agency policy requires it.	____	____	____	____________
7. Identify patient's risk for foot or nail problems.	____	____	____	____________
8. Assess type of home remedies patient uses for existing foot problems.	____	____	____	____________
9. Assess patient's ability to care for nails or feet: visual alterations, fatigue, musculoskeletal weakness.	____	____	____	____________
10. Assess patient's knowledge of foot and nail care practices.	____	____	____	____________
Planning				
1. Explain procedure to patient, including fact that proper soaking requires several minutes.	____	____	____	____________
2. Perform hand hygiene. Arrange equipment on over-bed table.	____	____	____	____________
3. Pull curtain around bed, or close room door (if desired).	____	____	____	____________
Implementation				
1. Assist ambulatory patient to sit in bedside chair. Help bed-bound patient to supine position with head of bed elevated. Place disposable bath mat on floor under patient's feet or place towel on mattress.	____	____	____	____________
2. Fill washbasin with warm water. Test water temperature.	____	____	____	____________

	S	U	NP	Comments
3. Place basin on bath mat or towel, and help patient place feet in basin. Place call light within patient's reach.	_____	_____	_____	_____
4. Adjust over-bed table to low position, and place it over patient's lap. (Patient sits in chair or lies in bed.)	_____	_____	_____	_____
5. Fill emesis basin with warm water, and place basin on paper towels on over-bed table.	_____	_____	_____	_____
6. Instruct patient to place fingers in emesis basin and place arms in comfortable position.	_____	_____	_____	_____
7. Allow patient's feet and fingernails to soak for 10 to 20 minutes. Rewarm water in basin after 10 minutes.	_____	_____	_____	_____
8. Clean gently under fingernails with orange stick while fingers are immersed. Remove emesis basin and dry fingers thoroughly.	_____	_____	_____	_____
9. With nail clippers, clip fingernails straight across and even with tops of fingers. Shape nails with emery board or file. If patient has circulatory problems, do not cut nail; file the nail only.	_____	_____	_____	_____
10. Push cuticle back gently with orange stick.	_____	_____	_____	_____
11. Move over-bed table away from patient.	_____	_____	_____	_____
12. Put on disposable gloves, and scrub callused areas of feet with washcloth.	_____	_____	_____	_____
13. Clean gently under nails with orange stick. Remove feet from basin, and dry thoroughly.	_____	_____	_____	_____
14. Clean and trim toenails using procedures stated previously for fingernails. Do not file corners of toenails.	_____	_____	_____	_____
15. Apply lotion to feet and hands, and assist patient back to bed and into comfortable position.	_____	_____	_____	_____
16. Remove disposable gloves, and place in receptacle. Clean and return equipment and supplies to proper place. Dispose of soiled linen in hamper. Perform hand hygiene.	_____	_____	_____	_____

	S	U	NP	Comments
Evaluation				
1. Inspect nails and surrounding skin surfaces after soaking and nail trimming.	_____	_____	_____	_____
2. Ask patient to explain or demonstrate nail care.	_____	_____	_____	_____
3. Observe patient's walk after toenail care.	_____	_____	_____	_____
4. Record procedure and observations.	_____	_____	_____	_____
5. Report any breaks in skin or ulcerations to nurse in charge or physician.	_____	_____	_____	_____

Name ____________________ **Date** __________ **Instructor's Name** ________________________

Performance Checklist: Skill 27-3 Providing Oral Hygiene

	S	U	NP	Comments
Assessment				
1. Perform hand hygiene, and apply disposable gloves.	____	____	____	____________________
2. Inspect integrity of lips, teeth, buccal mucosa, gums, palate, and tongue.	____	____	____	____________________
3. Identify presence of common oral problems.	____	____	____	____________________
4. Remove gloves, and perform hand hygiene.	____	____	____	____________________
5. Assess risk for oral hygiene problems.	____	____	____	____________________
6. Determine patient's oral hygiene practices.	____	____	____	____________________
7. Assess patient's ability to grasp and manipulate toothbrush.	____	____	____	____________________
Planning				
1. Place paper towels on over-bed table, and arrange other equipment within easy reach.	____	____	____	____________________
Implementation				
1. Raise bed to comfortable working position. Raise head of bed (if allowed) and lower side rail. Move patient, or help patient move closer. Side-lying position can be used.	____	____	____	____________________
2. Place towel over patient's chest.	____	____	____	____________________
3. Apply gloves.	____	____	____	____________________
4. Apply enough toothpaste to cover length of bristles. Holding brush over emesis basin. Pour small amount of water over toothpaste.	____	____	____	____________________
5. Patient assists by brushing. Hold toothbrush bristles at 45-degree angle to gum line. Be sure tips of bristles rest against and penetrate under gum line. Brush inner and outer surfaces of upper and lower teeth by brushing from gum to crown of each tooth. Clean biting surfaces of teeth by holding top of bristles parallel with teeth and brushing gently back and forth. Brush sides of teeth by moving bristles back and forth.	____	____	____	____________________

	S	U	NP	Comments
6. Have patient hold brush at 45-degree angle and lightly brush over surface and sides of tongue. Avoid initiating gag reflex.				
7. Allow patient to rinse mouth thoroughly by taking several sips of water, swishing water across all tooth surfaces, and spitting into emesis basin.				
8. Have patient to rinse mouth with antiseptic mouth rinse for 30 seconds. Then have patient spit rinse into emesis basin.				
9. Assist in wiping patient's mouth.				
10. Allow patient to floss.				
11. Allow patient to rinse mouth thoroughly with cool water and spit into emesis basin. Assist in wiping patient's mouth.				
12. Assist patient to comfortable position, remove emesis basin and bedside table, raise side rail, and lower bed to original position.				
13. Wipe off over-bed table, discard soiled linen and paper towels in appropriate containers, remove soiled gloves, and return equipment to proper place.				
14. Perform hand hygiene.				
Evaluation				
1. Ask patient if any area of oral cavity feels uncomfortable or irritated.				
2. Apply gloves, and inspect condition of oral cavity.				
3. Ask patient to describe proper hygiene techniques.				
4. Observe patient brushing.				
5. Record procedure, noting condition of oral cavity.				
6. Report bleeding or presence of lesions to nurse in charge or physician.				

Name ____________________ Date __________ Instructor's Name ________________________

Performance Checklist: Skill 27-4 Performing Mouth Care for an Unconscious or Debilitated Patient

	S	U	NP	Comments
Assessment				
1. Perform hand hygiene. Apply disposable gloves.	____	____	____	____________
2. Test for presence of gag reflex by placing blade on back half of tongue.	____	____	____	____________
3. Inspect condition of oral cavity.	____	____	____	____________
4. Remove gloves. Perform hand hygiene.	____	____	____	____________
5. Assess patient's risk for oral hygiene problems.	____	____	____	____________
Planning				
1. Unless contraindicated lower side rail and position patient on side (Sims' position) with head turned well toward dependent side and head of bed lowered. Raise side rail.	____	____	____	____________
2. Explain procedure to patient.	____	____	____	____________
Implementation				
1. Apply disposable gloves.	____	____	____	____________
2. Place paper towels on over-bed table, and arrange equipment. If needed, turn on suction machine, and connect tubing to suction catheter.	____	____	____	____________
3. Pull curtain around bed, or close room door.	____	____	____	____________
4. Raise bed to its highest horizontal level; lower side rail.	____	____	____	____________
5. Position patient close to side of bed; turn patient's head toward mattress.	____	____	____	____________
6. Remove dentures or partial plates if present.	____	____	____	____________
7. Place towel under patient's head and emesis basin under chin.	____	____	____	____________
8. If patient is unconscious, uncooperative, or having difficulty keeping mouth open, insert an oral airway. Insert upside down, then turn the airway sideways and then over tongue to keep teeth apart. Insert when patient is relaxed, if possible. Do not use force.	____	____	____	____________

	S	U	NP	Comments
9. Brush teeth with toothpaste using an up-and-down gentle motion. Clean chewing and inner tooth surfaces first. Clean outer tooth surfaces. Brush roof of mouth, gums, and inside cheeks. Gently brush tongue but avoid stimulating gag reflex (if present). Moisten brush with water to rinse. (Bulb syringe also may be used to rinse.) Repeat rinse several times.	____	____	____	____
10. For patients without teeth, use a tooth ette moistened in water or normal saline to clean oral cavity.	____	____	____	____
11. Suction secretions as they accumulate.	____	____	____	____
12. Apply thin layer of water-soluble jelly to lips	____	____	____	____
13. Inform patient that procedure is completed.	____	____	____	____
14. Raise side rails as appropriate or ordered. Remove gloves, and dispose in proper receptacle.	____	____	____	____
15. Lower side rails. Reposition patient comfortably, raise side rail, and return bed to original position.	____	____	____	____
16. Clean equipment and return to its proper place. Place soiled linen in proper receptacle.	____	____	____	____
17. Perform hand hygiene.	____	____	____	____
Evaluation				
1. Apply gloves, and inspect oral cavity.	____	____	____	____
2. Ask debilitated patient if mouth feels clean.	____	____	____	____
3. Evaluate patient's respirations, and auscultate lung sounds on an ongoing basis.	____	____	____	____
4. Record procedure, including pertinent observations.	____	____	____	____
5. Report any unusual findings to nurse in charge or physician.	____	____	____	____

	S	U	NP	Comments
14. Miter bottom flat sheet at head of bed:				
a. Face head of bed diagonally. Place hand away from head of bed under top corner of mattress, near mattress edge, and lift.	_____	_____	_____	_____
b. With other hand, tuck top edge of bottom sheet smoothly under mattress so that side edges of sheet above and below mattress meet if brought together.	_____	_____	_____	_____
c. Face side of bed and pick up top edge of sheet at approximately 45 cm (18 inches) from top of mattress.	_____	_____	_____	_____
d. Lift sheet, and lay it on top of mattress to form a neat triangular fold, with lower base of triangle even with mattress side edge.	_____	_____	_____	_____
e. Tuck lower edge of sheet, which is hanging free below the mattress, under mattress. Tuck with palms down, without pulling triangular fold.	_____	_____	_____	_____
f. Hold portion of sheet covering side of mattress in place with one hand. With the other hand, pick up top of triangular linen fold and bring it down over side of mattress. Tuck this portion under mattress.	_____	_____	_____	_____
15. Tuck remaining portion of sheet under mattress, moving toward foot of bed. Keep linen smooth.	_____	_____	_____	_____
16. *(Optional)* Open clean drawsheet so that it unfolds in half. Lay centerfold along middle of bed lengthwise, and position sheet so that it will be under the patient's buttocks and torso. Fanfold top layer toward patient, with edge along patient's back. Smooth bottom layer out over mattress, and tuck excess edge under mattress (keep palms down).	_____	_____	_____	_____
17. Place waterproof pad over drawsheet, with centerfold against patient's side. Fanfold top layer toward patient.	_____	_____	_____	_____

	S	U	NP	Comments
18. Have patient roll slowly toward you, over the layers of linen. Raise side rail on working side, and go to other side.	____	____	____	____
19. Lower side rail. Assist patient in positioning on other side, over folds of linen. Loosen edges of soiled linen from under mattress.	____	____	____	____
20. Remove soiled linen by folding it into a bundle or square, with soiled side turned in. Discard in linen bag. If necessary, wipe mattress with antiseptic solution, and dry mattress surface before applying new linen.	____	____	____	____
21. Pull clean, fanfolded linen smoothly over edge of mattress from head to foot of bed.	____	____	____	____
22. Assist patient in rolling back into supine position. Reposition pillow.	____	____	____	____
23. Pull fitted sheet smoothly over mattress ends. Miter top corner of bottom sheet (see step 11). When tucking corner, be sure that sheet is smooth and free of wrinkles.	____	____	____	____
24. Facing side of bed, grasp remaining edge of bottom flat sheet. Lean back, keep back straight, and pull while tucking excess linen under mattress. Proceed from head to foot of bed. (Avoid lifting mattress during tucking to ensure fit.)	____	____	____	____
25. Smooth fanfolded drawsheet out over bottom sheet. Grasp edge of sheet with palms down, lean back, and tuck sheet under mattress. Tuck from middle to top and then to bottom.	____	____	____	____
26. Place top sheet over patient with centerfold lengthwise down middle of bed. Open sheet from head to foot, and unfold over patient.	____	____	____	____
27. Ask patient to hold clean top sheet, or tuck sheet around patient's shoulders. Remove bath blanket and discard in linen bag.	____	____	____	____
28. Place blanket on bed, unfolding it so that crease runs lengthwise along middle of bed. Unfold blanket to cover patient. Make sure top edge is parallel with edge of top sheet and 15 to 20 cm (6 to 8 inches) from top sheet's edge.	____	____	____	____

	S	U	NP	Comments
29. Place spread over bed according to step 28. Be sure that top edge of spread extends about 2.5 cm (1 inch) above blanket's edge. Tuck top edge of spread over and under top edge of blanket.	____	____	____	________________
30. Make cuff by turning edge of top sheet down over top edge of blanket and spread.	____	____	____	________________
31. Standing on one side at foot of bed, lift mattress corner slightly with one hand and tuck linens under mattress. Top sheet and blanket are tucked under together. Be sure that linens are loose enough to allow movement of patient's feet. Making a horizontal toe pleat is an option.	____	____	____	________________
32. Make modified mitered corner with top sheet, blanket, and spread.				
a. Pick up side edge of top sheet, blanket, and spread approximately 45 cm (18 inches) from foot of mattress. Lift linen to form triangular fold, and lay it on bed.	____	____	____	________________
b. Tuck lower edge of sheet, which is hanging free below mattress, under mattress. Do not pull triangular fold.	____	____	____	________________
c. Pick up triangular fold, and bring it down over mattress while holding linen in place along side of mattress. Do not tuck tip of triangle.	____	____	____	________________
33. Raise side rail. Make other side of bed; spread sheet, blanket, and bedspread out evenly. Fold top edge of spread over blanket and make cuff with top sheet (see step 30); make modified mitered corner at foot of bed (see step 32).	____	____	____	________________
34. Change pillowcase:				
a. Have patient raise head. While supporting neck with one hand, remove pillow. Allow patient to lower head.	____	____	____	________________
b. Remove soiled case by grasping pillow at open end with one hand and pulling case back over pillow with the other hand. Discard case in linen bag.	____	____	____	________________

	S	U	NP	Comments
c. Grasp clean pillowcase at center of closed end. Gather case, turning it inside out over the hand holding it. With the same hand, pick up middle of one end of the pillow. Pull pillowcase down over pillow with the other hand.	____	____	____	____________
d. Be sure pillow corners fit evenly into corners of pillowcase. Place pillow under patient's head.	____	____	____	____________
35. Place call light within patient's reach, and return bed to comfortable position.	____	____	____	____________
36. Open room curtains, and rearrange furniture. Place personal items within easy reach on over-bed table or bedside stand. Return bed to a comfortable height.	____	____	____	____________
37. Discard dirty linen in hamper or chute and wash hands.	____	____	____	____________
38. Ask if patient feels comfortable.	____	____	____	____________
Evaluation				
1. Inspect skin for areas of irritation.	____	____	____	____________
2. Observe patient for signs of fatigue, dyspnea, pain, or discomfort.	____	____	____	____________

Name ____________________ Date __________ Instructor's Name ______________________

Procedural Guidelines 27-1 Cleaning Dentures

	S	U	NP	Comments
1. Perform hand hygiene.	____	____	____	____________
2. Clean dentures for patient during routine mouth care. Dentures need to be cleansed as often as natural teeth.	____	____	____	____________
3. Fill emesis basin with tepid water. (If using sink, place washcloth in bottom of sink, and fill sink with approximately 1 inch of water.)	____	____	____	____________
4. Remove dentures: If patient is unable to do this independently, don gloves, grasp upper plate at front with thumb and index finger wrapped in gauze, and pull downward. Gently lift lower denture from jaw, and rotate one side downward to remove from patient's mouth. Place dentures in emesis basin or sink.	____	____	____	____________
5. Apply dentifrice or toothpaste to denture, and brush surfaces of dentures. Hold dentures close to water. Hold brush horizontally, and use back and forth motion to cleanse biting surfaces. Use short strokes from top of denture to biting surfaces of teeth to clean outer tooth surface. Hold brush vertically, and use short strokes to clean inner tooth surfaces. Hold brush horizontally, and use back and forth motion to clean undersurface of dentures.	____	____	____	____________
6. Rinse dentures thoroughly in tepid water.	____	____	____	____________
7. Return dentures to patient, or store in tepid water in denture cup.	____	____	____	____________

Name ____________________ Date __________ Instructor's Name ____________________

Procedural Guidelines 27-2 Shampooing Hair of Bed-Bound Patient

	S	U	NP	Comments
1. Before washing patient's hair, determine that there are no contraindications to this procedure. Certain medical conditions, such as head and neck injuries, spinal cord injuries, and arthritis, place the patient at risk for injury during shampooing because of positioning and manipulation of patient's head and neck.	____	____	____	____________
2. Perform hand hygiene. Apply disposable gloves if open lesions present.	____	____	____	____________
3. Inspect the hair and scalp before initiating the procedure. This determines the presence of any conditions that require the use of special shampoos or treatments.	____	____	____	____________
4. Place waterproof pad under patient's shoulders, neck, and head. Position patient supine, with head and shoulders at top edge of bed. Place plastic trough under patient's head and washbasin at end of trough spout. Be sure trough spout or tubing extends beyond edge of mattress.	____	____	____	____________
5. Place rolled towel under patient's neck and bath towel over patient's shoulders.	____	____	____	____________
6. Brush and comb patient's hair.	____	____	____	____________
7. Obtain warm water.	____	____	____	____________
8. Ask patient to hold face towel or washcloth over eyes.	____	____	____	____________
9. Slowly pour water from water pitcher over hair until it is completely wet. If hair contains matted blood, put on gloves, apply peroxide to dissolve clots, and then rinse hair with saline. Apply small amount of shampoo.	____	____	____	____________
10. Work up lather with both hands. Start at hairline, and work toward back of neck. Lift head slightly with one hand to wash back of head. Shampoo sides of head. Massage scalp by applying pressure with fingertips.	____	____	____	____________

	S	U	NP	Comments
11. Rinse hair with water. Make sure water drains into basin. Repeat rinsing until hair is free of soap.	_____	_____	_____	_____
12. Apply conditioner or cream rinse if requested, and rinse hair thoroughly.	_____	_____	_____	_____
13. Wrap patient's head in bath towel. Dry patient's face with cloth used to protect eyes. Dry off any moisture along neck or shoulders.	_____	_____	_____	_____
14. Dry patient's hair and scalp. Use second towel if first becomes saturated.	_____	_____	_____	_____
15. Comb hair to remove tangles and dry with dryer if desired.	_____	_____	_____	_____
16. Apply oil preparation or conditioning product to hair, if desired by patient.	_____	_____	_____	_____
17. Assist patient to comfortable position and complete styling of hair.	_____	_____	_____	_____

Name ____________________ Date __________ Instructor's Name ____________________

Procedural Guidelines 27-3 Making an Unoccupied Bed

	S	U	NP	Comments
1. Perform hand hygiene.	____	____	____	____________
2. Determine if patient has been incontinent or if excess drainage is on linen. Gloves will be necessary.	____	____	____	____________
3. Assess activity orders or restrictions in mobility to determine if patient can get out of bed for procedure. Assist to bedside chair or recliner.	____	____	____	____________
4. Lower side rails on both sides of bed and raise bed to comfortable working position.	____	____	____	____________
5. Remove soiled linen and place in laundry bag. Avoid shaking or fanning linen.	____	____	____	____________
6. Reposition mattress and wipe off any moisture using a washcloth moistened in antiseptic solution. Dry thoroughly.	____	____	____	____________
7. Apply all bottom linen on one side of bed before moving to opposite side. Apply bottom sheet, flat or fitted.	____	____	____	____________
8. Be sure to place fitted sheet smoothly over mattress. To apply a flat unfitted sheet, allow about 25 cm (10 inches) to hang over mattress edge. Lower hem of sheet lies seam-down, even with bottom edge of mattress. Pull remaining top portion of sheet over top edge of mattress.	____	____	____	____________
9. While standing at head of bed, miter top corner of bottom flat sheet.	____	____	____	____________
10. Tuck remaining portion of unfitted sheet under mattress.	____	____	____	____________
11. Optional: Apply drawsheet, laying center fold along middle of bed lengthwise. Smooth drawsheet over mattress and tuck excess edge under mattress, keeping palms down.	____	____	____	____________
12. Move to opposite side of bed and spread bottom sheet smoothly over edge of mattress from head to foot of bed.	____	____	____	____________

	S	U	NP	Comments
13. Apply fitted sheet smoothly over each mattress corner. For an unfitted sheet, miter top corner of bottom sheet (see step 8), making sure corner is stretched tight.	_____	_____	_____	_____
14. Grasp remaining edge of unfitted bottom sheet and tuck tightly under mattress while moving from head to foot of bed. Smooth folded drawsheet over bottom sheet and tuck under mattress, first at middle, then at top, and then at bottom.	_____	_____	_____	_____
15. If needed, apply waterproof pad over bottom sheet or drawsheet.	_____	_____	_____	_____
16. Place top sheet over bed with vertical center fold lengthwise down middle of bed. Open sheet out from head to foot, being sure top edge of sheet is even with top edge of mattress.	_____	_____	_____	_____
17. Make horizontal toe pleat: stand at foot of bed and fanfold top sheet 5 to 10 cm (2 to 4 inches) across bed. Pull sheet up from bottom to make fold approximately 15 cm (6 inches) from bottom edge of mattress.	_____	_____	_____	_____
18. Tuck in remaining portion of sheet under foot of mattress. Then place blanket over bed with top edge parallel to top edge of sheet and 15 to 20 cm (6 to 8 inches) down from edge of sheet. (Optional: Apply additional spread over bed.)	_____	_____	_____	_____
19. Make cuff by turning edge of top sheet down over top edge of blanket and spread.	_____	_____	_____	_____
20. Standing on one side at foot of bed, lift mattress corner slightly with one hand, and with other hand tuck top sheet, blanket, and spread under mattress. Be sure toe pleats are not pulled out.	_____	_____	_____	_____
21. Make modified mitered corner with top sheet, blanket, and spread. After making triangular fold, do not tuck tip of triangle.	_____	_____	_____	_____
22. Go to other side of bed. Spread sheet, blanket, and spread out evenly. Make cuff with top sheet and blanket. Make modified corner at foot of bed.	_____	_____	_____	_____

	S	U	NP	Comments
23. Apply clean pillowcase.	_____	_____	_____	_____
24. Place call light within patient's reach on bed rail or pillow and return bed to height allowing for patient transfer. Assist patient to bed.	_____	_____	_____	_____
25. Arrange patient's room. Remove and discard supplies. Perform hand hygiene.	_____	_____	_____	_____

Oxygenation 28

Case Study

1. You are the nurse in an outpatient clinic where a 32-year-old female patient has come for ongoing medical treatment. She tells you that she has had asthma since she was a young child. While speaking with the patient, you notice that she is exhibiting mild wheezing and a productive cough. She appears slightly pale.
   a. What additional assessment questions should be asked of this patient?
   b. Identify a possible nursing diagnosis for this patient.
   c. What nurse-initiated actions may be taken at this time?
   d. Identify general information that should be included in patient teaching for promoting oxygenation.

Chapter Review

Match the description/definition in Column A with the correct term in Column B.

	Column A	*Column B*
________	1. Collapse of alveoli, preventing exchange of oxygen and carbon dioxide	a. Hypoxia
________	2. Tachypnea pattern of breathing associated with metabolic acidosis	b. Pneumothorax
________	3. Need to sit upright to breathe easier	c. Atelectasis
________	4. Blue discoloration of the skin and mucous membranes	d. Cyanosis
________	5. Collection of air in the pleural space	e. Kussmaul's respiration
________	6. Bloody sputum	f. Orthopnea
________	7. Inadequate tissue oxygenation at the cellular level	g. Hemothorax
________	8. Amount of blood in the ventricles at the end of diastole	h. Preload
________	9. Collection of blood in the pleural space	i. Afterload
________	10. Resistance of ejection of blood from the left ventricle	j. Apneustic
		k. Hemoptysis

Complete the following:

11. The average resting heart rate for an adult is ________ beats per minute.
12. Chest movement is affected by the following conditions:

13. Identify whether the following signs and symptoms are associated with left ventricular or right ventricular heart failure:
    a. Distended neck veins

    b. Ankle edema

    c. Pulmonary congestion

d. Increased arterial blood pressure

14. Select all of the following that may cause hyperventilation:
    a. Anxiety _______
    b. Fever _______
    c. Severe atelectasis _______
    d. Aspirin poisoning _______
    e. Excessive administration of oxygen _______

15. Provide an example of a physiological alteration that may result in each of the following:
    a. Decreased oxygen carrying capacity
    b. Decreased inspired oxygen concentration
    c. Hypovolemia
    d. Increased metabolic rate

16. A premature infant has a deficiency of ________________________ and is at risk for hyaline membrane disease.

17. An example of a modifiable risk factor for cardiopulmonary disease is:

18. Select all the expected pathophysiological changes in the heart and lungs that occur with aging:
    a. Thinning of the ventricular wall of the heart _______
    b. SA node becoming fibrotic from calcification _______
    c. Increased elastin in the arterial vessel walls _______
    d. Increased chest wall compliance and elastic recoil _______
    e. Decreased alveolar surface area _______
    f. Increased responsiveness of central and peripheral chemoreceptors _______
    g. Decreased number of cilia _______
    h. Increased respiratory drive _______

19. The patient awakes in a panic and feels as though he or she is suffocating. This is noted by the nurse as:

20. A musical, high-pitched lung sound that may be heard on inspiration or expiration is:

21. Identify the following two cardiac rhythms:

a.

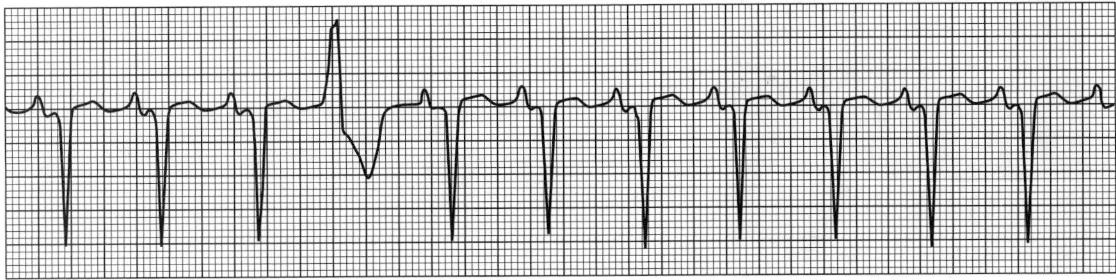

b.

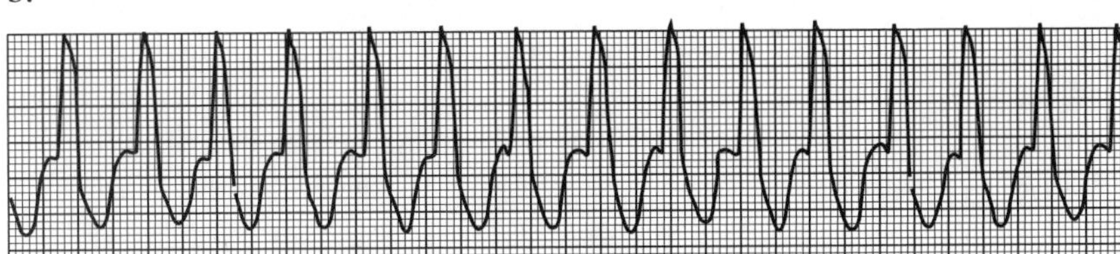

22. Briefly define the following abnormal chest wall movements:
    a. Retraction:

    b. Paradoxical breathing:

23. Which type of asepsis is used for tracheal suctioning?

24. Continuous bubbling in the chest tube water-seal chamber indicates:

25. Identify an example of a nursing intervention for promotion of each of the following:
    a. Dyspnea management:

    b. Patent airway:

    c. Lung expansion:

    d. Mobilization of secretions:

26. Identify the following types of oxygen delivery systems and the flow rate for each:
    a.

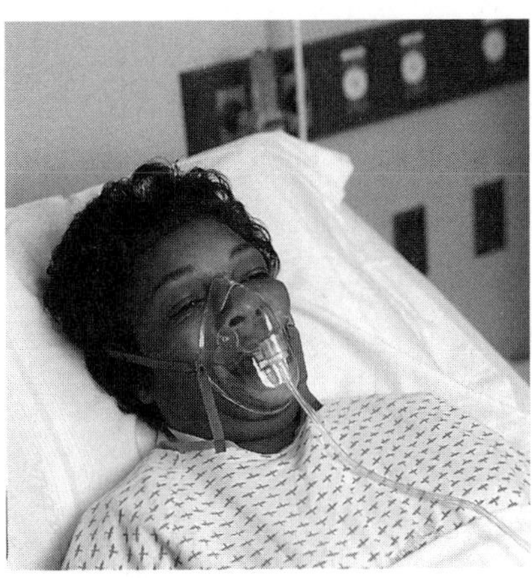

b.

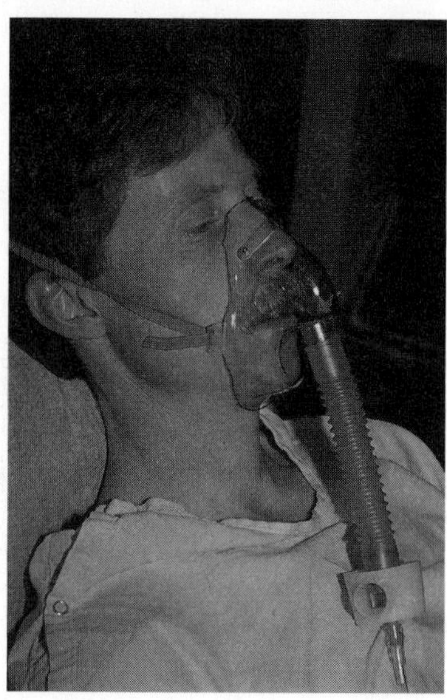

27. Identify the following for tuberculin (Mantoux) testing:
    a. The skin test is administered on the patient's:
    b. The test is read after ________ hours.
    c. A reddened, flat area is a(n) ________________ reaction.
28. For chest percussion, vibration, and postural drainage:
    a. Chest percussion is contraindicated for a patient with:
    b. Vibration is used only during:
    c. The position for a 2-year-old for postural drainage is:
29. For continuous positive airway pressure (CPAP):
    a. CPAP is used for:
    b. The usual pressure setting is:
    c. A disadvantage of CPAP is:
30. An indication for home oxygen therapy is an SaO_2 value of:
31. The ABCs of CPR are:
    A:
    B:
    C:
32. Defibrillation is recommended within ________________(time) for an out-of-hospital sudden cardiac arrest and within ________________(time) for an inpatient.
33. The prevalence of atrial fibrillation increases with age and is the leading contributing factor for stroke in the older adult.
    True _____ False _____
34. Identify an example of a safety measure that should be implemented when the patient is using home oxygen therapy.
35. For the nursing diagnosis *Ineffective airway clearance related to the presence of tracheobronchial secretions,* identify a patient outcome and a nursing intervention to assist the patient to meet the outcome.

Select the best answer for each of the following questions:

36. Individuals have come to the health fair to receive their free influenza vaccine. The nurse briefly discusses the medical backgrounds of the patients. The influenza vaccine will be withheld from the:
    1. HIV-positive male
    2. Older adult female
    3. Male with chronic arthritis
    4. Female with a hypersensitivity to eggs

37. The patient has a chest tube in place to drain bloody secretions from the chest cavity. When caring for a patient with a chest tube, the nurse should:
    1. Keep the drainage device above chest level
    2. Clamp the chest tube when the patient is ambulating
    3. Have the patient cough if the tubing becomes disconnected
    4. Leave trapped fluid in the tubing and estimate the amount
38. The nurse is making a home visit to a patient who has emphysema. Specific instruction to control exhalation pressure for this patient with an increased residual volume of air should include:
    1. Coughing
    2. Deep breathing
    3. Pursed-lip breathing
    4. Diaphragmatic breathing
39. The patient has been admitted to the medical center with a respiratory condition and dyspnea. A number of medications are prescribed for the patient. For a patient with this difficulty, the nurse should question the order for:
    1. Steroids
    2. Mucolytics
    3. Bronchodilators
    4. Narcotic analgesics
40. Following a patient assessment, the nurse suspects hypoxemia. This is based on the nurse finding that the patient is experiencing:
    1. Restlessness
    2. Bradypnea
    3. Bradycardia
    4. Hypotension
41. The patient has experienced some respiratory difficulty and is placed on oxygen via nasal cannula. The nurse assists the patient with this form of oxygen delivery by:
    1. Changing the tubing every 4 hours
    2. Assessing the nares for breakdown
    3. Inspecting the back of the mouth q8h
    4. Securing the cannula to the nose with nonallergic tape
42. The patient is being seen in the outpatient medical clinic. The nurse has reviewed the patient's chart and finds that there is a history of a cardiopulmonary abnormality. This is supported by the nurse's assessment of the patient having:
    1. Scleral jaundice
    2. Reddened conjunctivae
    3. Symmetrical chest movement
    4. Splinter hemorrhages in the nails
43. A 65-year-old patient is seen in the physician's office for a routine annual checkup. As part of the physical examination, an ECG is performed. The ECG reveals a normal P wave, P-R interval, and QRS complex and a heart rate of 58 beats per minute. The nurse evaluates this finding as:
    1. Sinus tachycardia
    2. Sinus bradycardia
    3. Sinus dysrhythmia
    4. Supraventricular bradycardia
44. The patient is admitted to the medical center with a diagnosis of left ventricular congestive heart failure. The nurse is completing the physical assessment and is anticipating finding that the patient has:
    1. Liver enlargement
    2. Peripheral edema
    3. Pulmonary congestion
    4. Jugular neck vein distention
45. A patient has just returned to the unit after abdominal surgery. The nurse is planning care for this patient and is considering interventions to promote pulmonary function and prevent complications. The nurse:
    1. Teaches the patient leg exercises to perform
    2. Asks the physician to order nebulizer treatments
    3. Demonstrates the use of a flow-oriented incentive spirometer
    4. Informs the patient that his secretions will need to be suctioned
46. The nurse manager is evaluating the care that is provided by the new staff nurse during the orientation period. One of the

patients requires nasotracheal suctioning, and the nurse manager determines that the appropriate technique is used when the new staff nurse:
1. Places the patient in the supine position
2. Prepares for a clean or nonsterile procedure
3. Suctions the oropharyngeal area first, then moves to the nasotracheal area
4. Applies intermittent suction for 10 seconds while the suction catheter is being removed

47. Chest tubes have been inserted into the patient following thoracic surgery. In working with this patient, the nurse should:
1. Coil and secure excess tubing next to the patient
2. Clamp off the chest tubes except during respiratory assessments
3. Milk or strip the tubing every 15 to 30 minutes to maintain drainage
4. Remove the tubing from the connection to check for adequate suction

48. The patient is being discharged home with an order for oxygen PRN. In preparing to teach the patient and family, a priority for the nurse is to provide information on the:
1. Use of the oxygen delivery equipment
2. Physiology of the respiratory system
3. Use of PaO_2 levels to determine oxygen demand
4. Length of time that the oxygen is to be used by the patient

49. In the discrimination of types of chest pain that the patient may experience, the nurse recognizes that pain associated with inflammation of the pericardial sac is noted by the patient experiencing:
1. Knifelike pain to the upper chest
2. Constant, substernal pain
3. Pain with inspiration
4. Pain aggravated by coughing

50. The nurse is checking the patient who has a chest tube in place and finds that there is constant bubbling in the water-seal chamber. The nurse should:
1. Tighten loose connections
2. Leave the chest tube clamped
3. Raise the tubing above the level of the insertion site
4. Prepare the patient for the removal of the tube

51. For a patient who is receiving noninvasive ventilation and states that he feels claustrophobic, the nurse should:
1. Discontinue the treatment
2. Lower the pressure settings
3. Notify the health care provider immediately
4. Demonstrate use of the quick-release straps

52. The nurse instructs the community group that pneumococcal vaccine is recommended for administration to low-risk individuals:
1. Yearly
2. Every 2 years
3. Every 5 years
4. Every 10 years

53. The nurse is completing a physical assessment of the patient with a history of a cardiopulmonary abnormality. A finding associated with hyperlipidemia is the patient having:
1. Clubbing
2. Xanthelasma
3. Pale conjunctivae
4. Periorbital edema

Study Group Questions

- How do the anatomy and physiology of the cardiovascular and respiratory systems promote oxygenation?
- What physiological factors affect oxygenation?
- How do growth and development influence oxygenation?
- How do behavioral and environmental factors influence oxygenation?
- What are some common alterations in cardiovascular and pulmonary functioning?

- How are the critical thinking and nursing processes applied to patients having difficulty with oxygenation?
- What assessment information should be obtained to determine the patient's oxygenation status?
- What findings are usually seen in a patient who has inadequate oxygenation?
- How can the nurse promote oxygenation for patients in the health promotion, acute care, and restorative care settings?
- What specific measures and procedures should be implemented by the nurse to manage dyspnea, maintain a patent airway, mobilize secretions, and expand the lungs?
- What should be included in patient/family teaching for promotion and maintenance of oxygenation?
- What safety measures should be implemented for the use of oxygen in the home?

Name ____________________ **Date** __________ **Instructor's Name** ______________________

Performance Checklist: Skill 28-1 Suctioning

	S	U	NP	Comments
Assessment				
1. Assess signs and symptoms of upper and lower airway obstruction requiring nasal or oral tracheal suctioning.	_____	_____	_____	______________________
2. Determine the presence of hypoxemia.	_____	_____	_____	______________________
3. Assess for risk factors for upper or lower airway obstruction.	_____	_____	_____	______________________
4. Determine additional factors that normally influence upper or lower airway function.	_____	_____	_____	______________________
5. Assess factors that influence character of secretions.	_____	_____	_____	______________________
6. Identify contraindications to nasotracheal suctioning.	_____	_____	_____	______________________
7. Examine sputum microbiology data.	_____	_____	_____	______________________
8. Obtain patient's vital signs and oxygen saturation via pulse oximetry. Keep oximeter probe in during procedure.	_____	_____	_____	______________________
9. Assess patient's understanding of procedure.	_____	_____	_____	______________________
Planning				
1. Explain to patient how procedure will help clear airway and relieve breathing problems. Explain that temporary coughing, sneezing, gagging, or shortness of breath is normal during the procedure. Encourage patient to cough out secretions. Practice coughing, if able. Splint surgical incisions, if necessary.	_____	_____	_____	______________________
2. Explain importance of coughing during procedure.	_____	_____	_____	______________________
3. Assist patient with assuming position comfortable for nurse and patient (usually semi-Fowler's or sitting upright with head hyperextended, unless contraindicated).	_____	_____	_____	______________________
4. Place towel across patient's chest, if needed.	_____	_____	_____	______________________

	S	U	NP	Comments
Implementation				
1. Perform hand hygiene, and apply face shield if splashing is likely.	____	____	____	____________
2. Connect one end of connecting tubing to suction machine, and place other end in convenient location near patient. Turn suction device on, and set vacuum regulator to appropriate negative pressure.	____	____	____	____________
3. If indicated, increase supplemental oxygen therapy to 100% or as ordered by physician or health care provider. Encourage patient to breathe deeply.	____	____	____	____________
4. Prepare suction catheter.	____	____	____	____________
a. One-time-use catheter				
(1) Open suction kit or catheter using aseptic technique. If sterile drape is available, place it across patient's chest or on the over-bed table. Do not allow the suction catheter to touch any nonsterile surfaces.	____	____	____	____________
(2) Unwrap or open sterile basin, and place on bedside table. Be careful not to touch inside of basin. Fill basin with about 100 ml of sterile normal saline solution or water.	____	____	____	____________
(3) Open lubricant. Squeeze small amount onto open sterile catheter package without touching package. NOTE: Lubricant is not necessary for artificial airway suctioning.	____	____	____	____________
b. Closed (in-line) suction catheter	____	____	____	____________
5. Turn on suction device, and set regulator to appropriate pressure.	____	____	____	____________
6. Apply a pair of clean gloves for oropharyngeal suction. Apply sterile glove to each hand, or clean glove to nondominant hand and sterile glove to dominant hand for all other suction techniques.	____	____	____	____________
7. Pick up suction catheter with dominant hand without touching nonsterile surfaces. Pick up connecting tubing with nondominant hand. Secure catheter to tubing.	____	____	____	____________
8. Check that the equipment is functioning properly by suctioning small amount of normal saline solution from basin.	____	____	____	____________

	S	U	NP	Comments
9. Suction airway.				
a. **Oropharyngeal suctioning**				
(1) Remove oxygen mask if present. Insert Yankauer catheter along gum line to pharynx. With suction applied, move catheter around mouth until you clear the secretions. Encourage patient to cough. Replace oxygen mask, as appropriate.	____	____	____	____________
(2) Rinse catheter with water in basin until catheter and connecting tube are cleared of secretions.	____	____	____	____________
(3) Place catheter or Yankauer in a clean, dry area for reuse with suction turned off. If patient able to suction self, place within patient's reach with suction on.	____	____	____	____________
b. **Nasopharyngeal and nasotracheal suctioning**				
(1) Lightly coat distal 6 to 8 cm (2 to 3 inches) of catheter tip with water-soluble lubricant.	____	____	____	____________
(2) Remove oxygen delivery device, if applicable, with nondominant hand. Without applying suction and using dominant thumb and forefinger, gently but quickly insert catheter into naris during inhalation. Following the natural course of the naris, slightly slant the catheter downward or through mouth. Do not force through naris.	____	____	____	____________
(a) *Nasopharyngeal suctioning:* In adults, insert catheter about 16 cm (6 inches); in older children, 8 to 12 cm (3 to 5 inches); in infants and young children, 4 to 8 cm (2 to 3 inches). Rule of thumb is to insert catheter distance from tip of nose (or mouth) to base of earlobe.	____	____	____	____________

	S	U	NP	Comments
(b) *Nasotracheal suctioning:* In adults, insert catheter about 20 cm (8 inches); in older children, 14 to 20 cm (5.5 to 8 inches); and in young children and infants, 8 to 14 cm (3 to 5.5 inches).	____	____	____	____
[1] *Positioning:* In some instances turning patient's head to right helps nurse suction left mainstem bronchus; turning head to left helps nurse suction right mainstem bronchus. If resistance felt after insertion of catheter maximum recommended distance, catheter has probably hit carina. Pull catheter back 1 to 2 cm before applying suction.	____	____	____	____
(3) With catheter tip in position, apply intermittent suction for up to 10 seconds by placing and releasing nondominant thumb over vent of catheter and slowly withdrawing catheter while rotating it back and forth between dominant thumb and forefinger. Encourage patient to cough. Replace oxygen device, if applicable.	____	____	____	____
(4) Rinse catheter and connecting tubing with normal saline or water until cleared.	____	____	____	____
(5) Assess for need to repeat suctioning procedure. Observe for alterations in cardiopulmonary status. When possible, allow adequate time (1 to 2 minutes) between suction passes for ventilation and oxygenation. Assist patient to deep breathe and cough.	____	____	____	____

	S	U	NP	Comments
c. Artificial airway suctioning				
(1) Hyperinflate and/or hyperoxygenate patient before suctioning, using manual resuscitation Ambu-bag connected to oxygen source or sigh mechanism on mechanical ventilator.	____	____	____	____
(2) If patient is receiving mechanical ventilation, open swivel adapter, or if necessary remove oxygen or humidity delivery device with nondominant hand.	____	____	____	____
(3) Without applying suction, gently but quickly insert catheter using dominant thumb and forefinger into artificial airway (it is best to try to insert catheter into the artificial airway while patient is inhaling) until you meet resistance or until patient coughs; then pull back 1 cm (½ inch).	____	____	____	____
(4) Apply intermittent suction by placing and releasing nondominant thumb over vent of catheter; slowly withdraw catheter while rotating it back and forth between dominant thumb and forefinger. Encourage patient to cough. Watch for respiratory distress.	____	____	____	____
(5) If patient is receiving mechanical ventilation, close swivel adapter, or replace oxygen delivery device.	____	____	____	____
(6) Encourage patient to deep breathe, if able. Some patients respond well to several manual breaths from the mechanical ventilator or bag-valve-mask.	____	____	____	____
(7) Rinse catheter and connecting tubing with normal saline until clear. Use continuous suction.	____	____	____	____

	S	U	NP	Comments
(8) Assess patient's cardiopulmonary status for secretion clearance. Repeat steps (1) through (7) once or twice more to clear secretions. Allow at least 1 full minute between suction passes.	____	____	____	____
(9) When you have cleared pharynx and trachea sufficiently of secretions, perform oropharyngeal suctioning to clear mouth of secretions. Do not suction nose again after suctioning mouth.	____	____	____	____
10. When you have completed suctioning, disconnect catheter from connecting tubing. Roll catheter around fingers of dominant hand. Pull glove off inside out so that catheter remains coiled in glove. Pull off other glove over first glove in same way to seal in contaminants. Discard in appropriate receptacle. Turn off suction device.	____	____	____	____
11. Remove towel, place in laundry or appropriate receptacle, and reposition patient.	____	____	____	____
12. If indicated, readjust oxygen to original level because patient's blood oxygen level should have returned to baseline.	____	____	____	____
13. Discard remainder of normal saline into appropriate receptacle. If basin is disposable, discard into appropriate receptacle. If basin is reusable, rinse it out and place it in soiled utility room.	____	____	____	____
14. Remove face shield, and discard into appropriate receptacle. Perform hand hygiene.	____	____	____	____
15. Place unopened suction kit on suction machine table or at head of bed.	____	____	____	____
16. Assist patient to a comfortable position, and provide oral hygiene as needed.	____	____	____	____
Evaluation				
1. Compare patient's respiratory assessment before and after suctioning.	____	____	____	____
2. Observe airway secretions.	____	____	____	____
3. Ask patient if breathing is easier and if there is less congestion.	____	____	____	____

	S	U	NP	Comments
4. Record the amount, consistency, color, and odor of secretions.	_____	_____	_____	__________
5. Record the patient's response to the suction procedure.	_____	_____	_____	__________
6. Record and report the presuctioning and postsuctioning cardiopulmonary status.	_____	_____	_____	__________

Name ____________ Date ________ Instructor's Name ______________

Performance Checklist: Skill 28-2 Care of Patients With Chest Tubes

	S	U	NP	Comments
Assessment				
1. Perform hand hygiene.	____	____	____	____________
2. Assess pulmonary status.	____	____	____	____________
3. Obtain vital signs, oxygen saturation level, and level of cognition.	____	____	____	____________
4. Ask patient to rate level of comfort.	____	____	____	____________
5. Observe:				
a. Chest tube dressing.	____	____	____	____________
b. Tubing for kinks, dependent loops, or clots.	____	____	____	____________
c. Chest drainage system, which should be upright and below level of tube insertion.	____	____	____	____________
Planning				
1. Provide two shodded hemostats for each chest tube, attached to top of patient's bed with adhesive tape. Chest tubes are only clamped under specific circumstances per physician order or nursing policy and procedure.	____	____	____	____________
2. Position the patient.				
a. Semi-Fowler's position to evacuate air (pneumothorax)	____	____	____	____________
b. High-Fowler's position to drain fluid (hemothorax)	____	____	____	____________
Implementation				
1. Be sure tube connection between chest and drainage tubes is intact and taped.	____	____	____	____________
a. Make sure water-seal vent is not occluded.	____	____	____	____________
b. Make sure suction-control chamber vent is not occluded when using suction.	____	____	____	____________
2. Coil excess tubing on mattress next to patient. Secure with rubber band, safety pin, or plastic clamp.	____	____	____	____________
3. Adjust tubing to hang in straight line from top of mattress to drainage chamber.	____	____	____	____________
4. If chest tube is draining fluid, indicate time that you began drainage on drainage bottle's adhesive tape or on write-on surface of disposable commercial system.	____	____	____	____________
5. Strip or milk chest tube only if indicated.	____	____	____	____________
6. Perform hand hygiene.	____	____	____	____________

	S	U	NP	Comments
Evaluation				
1. Monitor vital signs and pulse oximetry.	_____	_____	_____	_____
2. Observe:				
a. Chest tube dressing.	_____	_____	_____	_____
b. Tubing, which should be free of kinks and dependent loops.	_____	_____	_____	_____
c. The chest drainage system, which should be upright and below level of tube insertion. Note presence of clots or debris in tubing.	_____	_____	_____	_____
d. Water seal for fluctuations with patient's inspirations and expirations.	_____	_____	_____	_____
(1) Waterless system: diagnostic indicator for fluctuations with patient's inspirations and expirations	_____	_____	_____	_____
(2) Water-seal system: bubbling in the water-seal chamber	_____	_____	_____	_____
e. Waterless system: bubbling is diagnostic indicator.	_____	_____	_____	_____
f. Type and amount of fluid drainage. Note color and amount of drainage, patient's vital signs, and skin color.	_____	_____	_____	_____
g. Waterless system: the suction control (float ball) indicates the amount of suction the patient's intrapleural space is receiving.	_____	_____	_____	_____
3. Ask patient to rate comfort level.	_____	_____	_____	_____
4. Record patency of chest tubes, presence of drainage, presence of fluctuations, patient's vital signs, chest dressing status, type of suction, and level of comfort.	_____	_____	_____	_____

Name ____________ Date ________ Instructor's Name ____________

Performance Checklist: Skill 28-3 Care of the Patient With Noninvasive Ventilation

	S	U	NP	Comments
Assessment				
1. Assess patient's respiratory status and observe for signs and symptoms associated with hypoxia.	____	____	____	____________
2. Observe patient's ability to clear and remove airway secretions.	____	____	____	____________
3. If available, note patient's most recent arterial blood gas (ABG) results or arterial oxygen saturation.	____	____	____	____________
4. Obtain vital signs before initiation of therapy.	____	____	____	____________
5. Review patient's medical record for medical order for CPAP/BiPAP and appropriate settings.	____	____	____	____________
Planning				
1. Explain to patient and family the purpose and reasons for CPAP/BiPAP.	____	____	____	____________
Implementation				
1. Perform hand hygiene; apply gloves and goggles. Apply barrier gown if secretions are projectile.	____	____	____	____________
2. Determine correct mask size. Use supplied masking charts to determine correct size.	____	____	____	____________
3. Connect CPAP/BiPAP device delivery tubing to pressure generator.	____	____	____	____________
4. Connect patient to pulse oximetry.	____	____	____	____________
5. Set CPAP/BiPAP initial settings:				
CPAP: 4 to 8 cm H_2O	____	____	____	____________
BiPAP:				
Inspiratory usually set at 8 cm H_2O	____	____	____	____________
Expiratory usually set at 4 cm H_2O	____	____	____	____________
6. Perform frequent skin assessment to determine the presence of pressure, skin irritation, or skin breakdown.	____	____	____	____________
7. Dispose of supplies as appropriate and perform hand hygiene.	____	____	____	____________
Evaluation				
1. Evaluate patient's response to noninvasive ventilation. Observe for decreased anxiety; improved LOC and cognitive abilities; decreased fatigue; absence of dizziness; decreased pulse rate, regular rhythm; decreased respiratory rate and work of breathing; return to normal blood pressure; improved color.	____	____	____	____________

	S	U	NP	Comments
2. Monitor ABG levels—observe pulse oximetry.	_____	_____	_____	_____
3. Observe skin integrity over the bridge of patient's nose.	_____	_____	_____	_____
4. Monitor patient's and family's ability to manipulate device and face mask.	_____	_____	_____	_____
5. Record respiratory assessment findings; CPAP/BiPAP settings; SpO_2; patient's response to noninvasive ventilation.	_____	_____	_____	_____
6. Report any sudden change in patient's respiratory status or worsening ABGs or pulse oximetry.	_____	_____	_____	_____

Name ____________________ Date __________ Instructor's Name ____________________

Procedural Guidelines 28-1 Closed (In-Line) Suction Catheter

	S	U	NP	Comments
1. Perform respiratory assessment.	____	____	____	____________
2. Explain the procedure to the patient and the importance of coughing during the suctioning procedure.	____	____	____	____________
3. Assist patient with assuming a position of comfort for both patient and nurse, usually semi-Fowler's or high-Fowler's position. Place towel across the patient's chest.	____	____	____	____________
4. Perform hand hygiene and attach suction.	____	____	____	____________
a. If catheter is not already in place, open suction catheter package using aseptic technique, attach closed suction catheter to ventilator circuit by removing swivel adapter and placing closed suction catheter apparatus on ET or tracheostomy tub, and connect Y on mechanical ventilator circuit to closed suction catheter with flex tubing.	____	____	____	____________
b. Connect one end of connecting tubing to suction machine, and connect other to the end of a closed system or in-line suction catheter, if not already done. Turn suction device on, and set vacuum regulator to appropriate negative pressure (see manufacturer's directions). Many closed system suction catheters require slightly higher suction; consult manufacturer's guidelines.	____	____	____	____________
5. Hyperinflate and/or hyperoxygenate patient with bag-valve-mask or manual breathing mechanism on mechanical ventilator according to institution protocol and clinical status (usually 100% oxygen).	____	____	____	____________
6. Unlock suction control mechanism if required by manufacturer. Open saline port, and attach saline syringe or vial.	____	____	____	____________
7. Pick up suction catheter enclosed in plastic sleeve with dominant hand.	____	____	____	____________

	S	U	NP	Comments
8. Insert catheter; use a repeating maneuver of pushing catheter and sliding (or pulling) plastic sleeve back between thumb and forefinger until you feel resistance or patient coughs.	_____	_____	_____	____________________
9. Encourage patient to cough, and apply suction by squeezing on suction control mechanism while withdrawing catheter. It is difficult to apply intermittent pulses of suction and nearly impossible to rotate the catheter compared with a standard catheter. Be sure to withdraw catheter completely into plastic sheath so it does not obstruct airflow.	_____	_____	_____	____________________
10. Reassess cardiopulmonary status, including pulse oximetry, to determine need for subsequent suctioning or presence of complications. Repeat steps 5 through 9 one to two more times to clear secretions. Allow adequate time (at least 1 full minute) between suction passes for ventilation and reoxygenation.	_____	_____	_____	____________________
11. When airway is clear, withdraw catheter completely into sheath. Be sure that colored indicator line on catheter is visible in the sheath. Squeeze vial or push syringe while applying suction to rinse inner lumen of catheter. Use at least 5 to 10 ml of saline to rinse the catheter. Lock suction mechanism, if applicable, and turn off suction.	_____	_____	_____	____________________
12. If patient requires oral or nasal suctioning, perform Skill 28-1 with separate standard suction catheter.	_____	_____	_____	____________________
13. Reposition patient.	_____	_____	_____	____________________
14. Remove gloves and discard them, and perform hand hygiene.	_____	_____	_____	____________________
15. Compare patient's cardiopulmonary assessments before and after suctioning and observe airway secretions.	_____	_____	_____	____________________

Sleep 29

Case Study

1. A middle adult patient has come to the physician's office to obtain a prescription for a "sleeping pill" because she has been having difficulty either falling or staying asleep. You are completing the initial nursing assessment and discover that the patient is recently divorced and trying to juggle extensive work and child care responsibilities.
   a. Identify a possible nursing diagnosis and outcome for this patient.
   b. Indicate nursing interventions and teaching areas for this patient.

Chapter Review

Match the description/definition in Column A with the correct term in Column B.

	Column A	Column B
_______	1. Cessation of breathing for periods of time during sleep	a. Cataplexy
_______	2. A decrease in the amount, quality, and consistency of sleep	b. Sleep deprivation
_______	3. Sleepwalking	c. Circadian rhythm
_______	4. Sudden muscle weakness during intense emotions	d. Nocturnal enuresis
_______	5. Difficulty falling or staying asleep	e. Narcolepsy
_______	6. 24-hour day/night cycle	f. Sleep apnea
_______	7. Bedwetting	g. Somnambulism
_______	8. Excessive sleepiness during the day	h. Insomnia

Complete the following:

9. An example of a factor that may affect sleep is:

10. Select all of the appropriate nursing interventions to assist the older adult patient to achieve adequate sleep:
    a. Alter the daily sleep and wake times. _______
    b. Encourage the patient to stay in bed even if not feeling sleepy. _______
    c. Limit caffeine intake in the late afternoon or evening. _______
    d. Lower the head of the bed as flat as possible. _______
    e. Encourage increased fluid intake 2 to 4 hours before sleep. _______
    f. Avoid use of sedatives and hypnotics, if possible. _______

11. Identify a way in which the nurse can promote a restful environment:

12. It is expected that during sleep the heart rate will decrease by 10 beats per minute from the daytime average rate.
    True _____ False _____

13. Very few older adults experience sleep problems.
    True _____ False _____

14. The nurse tells the patient to include what information in a sleep log?

Select the best answer for each of the following questions:

15. Individuals experience changes in their sleep patterns as they progress through the life cycle. The nurse assesses that the patient is experiencing bedtime fears, restlessness during the night, and nightmares. These behaviors are associated with:
    1. Infants
    2. Toddlers
    3. Preschoolers
    4. School-age children
16. The nurse is making rounds during the night to check on her patients. When she enters one of the rooms at 3:00 AM, she finds that the patient is sitting up in a chair. The patient tells the nurse that she is not able to sleep. The nurse should first:
    1. Obtain an order for a hypnotic
    2. Assist the patient back to bed
    3. Provide a glass of warm milk and a back rub
    4. Ask about activities that have previously helped her sleep
17. The nurse is working on a pediatric unit at the local hospital. A 4-year-old boy is admitted to the unit. To assist this child to sleep, the nurse:
    1. Reads to him
    2. Teaches him relaxation activities
    3. Allows him to watch TV until he is tired
    4. Has him get ready for bed very quickly, without advance notice
18. The patient is found to be awakening frequently during the night. There are a number of medications prescribed for this patient. The nurse determines that the medication that may be creating this patient's particular sleep disturbance is the:
    1. Narcotic
    2. Beta blocker
    3. Antidepressant
    4. Antihistamine
19. The nurse suspects that the patient may be experiencing sleep deprivation. This suspicion is validated by the nurse's finding that the patient has:
    1. Increased reflex response
    2. Blurred vision
    3. Cardiac arrhythmia
    4. Increased response time
20. The nurse is working in a sleep clinic that is part of the local hospital. In preparing to work with patients with different sleep needs, the nurse understands that:
    1. Bedtime rituals are most important for adolescents
    2. Regular use of sleeping medications is appropriate
    3. Warm milk before bedtime may help the patient sleep
    4. Individuals are most easily aroused from sleep during stages 3 and 4
21. Parents take their 5-year-old child to the outpatient clinic for a checkup. They identify to the nurse that the child has been experiencing difficulty sleeping. The nurse recognizes that one of the possible causes may be an insomnia-producing food allergy. The nurse questions the parents about the child's intake of:
    1. Meat
    2. Eggs
    3. Seafood
    4. String beans
22. The nurse is visiting a patient in his home. While completing a patient history and home assessment, the nurse finds that there are many prescription medications kept in the bathroom cabinet. In determining possible areas that may influence the patient's sleep patterns, the nurse looks for a classification of medication that may suppress the patient's rapid eye movement (REM) sleep. The nurse looks in the cabinet for a:
    1. Diuretic
    2. Stimulant
    3. Beta blocker
    4. Nasal decongestant
23. A newborn is brought to the pediatrician's office for the first physical exam. The parents ask the nurse when they can expect the baby to sleep through the night. The

nurse responds that, although there may be individual differences, infants usually develop a nighttime pattern of sleep by the age of:
1. 6 weeks
2. 3 months
3. 6 months
4. 10 months

24. The nurse is working with older adults in the senior center. A group is discussing problems with sleep. The nurse recognizes that older adults:
1. Take less time to fall asleep
2. Are more difficult to arouse from sleep
3. Have a significant decline in stage 4 sleep
4. Require more sleep than a middle-aged adult

25. A patient with congestive heart failure is being discharged from the hospital to her home. The patient will be taking a diuretic daily. The nurse recognizes that, with this drug, the patient may experience:
1. Nocturia
2. Nightmares
3. Reduced REM sleep
4. Increased daytime sleepiness

26. During a home visit, the nurse discovers that the patient has been having difficulty sleeping. To assist the patient to achieve sufficient sleep, an appropriate question the nurse might ask is the following:
1. "Do you keep your bedroom completely dark at night?"
2. "Do you nap enough during the day?"
3. "Why don't you eat something right before you go to bed?"
4. "What kinds of things do you do right before bedtime?"

27. The patient has come to the sleep clinic to determine what may be creating his sleeping problems. In addition, his partner is having sleep pattern interruptions. If this patient is experiencing sleep apnea, the nurse may expect the partner to identify that the patient:
1. Snores excessively
2. Talks in his sleep
3. Is very restless
4. Walks in his sleep

28. The nurse anticipates that the patient who is in non–rapid eye movement (NREM) stage 1 sleep is:
1. Easily aroused
2. Completely relaxed
3. Having vivid, full-color dreams
4. Experiencing significantly reduced vital signs

29. The nurse is working with a patient who has a history of respiratory disease. This patient is specifically expected to demonstrate:
1. Longer time falling asleep
2. Decreased NREM sleep
3. Increased awakenings in the early morning
4. Need for extra pillows for comfort

30. To help promote sleep for a patient, the nurse recommends:
1. Exercise about 2 hours before bedtime
2. Intake of a large meal about 3 hours before bedtime
3. Drinking alcoholic beverages at bedtime
4. Napping frequently during the afternoon

31. An expected treatment for sleep apnea is:
1. Biofeedback
2. Full body massage
3. Administration of hypnotics
4. Continuous positive airway pressure (CPAP)

32. As sleep aids, medications that are considered relatively safe to use are:
1. Benzodiazepines
2. Barbiturates
3. Psychotropics
4. Antihistamines

33. An expected observation of a patient in REM sleep is:
1. Possible enuresis
2. Sleepwalking
3. Loss of skeletal muscle tone
4. Easy arousal from external noise

34. A parent asks the nurse what the appropriate amount of sleep is for her 11-year-old child. The nurse responds correctly by informing the parent that

children in this age-group should average:
1. 14 hours per night
2. 12 hours per night
3. 10 hours per night
4. 7 hours per night

Study Group Questions

- What is sleep?
- What are the physiological processes involved in sleep?
- How is sleep regulated by the body?
- What are the functions of sleep?
- What purpose do dreams serve?
- What are the normal requirements and patterns of sleep across the life span?
- What factors may influence sleep?
- What are some of the common sleep disorders and nursing interventions?
- What information should be included in a sleep history?
- How are the critical thinking and nursing processes applied with patients experiencing insufficient sleep or rest?
- What measures may be implemented by the nurse to promote sleep for patients/families?
- What information should be included in patient/family teaching for the promotion of rest and sleep?

Study Chart

Create a study chart to describe the Sleep Patterns Across the Life Span, *identifying the sleep patterns and needs for infants, toddlers, preschoolers, school-age children, adolescents, adults, and older adults.*

Promoting Comfort 30

Case Study

1. A patient is going to be using a PCA pump after surgery.
   a. What assessments need to be made before the patient uses the pump?
   b. What information is needed in the teaching plan for this patient?

Chapter Review

Match the description/definition in Column A with the correct term in Column B.

Column A

_______ 1. Local anesthesia, with minimal sedation, given between the vertebrae
_______ 2. Unpleasant, subjective sensory and emotional experience
_______ 3. Partial or complete disappearance of symptoms
_______ 4. Extends from the point of injury to another body area
_______ 5. Rapid onset, lasts briefly
_______ 6. Localized, sharp sensation resulting from stimulation of the skin
_______ 7. Increase in the severity of symptoms
_______ 8. Classification of medication used for pain relief
_______ 9. Prolonged, varying in intensity
_______ 10. Diffuse, radiating, and varying in intensity from dull to sharp

Column B

a. Pain
b. Analgesic
c. Exacerbation
d. Remission
e. Acute pain
f. Chronic pain
g. Superficial pain
h. Visceral pain
i. Placebo
j. Radiating pain
k. Epidural infusion

Complete the following:

11. The first structure in the brain to process pain impulses is the:

12. The gate control theory of pain suggests that pain can be reduced through the use of:

13. Select all of the correct physiological responses to acute pain as a result of sympathetic stimulation:
    a. Decreased respiratory rate _______
    b. Increased heart rate _______
    c. Peripheral vasodilation _______
    d. Increased blood glucose level _______
    e. Diaphoresis _______
    f. Pupil constriction _______
    g. Pallor _______
    h. Decreased blood pressure _______

14. Provide an example of a lifestyle response to chronic pain:

15. Identify two responses that an infant or child would have to pain:

16. The single most reliable indicator of pain is the:

17. Using the PQRSTU assessment guide, identify nursing interventions for the following:
   a. **Q**uality:

   b. **R**egion:

   c. **T**iming:

18. Identify how the nurse may assess the level of pain for the following patients:
   a. Toddler:

   b. Person whose second language is English:

19. To determine the location of the patient's pain, the nurse should ask the patient to:

20. A pain rating of _____ on a scale of 1 to 10 is an emergency and requires immediate action.
21. For the patient who experiences discomfort upon ambulation or during a dressing change, the nurse should plan to:

22. An example of how the nurse may individualize the patient's treatment for pain is:

23. Select all of the following that are correct statements regarding transcutaneous electrical nerve stimulation (TENS):
   a. It is an invasive procedure. _______
   b. It requires a health care provider's order. _______
   c. Skin preparation is required before electrode placement. _______
   d. Electrodes are applied directly onto dry skin. _______
   e. Controls are adjusted until the patient feels a buzzing sensation. _______
   f. Electrodes remain in the same area for the next treatment. _______
24. Select all of the following medications that are indicated for the treatment of mild to moderate pain:
   a. Ibuprofen (Motrin) _______
   b. Morphine _______
   c. Codeine _______
   d. Tramadol (Ultram) _______
   e. Fentanyl _______
   f. Acetaminophen (Tylenol) _______
   g. Propoxyphene (Darvon) _______
25. Identify two examples of non-pharmacological interventions that may be implemented to relieve pain:

26. An example of an adjuvant medication that may be used in conjunction with an analgesic to manage a patient's pain is:

27. The usual dosage of on-demand morphine in the PCA is:

28. A priority nursing intervention specifically for the patient with an epidural analgesic infusion is:

   A priority nursing assessment for all patients before and while receiving analgesics is:

29. Identify an intervention that the nurse should implement to adapt or alter the environment to promote a patient's comfort:

Select the best answer for each of the following questions:

30. Identify whether the following statements are true or false:
    a. Nurses can allow their own misconceptions about or interpretations of the pain experience to affect their willingness to intervene for their patient.
    True _____ False _____
    b. The degree and quality of pain are related to the patient's definition of pain.
    True _____ False _____
    c. When patients are experiencing pain, they will not hesitate to inform you.
    True _____ False _____
    d. Fatigue decreases a patient's perception of pain.
    True _____ False _____
    e. The nurse should provide descriptive words for the patient to assist in assessing the quality of the pain.
    True _____ False _____
    f. Pain assessment can be delegated to assistive personnel.
    True _____ False _____
    g. Large doses of opioids for the terminally ill patient will hasten the onset of death.
    True _____ False _____
    h. Health care providers will initially order higher doses than needed for patients with cancer pain.
    True _____ False _____
31. The patient is experiencing pain that is not being managed by analgesics given by the oral or intramuscular routes. Epidural analgesia is initiated. The nurse is alert for a complication of this treatment and observes the patient for:
    1. Diarrhea
    2. Hypertension
    3. Urinary retention
    4. An increased respiratory rate
32. The patient had a laparoscopic procedure this morning and is requesting a pain medication. The nurse assesses the patient's vital signs and decides to withhold the medication based on the finding of:
    1. Pulse rate = 90 beats per minute
    2. Respirations = 10 per minute
    3. Blood pressure = 130/80 mm Hg
    4. Temperature = 99° F, rectally
33. The nurse is working with an older adult population in the extended care facility. Many of the patients experience discomfort associated with arthritis and have analgesics prescribed. In administering an analgesic medication to an older adult patient, the nurse should:
    1. Give the medication when the pain increases in severity
    2. Combine narcotics for a greater effect
    3. Use the IM route whenever possible
    4. Give the medication before activities or procedures
34. One of the patients that the nurse is working with on an outpatient basis at the local clinic has rheumatoid arthritis. The patient has no known allergies to any medications, so the nurse anticipates that the physician will prescribe:
    1. Elavil (amitriptyline)
    2. Stadol (butorphanol)
    3. Indocin (indomethacin)
    4. MS Contin (morphine)
35. An adolescent has been carried to the sidelines of the soccer field after experiencing a twisted ankle. The level of pain is identified as low to moderate. The nurse observes that the patient has:
    1. Pupil constriction
    2. Diaphoresis
    3. A decreased heart rate
    4. A decreased respiratory rate
36. The nurse on the pediatric unit is finding that it is sometimes difficult to determine the presence and severity of pain in very young patients. The nurse recognizes that toddlers may be experiencing pain when they have:
    1. An increased appetite
    2. A relaxed posture
    3. An increased degree of cooperation
    4. Disturbances in their sleep patterns
37. A patient on the oncology unit is experiencing severe pain associated with

his cancer. Although analgesics have been prescribed and administered, the patient is having "breakthrough pain." The nurse anticipates that his treatment will include:
1. The use of a placebo
2. Experimental medications
3. An increase in the opioid dose
4. Administration of medications every hour

38. The patient is experiencing pain that is being treated with a fentanyl transdermal patch. The nurse advises this patient to:
    1. Avoid exposure to the sun
    2. Change the patch site every 2 hours
    3. Apply a heating pad over the site
    4. Expect immediate pain relief when the patch is applied
39. The patient is experiencing very severe pain and has been placed on a morphine drip. During the patient's assessment, the nurse finds that the patient's respiratory rate is 6 breaths per minute. The nurse anticipates that the patient will receive:
    1. Narcan (naloxone)
    2. Additional morphine
    3. Incentive spirometry
    4. No additional treatment for this expected response
40. A pain assessment tool that is used for cancer-related pain and is available in different languages is the:
    1. Brief Pain Inventory (BPI)
    2. Visual Analog Scale (VAS)
    3. Verbal Descriptor Scale (VDS)
    4. Critical Care Pain Observation Tool (CCPOT)
41. The nurse is working on an oncology unit in the medical center. All of the patients experience pain that requires management. The nurse should visit first with the patient who is also exhibiting signs of:
    1. Anxiety
    2. Fatigue
    3. Distraction
    4. Depression
42. For a patient with a consistent level of discomfort, the most effective pain relief is achieved with administration of analgesics:
    1. PRN
    2. Every 3 to 4 hours
    3. Every 12 hours
    4. Around the clock
43. The nurse anticipates that the patient with visceral pain will describe the pain as:
    1. Sharp
    2. Cramping
    3. Burning
    4. Shooting
44. Which of the following orders would the nurse question for the patient who has an epidural infusion for pain relief?
    1. Use of pulse oximetry
    2. Tubing changes every 24 hours
    3. An order for a sedative
    4. Use of fentanyl in the infusion
45. The patient will be using an ambulatory infusion pump at home for analgesia. Additional teaching is required if the patient is observed:
    1. Wearing the pump in the shower
    2. Flushing the catheter with saline
    3. Clamping the catheter after the infusion
    4. Using stool softeners

Study Group Questions

- How may the nurse use a holistic approach to assist the patient in achieving comfort?
- What is pain?
- What are the physiological components of the pain experience?
- How may the patient respond, physiologically and behaviorally, to the pain experience?
- What factors influence the pain experience?
- How are acute and chronic pain different?
- How should the nurse assess a patient's pain?
- How may the patient characterize pain?
- What nonpharmacological measures may be used to relieve pain?
- What interventions may the nurse implement to promote comfort and relieve pain?
- What pharmacological measures are available for pain relief?

- How is a back rub/massage performed in order to achieve an optimum effect?
- What actions should the nurse take if comfort or pain relief measures are not effective?
- What information should be included in patient/family teaching for pain control or relief?

Study Chart

Create a study chart to describe the Factors Influencing Pain and Comfort, *identifying how the age, gender, culture, meaning of pain, and prior experience of a patient alter the pain experience.*

Name ____________________ Date __________ Instructor's Name ________________________

Procedural Guidelines 30-1 Massage

	S	U	NP	Comments
1. Based on patient assessment, decide on performing massage on one or more body parts.	____	____	____	____________
2. Perform hand hygiene.	____	____	____	____________
3. Help patient to assume comfortable lying or sitting position.	____	____	____	____________
4. Dim room lights and/or turn on soft music.	____	____	____	____________
5. Use warm body lotion as lubricant.	____	____	____	____________
6. Massage each body part at least 10 minutes.	____	____	____	____________
Hands: Make contact with the patient's skin, first with one hand and then the other. Using both hands, slowly open the patient's palm, gliding your fingers over the palmar surface. While supporting the hand, use both thumbs to apply friction to the palm and use them in a circular motion to stretch the palm outward. Massage each finger outward and then separately, using a corkscrew-like motion from base of finger to the tip. With thumb and finger, knead each small muscle in the patient's fingers. Glide hands smoothly from fingertips to wrists. Repeat for other hand.	____	____	____	____________
Arms: Use a gliding stroke to massage from the patient's wrist to forearm. With thumb and forefinger of both hands, knead muscles from forearm to shoulder. Continue kneading biceps, deltoid, and triceps muscles. Finish with gliding strokes from the wrist to the shoulder.	____	____	____	____________
Neck: Support the neck at the hairline with one hand, and starting at the base of the neck, massage upward with a gliding stroke. Knead muscles on one side. Switch hands to support neck and knead other side. Stretch the neck slightly, with one hand at the top and the other at the bottom.	____	____	____	____________

	S	U	NP	Comments
Back: Begin at sacral area and massage in circular motion (see Figure 30-6) while moving upward from buttocks to shoulders. Use a firm, smooth stroke over the scapula. Continue in one smooth stroke to upper arms and laterally along sides of back down to iliac crests. Use long, gliding strokes along muscles of spine. Knead any muscles that feel tense or tight.	_____	_____	_____	______________________
7. At end of massage, have patient relax, taking slow, deep breaths.	_____	_____	_____	______________________

31 Nutrition

Case Study

1. You are working with a patient who is being discharged from the acute care unit after having had a heart attack (myocardial infarction). The patient's primary care provider has prescribed a diet that is low in sodium and saturated fat. The patient comes from a family that values some traditional cultural practices where food plays an important role.
   a. What do you need to know about the patient and the family to assist in dietary planning?
   b. How can you assist this patient to meet the prescribed dietary requirements?

Chapter Review

Match the description/definition in Column A with the correct term in Column B.

	Column A	*Column B*
________	1. Increase in blood glucose level	a. Anabolism
________	2. Breakdown of food products into smaller particles	b. Hypoglycemia
________	3. Production of more complex chemical substances through the synthesis of nutrients	c. Digestion
		d. Anthropometry
________	4. All biochemical and physiological processes by which the body maintains itself	e. Catabolism
		f. Nutrients
________	5. Organic substances in food that are present in small amounts and act as coenzymes in biochemical reactions	g. Minerals
		h. Metabolism
________	6. Inorganic elements that act as catalysts in biochemical reactions	i. Hyperglycemia
		j. Vitamins
________	7. Substances necessary for body functioning	
________	8. Breakdown of complex body substances into simpler substances	
________	9. Decrease in blood glucose level	
________	10. Measurement of size and makeup of body at specific sites	

Complete the following:

11. Identify an example of a nutrition objective from *Healthy People 2010:*

12. A vitamin that is synthesized by the body is:

13. Identify whether the following represent carbohydrates, proteins, or fats:
    a. Starches
    b. Meats
    c. Linoleic acid

d. Fiber

e. 9 kcal/g of energy

f. Amino acids

g. Fruits

14. What information can you provide to an individual at a health fair who is interested in general nutritional guidelines?

15. Provide an example of an alternative dietary pattern.

16. For each area of nutritional assessment, identify specific elements to pursue with the patient:
   a. Food and nutrient intake:

   b. Physical examination:

   c. Anthropometric measurements:

17. Select which of the following are indicators of malnutrition:
   a. Listlessness _______
   b. Straight arms and legs _______
   c. Some fat under the skin _______
   d. Paresthesia _______
   e. Loss of ankle reflexes _______
   f. Rapid heart rate _______
   g. No palpable masses _______
   h. Apathy _______
   i. Dry, scaly skin _______
   j. Reddish-pink mucous membranes _______
   k. Spongy gums with marginal redness _______
   l. Surface papillae present on the tongue _______
   m. Pale conjunctivae _______
   n. Corneal xerosis _______
   o. Firm, pink nails _______
   p. Calf tenderness and tingling _______

18. The nurse calculates the patient's body mass index (BMI) by dividing the weight in kilograms by the height in square meters. If the patient weights 180 lb and is 6 feet tall, what is the BMI?

19. A neurogenic cause of dysphagia is:

   A myogenic cause is:

20. A common sign or symptom of food-borne illnesses is:

21. The nurse on an acute care unit wishes to promote a patient's appetite. What is an intervention that should be implemented by the nurse?

22. The patient who is experiencing dysphagia should be positioned:

23. An advantage of enteral nutrition over parenteral nutrition is that enteral nutrition:

24. The most serious complication of tube feedings is:

To avoid this complication, the nurse should:

25. The method of choice for long-term enteral feeding is:

26. The pH of the gastric aspirate for a patient who has been fasting is:

27. A parenteral nutrition formula that is hyperosmolar (greater than 10% dextrose) should be administered through a(n) ________________________ venous line.

28. The patient will be receiving parenteral nutrition (PN). Identify the following:
    a. The main reason for use of PN:

    b. A major nursing goal for the patient receiving PN:

    c. A nursing intervention to assist the patient in the prevention of metabolic complications related to PN therapy:

    d. Guidelines and precautions for lipid infusions:

29. Identify a dietary measure that should be implemented for a patient without teeth or with ill-fitting dentures:

30. Identify a nursing diagnosis and expected outcome for a patient who is underweight:

Select the best answer for each of the following questions:

31. The nurse is working with a patient who requires an increase in complete proteins in the diet. The nurse recommends:
    1. Milk
    2. Cereals
    3. Legumes
    4. Vegetables
32. The nurse is talking with a community resident who has come to the health fair. The resident tells the nurse that he takes a lot of extra vitamins every day. Because of the potential for toxicity, the resident is advised not to exceed the dietary guidelines for:
    1. Vitamin A
    2. Vitamin B_1
    3. Vitamin B_{12}
    4. Folic acid
33. The nurse is working with a patient who is a lactovegetarian. The food that is selected as appropriate for this dietary pattern is:
    1. Fish
    2. Milk
    3. Eggs
    4. Poultry
34. The patient states that he does not eat fish anymore. An appropriate follow-up question by the nurse is the following.
    1. "Why don't you eat fish anymore?"
    2. "What caused you to lose interest in fish?"
    3. "Fish makes you feel ill in some way?"
    4. "Aren't you aware that fish is a valuable source of nutrients?"
35. The nurse is preparing to insert a nasogastric tube for enteral feedings. The nurse recognizes that this intervention is used when the patient:
    1. Has a gag reflex
    2. Is not able to chew foods
    3. Is slow to eliminate food
    4. Is not able to ingest foods
36. The nurse is preparing the enteral feeding for a patient who has a nasogastric tube in place. The most effective method that the

nurse can use to check for placement of a nasogastric tube is to:

1. Perform a pH analysis of aspirated secretions
2. Measure the visible tubing exiting from the nose
3. Inject air into the tube and auscultate over the stomach
4. Place the end of the tube into water and observe for bubbling

37. A female patient who has come to the family planning center is taking an oral contraceptive. This patient should increase vitamin B_6 and niacin intake. The nurse recommends that the patient consume more:
    1. Tomatoes
    2. Whole grains
    3. Citrus fruits
    4. Green, leafy vegetables
38. The patient has heard on television that zinc is an important element in the body's immune response. The patient asks the nurse what foods contain zinc. Because of its zinc content, the nurse recommends:
    1. Fish
    2. Liver
    3. Whole grains
    4. Green, leafy vegetables
39. The nurse is assigned to make home visits to a number of patients. Of all the patients that the nurse visits, the patient with the greatest risk of a nutritional deficiency is the patient with:
    1. Decreased metabolic requirements
    2. An alteration in dietary schedule
    3. A body weight that is 5% over the ideal weight
    4. A weight loss of 3% within the past 6 months
40. Following surgery, the patient is having her dietary intake advanced. After a period of NPO, the patient is placed on a clear liquid diet. What food does the nurse request for the patient?
    1. Milk
    2. Soup
    3. Custard
    4. Popsicles
41. While completing an assessment during a home visit, the nurse discovers that the patient has a history of congestive heart failure and is taking digoxin 0.25 mg daily. Being aware that medications may influence the patient's dietary patterns, the nurse is alert to the patient experiencing:
    1. Anorexia
    2. Gastric distress
    3. An alteration in taste
    4. An alteration in smell
42. A patient on the unit has an enteral tube in place for feedings. When the nurse enters the room, the patient says that he is experiencing cramps and nausea. The nurse should:
    1. Cool the formula
    2. Remove the tube
    3. Use a more concentrated formula
    4. Decrease the administration rate
43. The nurse is completing a physical assessment on a patient who has just been admitted to the rehabilitation facility. The nurse suspects a nutritional alteration as a result of finding:
    1. Shiny hair
    2. Spoon-shaped, ridged nails
    3. Moist conjunctival membranes
    4. A pink tongue with papillae present
44. The nurse instructs the patient who is a vegan to specifically include which supplement in the diet?
    1. Vitamin A
    2. Vitamin C
    3. Vitamin B_{12}
    4. Niacin
45. The individual with the highest percentage of water in the body is a(n):
    1. Infant
    2. Obese patient
    3. Lean patient
    4. Older adult
46. The patient with a gastrostomy has an excessive residual volume. The nurse should:
    1. Request an order for a chest x-ray
    2. Alter the type of feeding being given
    3. Request an order for an antidiarrheal agent
    4. Maintain the patient in high-Fowler's position

47. The nurse is monitoring the patient's laboratory reports. Which of the following, if decreased, is indicative of anemia?
    1. BUN level
    2. Creatinine level
    3. Albumin level
    4. Hemoglobin level
48. The nurse is instructing the family of a patient who is on an NDD-dysphagia puree diet to include:
    1. Mashed potatoes
    2. Moistened breads
    3. Well-cooked noodles
    4. Soft fruits
49. The nurse recognizes that the patient on a low cholesterol diet requires additional teaching if he indicates that he eats which of the following?
    1. Oatmeal
    2. Pastries
    3. Dried fruits
    4. Green peppers
50. A realistic weight loss goal for the patient who is overweight is:
    1. 1 pound per week
    2. 3 pounds per week
    3. 5 pounds per week
    4. 7 pounds per week
51. To prevent the presence of *E. coli* in food, the nurse specifically instructs the patient and family to:
    1. Carefully can foods at home
    2. Boil shellfish completely
    3. Cook ground beef well
    4. Keep dairy products refrigerated
52. The nurse is visiting the patient in the home and notes that additional teaching is required if the patient is observed:
    1. Cooking poultry to 180° F
    2. Thawing frozen foods at room temperature
    3. Discarding all foods that may be spoiled
    4. Cleaning the inside of the refrigerator with bleach
53. Tube feedings are ordered for a patient with a nasogastric tube. Unless the agency specifies otherwise, the nurse should:
    1. Dilute the feedings with water
    2. Infuse the feedings over 1 to 2 hours
    3. Begin with 150 to 250 ml at a time
    4. Increase feedings by 100 to 150 ml per feeding every 8 hours

Study Group Questions

- What are the basic principles of nutrition?
- What body processes are involved in the intake, use, and elimination of foods?
- What are the six major nutrients, their purposes, and food sources?
- What are the current recommendations for daily nutritional intake?
- How do nutritional needs change across the life span?
- How does culture/ethnicity influence dietary intake?
- What are some common alternative food patterns?
- How should the nurse assess the patient's nutritional status?
- What patients are at a greater risk for nutritional deficiencies?
- What nursing diagnoses may be appropriate for patients with nutritional alterations?
- How does the nurse assist patients to meet nutritional needs in the health promotion, acute care, and restorative care setting?
- What special diets may be prescribed for individuals?
- What are the nursing procedures for implementation of enteral and parenteral nutrition?
- What guidelines and precautions should be considered by the nurse in assisting the patient with enteral or parenteral nutrition?
- What general information should be included for patients/families for promotion or restoration of an adequate nutritional intake?

Study Chart

Create a study chart to describe the Six Nutrients, *identifying uses of each in the body and their food sources: carbohydrates, proteins, lipids, vitamins, minerals, and water.*

Name ____________________ Date __________ Instructor's Name __________________________

Performance Checklist: Skill 31-1 Aspiration Precautions

	S	U	NP	Comments
Assessment				
1. Perform nutritional screening.	_____	_____	_____	____________________
2. Assess patients who are at increased risk of aspiration for signs and symptoms of dysphagia.	_____	_____	_____	____________________
3. Observe patient during mealtime for signs of dysphagia, and allow patient to attempt to feed self. Note at end of meal if patient fatigues.	_____	_____	_____	____________________
4. Ask patient about any difficulties with chewing or swallowing various textures of food.	_____	_____	_____	____________________
5. Report signs and symptoms of dysphagia to the physician or health care provider.	_____	_____	_____	____________________
6. Place identification on patient's chart or Kardex indicating that dysphagia is present.	_____	_____	_____	____________________
Planning				
1. Instruct patient about what you are going to do and why.	_____	_____	_____	____________________
2. Explain to patient why you are observing him or her while he or she eats.	_____	_____	_____	____________________
Implementation				
1. Perform hand hygiene.	_____	_____	_____	____________________
2. Using penlight and tongue blade, gently inspect mouth for pockets of food.	_____	_____	_____	____________________
3. Elevate head of patient's bed so that hips are flexed at a 90-degree angle and head is flexed slightly forward, or help patient to same position in a chair.	_____	_____	_____	____________________
4. Observe patient consume various consistencies of foods and liquids.	_____	_____	_____	____________________
5. Add thickener to thin liquids to create the consistency of mashed potatoes, or serve patient pureed foods.	_____	_____	_____	____________________
6. Place ½ to 1 teaspoon of food on unaffected side of the mouth, allowing utensils to touch the mouth or tongue.	_____	_____	_____	____________________
7. Place hand on throat to gently palpate swallowing event as it occurs. Swallowing twice is often necessary to clear the pharynx.	_____	_____	_____	____________________

	S	U	NP	Comments
8. Provide verbal coaching while feeding patient and positive reinforcement to patient.	____	____	____	____________
9. Observe for coughing, choking, gagging, and drooling of food; suction airway as necessary.	____	____	____	____________
10. Provide rest periods as necessary during meal.				
11. Ask patient to remain sitting upright for at least 30 minutes after the meal.	____	____	____	____________
12. Help patient to perform hand hygiene and mouth care.	____	____	____	____________
13. Return patient's tray to appropriate place and perform hand hygiene.	____	____	____	____________
Evaluation				
1. Observe patient's ability to ingest foods of various textures and thickness.	____	____	____	____________
2. Monitor patient's food and fluid intake.	____	____	____	____________
3. Weigh patient weekly.	____	____	____	____________
4. Observe patient's oral cavity after meal to detect pockets of food.	____	____	____	____________
5. Record patient's tolerance of food textures, amount of assistance required, patient position during meal, symptoms of dysphagia, and amount eaten.	____	____	____	____________
6. Report any coughing, gagging, choking, or swallowing difficulties.	____	____	____	____________

Name ____________________ **Date** __________ **Instructor's Name** ____________________________

Performance Checklist: Skill 31-2 Intubating the Patient With a Nasogastric (NG) or Nasointestinal (NI) Feeding Tube

	S	U	NP	Comments
Assessment				
1. Verify patient's need for enteral tube feeding.	____	____	____	____________
2. Assess patency of nares. Have patient close each nostril alternately and breathe. Examine each naris for patency and skin breakdown.	____	____	____	____________
3. Assess patient's medical history for nasal problems and risk of aspiration.	____	____	____	____________
4. Assess patient for gag reflex.	____	____	____	____________
5. Assess patient's mental status.	____	____	____	____________
6. Assess for bowel sounds.	____	____	____	____________
7. Determine if health care provider wants a prokinetic agent administered before placement of an NI tube.	____	____	____	____________
Planning				
1. Explain procedure to patient.	____	____	____	____________
2. Explain to patient how to communicate during intubation by raising index finger to indicate gagging or discomfort.	____	____	____	____________
3. Position patient in sitting or high-Fowler's position. If patient is comatose, place in semi-Fowler's position with head propped forward with a pillow.	____	____	____	____________
4. Examine feeding tube for flaws: rough or sharp edges on distal end and closed or clogged outlet holes.	____	____	____	____________
5. Determine length of tube you will insert, and mark with tape or indelible ink.	____	____	____	____________
6. Prepare NG or NI tube for intubation:				
a. Perform hand hygiene.	____	____	____	____________
b. If the tube has a guide wire or stylet, inject 10 ml of water from 60-ml Luer-Lok or catheter-tip syringe into the tube.	____	____	____	____________
c. Make certain that you position guide wire securely position against weighted tip and that both Luer-Lok connections are snugly fitted together.	____	____	____	____________
7. Cut adhesive tape 10 cm (4 inches) long, or prepare tube fixation device.	____	____	____	____________

	S	U	NP	Comments
Implementation				
1. Put on clean gloves.	____	____	____	____
2. Dip tube with surface lubricant into glass of room temperature water or apply water-soluble lubricant.	____	____	____	____
3. Hand patient a glass of water with a straw or a glass with crushed ice (if able to swallow).	____	____	____	____
4. Gently insert tube through nostril to back of throat (posterior nasopharynx). May cause patient to gag. Aim back and down toward ear.	____	____	____	____
5. Check for position of tube in back of throat with penlight and tongue blade.	____	____	____	____
6. Have patient flex head toward chest after tube has passed through nasopharynx.	____	____	____	____
7. Emphasize need to mouth breathe and swallow during the procedure.	____	____	____	____
8. When you insert the tip of tube approximately 10 inches (in the adult), stop and listen for air exchange from the distal portion of the tube.	____	____	____	____
9. Advance tube each time patient swallows until desired length has been passed.	____	____	____	____
10. Check position of tube.	____	____	____	____
11. Temporarily anchor tube temporarily to the nose with a small piece of tape, and check tube placement.	____	____	____	____
12. After you obtain gastric aspirates, anchor tube to nose and avoid pressure on nares. Mark exit site with indelible ink. Use one of following options for anchoring:				
a. Apply tape				
(1) Apply tincture of benzoin or other skin adhesive on tip of patient's nose and allow it to become "tacky."	____	____	____	____
(2) Split one end of the adhesive tape strip lengthwise 5 cm (2 inches).	____	____	____	____
(3) Wrap each of the 5-cm strips around tube as it exits nose.	____	____	____	____

	S	U	NP	Comments
b. Apply tube fixation device using shaped adhesive patch				
(1) Apply wide end of patch to bridge of nose.	_____	_____	_____	_____
(2) Slip connector around feeding tube as it exits nose.	_____	_____	_____	_____
13. Fasten end of NG tube to patient's gown using a piece of tape.	_____	_____	_____	_____
14. Assist patient to a comfortable position.	_____	_____	_____	_____
15. Obtain x-ray film of chest/abdomen.	_____	_____	_____	_____
16. Change gloves, and administer oral hygiene. Cleanse tubing at nostril with washcloth dampened in soap and water.	_____	_____	_____	_____
17. Remove gloves, dispose of equipment, and perform hand hygiene.	_____	_____	_____	_____
Evaluation				
1. Observe patient to determine response to NG or NI tube intubation.	_____	_____	_____	_____
2. Confirm x-ray results.	_____	_____	_____	_____
3. Remove guide wire or stylet after x-ray confirmation.	_____	_____	_____	_____
4. Routinely assess location of external exit site marking on the tube.	_____	_____	_____	_____
5. Record and report type and size of tube placed, location of distal tip of tube, patient's tolerance of procedure, pH value of gastric aspirate, and confirmation of tube position by x-ray.	_____	_____	_____	_____

Name ____________________ Date __________ Instructor's Name ____________________

Performance Checklist: Skill 31-3 Verifying Feeding Tube Placement

	S	U	NP	Comments
Assessment				
1. Know the policy and procedures for frequency and method of checking tube placement in your facility.	____	____	____	____________
2. Identify signs and symptoms of coughing, chocking, or cyanosis.	____	____	____	____________
3. Identify conditions that increase the risk for spontaneous tube dislocation from the intended position.	____	____	____	____________
4. Observe the external portion of the tube for movement of the ink mark away from the mouth or nares.	____	____	____	____________
5. Review patient's medication record to determine if patient is receiving a gastric acid inhibitor or a proton pump.	____	____	____	____________
6. Review patient's record for history of prior tube displacement.	____	____	____	____________
Planning				
1. Explain procedure to patient.	____	____	____	____________
Implementation				
1. Perform hand hygiene and apply gloves.	____	____	____	____________
2. Measures to verify placement of tube should be conducted at the following times:				
a. For intermittently tube-fed patients, test placement immediately before each feeding and before administration of medications.	____	____	____	____________
b. For continuously tube-fed patients, test placement every 4 to 12 hours and before medication administration.	____	____	____	____________
c. Wait at least 1 hour after medication administration by tube or mouth.	____	____	____	____________
3. Unplug end of feeding tube. Draw up 10 to 30 ml of air into a 60-ml syringe; then attach to end of feeding tube. Flush tube with 30 ml of air before attempting to aspirate fluid. Repositioning the patient from side to side is helpful. More than one bolus of air through the tube is necessary in some cases.	____	____	____	____________

	S	U	NP	Comments
4. Draw back on syringe slowly and obtain 5 to 10 ml of gastric aspirate. Observe appearance of aspirate to help assess the position of the tube.	_____	_____	_____	_______________
5. Gently mix aspirate in syringe and expel into medicine cup. Dip the pH strip into the fluid or apply a few drops of the fluid to the strip. Compare the color of the strip with the color on the chart to determine pH.	_____	_____	_____	_______________
6. If unable to aspirate fluid after repeated attempts, determine correct placement by verification of original x-ray examination of positioning, maintenance of tube in original taped position, absence of risk factors for tube dislocation, and no signs of the patient experiencing respiratory distress.	_____	_____	_____	_______________
7. Irrigate tube.	_____	_____	_____	_______________
8. Remove and dispose of gloves. Perform hand hygiene.	_____	_____	_____	_______________
Evaluation				
1. Observe patient for respiratory distress.	_____	_____	_____	_______________
2. Verify that color, pH, and appearance of aspirate are consistent with the initial tube placement according to x-ray results.	_____	_____	_____	_______________
3. Record and report pH and appearance of aspirate.	_____	_____	_____	_______________

Name ____________________ Date __________ Instructor's Name __________________________

Performance Checklist: Skill 31-4 Administering Enteral Nutrition via a Feeding Tube

	S	U	NP	Comments
Assessment				
1. Assess patient's need for enteral tube feeding.				
2. Assess for food allergies.				
3. Auscultate for bowel sounds.				
4. Obtain baseline weight and laboratory values. Assess patient for fluid volume excess or deficit, electrolyte abnormalities, and metabolic abnormalities such as hyperglycemia.				
5. Verify physician's order for formula, rate, route, and frequency.				
6. Assess stoma site for tubes placed through abdominal wall.				
Planning				
1. Explain procedure to patient.				
2. Perform hand hygiene.				
3. Prepare feeding container to administer formula continuously:				
a. Check expiration date on formula and integrity of container.				
b. Have tube feeding at room temperature.				
c. Connect tubing to container or prepare ready-to-hang container.				
d. Shake formula container well, and fill container with formula. Open stopcock on tubing, and fill tubing with formula to remove air. Hang formula on pole.				
4. For intermittent feeding, have syringe ready and be sure formula is at room temperature.				
5. Place patient in high-Fowler's position or elevate head of bed at least 30 degrees.				
Implementation				
1. Apply gloves.				
2. Determine tube placement.				

	S	U	NP	Comments
3. Check for gastric residual volume.				
a. Draw up 10 to 30 ml of air and connect syringe to end of feeding tube. Flush tube with air. Pull back slowly, and aspirate the total amount of gastric contents that may possibly be aspirated.	____	____	____	____
b. Return aspirated contents to stomach unless the volume is excessive.	____	____	____	____
4. Irrigate tubing.	____	____	____	____
5. Initiate feeding:				
a. Syringe or intermittent feeding				
(1) Pinch proximal end of feeding tube.	____	____	____	____
(2) Remove plunger from syringe and attach barrel of syringe to end of tube.	____	____	____	____
(3) Fill syringe with measured amount of formula. Release tube, elevate syringe to no more than 18 inches (45 cm) above insertion site, and allow it to empty gradually by gravity. Repeat steps (1) to (3) until you have prescribed amount delived to patient.	____	____	____	____
(4) If using feeding bag, prime tubing and attach gavage tubing to end of feeding tube. Set rate by adjusting roller clamp on tubing or placing on a feeding pump. Allow bag to empty gradually over 30 to 60 minutes. Label bag with tube-feeding type, strength, and amount. Include date, time, and initials.	____	____	____	____
b. Continuous-drip method				
(1) Prime and hang feeding bag and tubing on IV pole.	____	____	____	____
(2) Connect distal end of tubing to proximal end of feeding tube.	____	____	____	____
(3) Connect tubing through infusion pump, and set rate (see manufacturer's directions).	____	____	____	____
6. Advance rate of concentration of tube feeding gradually.	____	____	____	____

	S	U	NP	Comments
7. Following intermittent infusion or at end of infusion, irrigate feeding tube per hospital policy. Have registered dietitian recommend total free water requirement per day.	_____	_____	_____	__________
8. When you are not administering tube feedings, cap or clamp the proximal end of the feeding tube.	_____	_____	_____	__________
9. Rinse bag and tubing with warm water whenever feedings are interrupted. Use a new administration set every 24 hours.	_____	_____	_____	__________
10. For tubes placed through the abdominal wall, the exit site of the tube is usually left open to air.	_____	_____	_____	__________

Evaluation

	S	U	NP	Comments
1. Measure residual volume per agency policy.	_____	_____	_____	__________
2. Monitor finger-stick blood glucose level (usually at least every 6 hours until maximum administration rate is reached and maintained for 24 hours).	_____	_____	_____	__________
3. Monitor intake and output every 8 hours.	_____	_____	_____	__________
4. Weigh patient daily until patient reaches and maintains maximum administration rate for 24 hours; then weigh patient 3 times per week.	_____	_____	_____	__________
5. Monitor laboratory values.	_____	_____	_____	__________
6. Observe patient's respiratory status.	_____	_____	_____	__________
7. Observe patient's level of comfort.	_____	_____	_____	__________
8. Auscultate bowel sounds.	_____	_____	_____	__________
9. For tubes placed through the abdominal wall, observe stoma site for integrity.	_____	_____	_____	__________
10. Record patient's response to tube feeding, patency of tube, and any side effects.	_____	_____	_____	__________
11. Record and report type and amount of feeding, status of feeding tube, amount of water administered, patient's tolerance, and adverse effects.	_____	_____	_____	__________

Name ____________________ Date __________ Instructor's Name ____________________________

Procedural Guidelines 31-1 Administering Enternal Feedings via a Gastrostomy or Jejunostomy Tube

	S	U	NP	Comments
1. Assess appropriateness for initiation of enteral nutrition.	_____	_____	_____	____________________
2. Auscultate for bowel sounds before feeding. Consult physician if bowel sounds are absent.	_____	_____	_____	____________________
3. Obtain baseline weight and laboratory values.	_____	_____	_____	____________________
4. Verify physician's or health care provider's order for formula, rate, route, and frequency.	_____	_____	_____	____________________
5. Assess skin around gastrostomy/jejunostomy site for breakdown, irritation, or drainage.	_____	_____	_____	____________________
6. Explain procedure to patient and perform hand hygiene.	_____ _____	_____ _____	_____ _____	____________________ ____________________
7. Prepare feeding container to administer formula continuously:				
a. Check expiration date.	_____	_____	_____	____________________
b. Have tube feeding at room temperature.	_____	_____	_____	____________________
c. Connect tubing to container as needed or prepare ready-to-hang container.	_____	_____	_____	____________________
d. Shake formula well. Fill container and tubing with formula.	_____	_____	_____	____________________
8. For intermittent feeding, have syringe ready and be sure formula is at room temperature.	_____	_____	_____	____________________
9. Elevate head of bed at least 30 degrees.	_____	_____	_____	____________________
10. Apply gloves, and verify tube placement.	_____	_____	_____	____________________
11. Check gastric residual volume.				
a. *Gastrostomy tube:* Attach syringe and aspirate gastric secretions. Return aspirated contents to stomach unless the residual volume exceeds 100 ml. If the residual volume is greater than 100 ml on several consecutive occasions, hold feeding and notify physician.	_____	_____	_____	____________________
b. *Jejunostomy tube:* Aspirate intestinal secretions, observe volume, and return contents as described previously.	_____	_____	_____	____________________
12. Irrigate with 30 ml of water.	_____	_____	_____	____________________

	S	U	NP	Comments
13. Initiate feedings:				
A. **Syringe or Intermittent Feeding**				
(1) Pinch proximal end of the gastrostomy/jejunostomy tube.	____	____	____	____
(2) Remove plunger from syringe, and attach barrel of syringe to end of tube.	____	____	____	____
(3) Fill syringe with measured amount of formula. Release tube and elevate syringe. Allow syringe to empty gradually by gravity, refilling until prescribed amount has been delivered to the patient.	____	____	____	____
(4) If feeding bag is used, prime tubing and attach gavage tubing to end of feeding tube. Set rate by adjusting roller clamp on tubing or attaching a feeding pump. Allow bag to empty gradually over 30 to 60 minutes. Label bag with tube feeding type, strength, and amount. Include date, time, and initials. Change bag every 24 hours.	____	____	____	____
B. **Continuous-Drip Method**				
(1) Connect distal end of feeding tubing to proximal end of gastrostomy/jejunostomy tube.	____	____	____	____
(2) Connect tubing through feeding pump according to manufacturer's directions, and set rate.	____	____	____	____
14. Advance rate or concentration of tube feeding gradually.	____	____	____	____
15. Administer water via feeding tube as ordered with or between feedings.	____	____	____	____
16. Flush tube with 30 ml of water or normal saline every 4 to 6 hours around the clock and before and after administering medications via the tube.	____	____	____	____
17. When patient is not receiving tube feedings, cap or clamp the proximal end of the gastrostomy/jejunostomy tube.	____	____	____	____
18. Rinse container and tubing with warm water after all intermittent feedings.	____	____	____	____

	S	U	NP	Comments
19. The gastrostomy/jejunostomy exit site is usually left open to air. However, if patient needs a dressing because of drainage, change dressing daily or as needed and report the drainage to the physician or health care provider; inspect exit site every shift.	_____	_____	_____	__________
20. Dispose of supplies, and perform hand hygiene.	_____	_____	_____	__________
21. Evaluate patient's tolerance of tube feeding. Check amount of aspirate (residual) every 8 to 12 hours.	_____	_____	_____	__________
22. Monitor finger-stick blood glucose level every 6 hours until patient reaches and maintains maximum rate of administration for 24 hours.	_____	_____	_____	__________
23. Monitor intake and output every 8 hours.	_____	_____	_____	__________
24. Weigh patient daily until maximum administration rate is reached and maintained for 24 hours; then weigh patient 3 times per week.	_____	_____	_____	__________
25. Monitor laboratory values.	_____	_____	_____	__________
26. Observe stoma site for skin integrity.	_____	_____	_____	__________
27. Observe patient's level of comfort.	_____	_____	_____	__________
28. Auscultate bowel sounds.	_____	_____	_____	__________
29. Record amount and type of feeding, patient's response to tube feeding, patency of tube, and any side effects.	_____	_____	_____	__________
30. Report type and amount of feeding, status of feeding tube, patient's tolerance, and adverse effects.	_____	_____	_____	__________

32 Urinary Elimination

Case Studies

1. The patient is coming to the medical center for an intravenous pyelogram (IVP).
   a. What nursing assessments and patient teaching should be completed before this test is performed?
   b. What are the nurse's responsibilities for the patient following an IVP?
2. You will be working with unlicensed assistive personnel in an extended care setting.
   a. What urinary care may be safely delegated by the nurse?
3. On an acute care unit, the patient is to have her catheter removed. The primary nurse tells you that all that is necessary is to "cut it, wait for the balloon to deflate, and pull it out."
   a. How will you proceed with this catheter removal?
4. A clean-voided or midstream urine specimen is required from your male patient. He is able to perform activities of daily living, including hygienic care.
   a. How will you teach this patient to obtain the specimen?

Chapter Review

Match the description/definition in Column A with the correct term in Column B.

	Column A	*Column B*
______	1. Accumulation of urine in the bladder because of inability to empty bladder completely	a. Urgency
______	2. Painful or difficult urination	b. Hematuria
______	3. Difficulty in initiating urination	c. Oliguria
______	4. Volume of urine remaining in the bladder after voiding	d. Retention
______	5. Feeling the need to void immediately	e. Nocturia
______	6. Voiding large amounts of urine	f. Frequency
______	7. Urination, particularly excessive, at night	g. Dysuria
______	8. Presence of blood in the urine	h. Residual urine
______	9. Voiding very often	i. Hesitancy
______	10. Diminished urinary output in relation to fluid intake	j. Polyuria

Complete the following:

11. An example of a noninvasive procedure that may be used to examine the urinary system is:

12. What are the indications for the use of intermittent and indwelling urinary catheterization?

13. What positions may be used for catheterization of a female patient?

14. The recommended daily fluid intake for dilution of urine, promotion of micturition, and flushing the urethra of microorganisms is:

The minimum urinary output for an adult is: _______ per hour.

15. Provide an example of how each of the following factors may influence urination:
    a. Sociocultural:
    b. Fluid intake:
    c. Pathological conditions:
    d. Medications:

16. The type of urinary incontinence that results from an increased intra-abdominal pressure, with leakage of a small amount of urine, is called:

17. Identify the expected characteristics of a normal urine specimen:
    a. pH 10
    b. Protein 4 mg
    c. Presence of glucose
    d. Specific gravity 1.2
    e. Amber color

18. What is a priority when managing a patient's condom catheter?

19. To maintain the patient's dignity and self-esteem when assisting with urinary elimination, the nurse makes sure to:

20. Manual compression of the bladder is called:

21. Select all of the following statements that are correct for urinary diversions:
    a. A ureterostomy is a continent diversion. _______
    b. A transureterostomy connects the ureters and repositions one ureter through the abdominal wall. _______
    c. Continent diversions have pouches created to store urine. _______
    d. Patients with urinary diversions need special clothing and have activity restrictions. _______

22. For a patient on strict intake and output, urinary output is measured with:

23. Identify a method that the nurse may implement to stimulate a patient to void:

24. To assist the patient to start and stop the urine stream, the nurse instructs the patient that a way to strengthen the pelvic floor muscles is by performing:

25. Identify the distance of catheter insertion:
    a. Female patient:
    b. Male patient:

26. Select all of the following appropriate techniques for indwelling catheter care:
    a. Keep the drainage bag below the level of the bladder. _______
    b. Provide perineal care daily. _______
    c. Cleanse in a direction toward the urinary meatus. _______
    d. Attach the drainage bag to the side rail of the bed. _______
    e. Open the connection at the drainage bag to obtain a urine specimen. _______
    f. Avoid having any dependent loops of tubing. _______
    g. Drain all urine in the bag before patient ambulation or exercise. _______
    h. For the immobile patient, empty the drainage bag every 24 hours. _______
27. Select all of the following statements that are correct regarding a cystoscopy:
    a. The procedure may be performed under general anesthesia. _______
    b. Fluids are restricted before and during the procedure. _______
    c. Antibiotics are often administered intravenously. _______
    d. An informed consent is not required. _______
    e. Bowel preparation is performed the evening before the test. _______
    f. The patient is NPO if the test is performed with local anesthesia. _______
    g. Bed rest is usually indicated immediately after the test. _______
    h. Bloody or cloudy urine may be observed after the test. _______
    i. Fluid intake is encouraged after the test is completed. _______

Select the best answer for each of the following questions:

28. The patient on the medical unit is scheduled to have a 24-hour urine collection to diagnose a urinary disorder. The nurse should:
    1. Note the start time on the container
    2. Have the patient void while defecating
    3. Start with the first voiding sample from the patient
    4. Continue with the test if a specimen is flushed away
29. One of the nurse's assigned patients is experiencing urinary retention. The nurse anticipates a medication that may be ordered for this difficulty is:
    1. Propantheline (Pro-Banthine)
    2. Oxybutynin (Ditropan)
    3. Bethanechol (Urecholine)
    4. Phenylpropanolamine
30. Several patients on the long-term care unit have indwelling urinary catheters in place. The nurse is delegating catheter care to the nursing assistant. The nurse includes instruction in:
    1. Using lotion on the perineal area
    2. Disinfecting the first 2 to 3 inches of the catheter every 2 hours
    3. Ensuring that the drainage bag is secured to the side rail
    4. Cleansing the length of the catheter in a circular motion, proximal to distal
31. The patient with recurrent urinary tract infections asks the nurse how they may be avoided. In addition to hygienic care, the nurse discusses with the patient that selected foods may help prevent infections, while other foods may not. The nurse recommends that the patient promote urinary acidity by avoiding:
    1. Eggs
    2. Prunes
    3. Orange juice
    4. Whole grain breads
32. Prevention of infection is a patient outcome that is identified for a patient with a urinary alteration and an indwelling catheter. The nurse assists the patient to attain this outcome by:
    1. Emptying the drainage bag daily
    2. Draining all urine after the patient ambulates
    3. Performing perineal care q8h and PRN
    4. Opening the drainage system only at the connector points to obtain specimens
33. A patient being seen at the urologist's office suffers from urge incontinence.

The nurse anticipates that treatment for this difficulty will include:
1. Biofeedback
2. Catheterization
3. Cholinergic drug therapy
4. Electrical stimulation

34. The nurse notes that there is an order on the patient's record for a sterile urine specimen. The patient has an indwelling urinary catheter. The nurse will proceed to obtain this specimen by:
1. Withdrawing the urine from a urinometer
2. Opening the drainage bag and removing urine
3. Disconnecting the catheter from the drainage tubing
4. Using a needle to withdraw urine from the catheter port

35. The patient had a laparoscopic procedure in the morning and is having difficulty voiding later that day. Before initiating invasive measures, the nurse intervenes by:
1. Administering a cholinergic agent
2. Applying firm pressure over the perineal area
3. Increasing the patient's daily fluid intake to 3000 ml
4. Rinsing the perineal area with warm water

36. To determine the possibility of a renal problem, the patient is scheduled to have an intravenous pyelogram (IVP). Immediately following the procedure, the nurse will need to evaluate the patient's response and will be alert to:
1. An infection in the urinary bladder
2. An allergic reaction to the contrast material
3. Urinary suppression from injury to kidney tissues
4. Incontinence from paralysis of the urinary sphincter

37. The unit manager is evaluating the care that has been given to the patient by the new nursing staff member. The manager determines that the staff member has implemented an appropriate technique for clean-voided urine specimen collection if:
1. Fluids were restricted before the collection
2. Sterile gloves were applied for the procedure
3. The specimen was collected after the initial stream of urine had passed
4. The specimen was placed in a clean container and then placed in the utility room

38. A patient at the urology clinic is diagnosed with reflex incontinence. This problem was identified by the patient's statement of experiencing:
1. A constant dribbling of urine
2. An urge to void and not enough time to reach the bathroom
3. An uncontrollable loss of urine when coughing or sneezing
4. No urge to void and an unawareness of the bladder being full

39. A female patient has an order for urinary catheterization. The nursing student will be evaluated by the instructor on the insertion technique. The student is identified as implementing appropriate technique if:
1. The catheter is advanced 7 to 8 inches
2. The balloon is inflated before insertion to test its patency
3. The catheter is reinserted if it is accidentally placed in the vagina
4. Both hands are kept sterile throughout the procedure

40. The patient is diagnosed with prostate enlargement. The nurse is alert to a specific indication of this problem when finding that the patient has:
1. Chills
2. Cloudy urine
3. Polyuria
4. Bladder distention

41. Stress incontinence is associated with:
1. Irritation of the bladder
2. Neurological trauma
3. Alcohol or caffeine ingestion
4. Coughing or sneezing

42. For patients with diabetes mellitus, the nurse anticipates that the patient will experience:
1. Dribbling

2. Hesitancy
3. Polyuria
4. Hematuria

43. The nurse recognizes that one of the specific purposes of intermittent catheterization is for:
    1. Prevention of obstruction
    2. Assessment of residual urine
    3. Urinary drainage during surgical procedures
    4. Recording of output for comatose patients
44. The nurse notes that there is no urine in the drainage bag since it was emptied 1½ hours ago. The nurse should first:
    1. Remove the catheter
    2. Provide additional fluids
    3. Check for kinks or bends in the tubing
    4. Apply external pressure on the patient's bladder
45. The best way to remove urine from a patient's skin is for the nurse to use:
    1. Alcohol
    2. Mild soap
    3. An antibacterial agent
    4. A hydrogen peroxide mix
46. The nurse manager is observing the new nurse staff member provide care for a patient with a condom catheter. The manager determines that correction and additional instruction are required for the new employee if the staff nurse is observed:
    1. Draping the patient and exposing only the genitalia
    2. Attaching the urinary drainage bag to the lower bed frame
    3. Using adhesive tape to secure the catheter to the patient's penis
    4. Clipping the hair at the base of the penile shaft
47. The nurse anticipates that a treatment option for a patient with functional incontinence will include:
    1. Catheterization
    2. Bladder training
    3. Electrical stimulation
    4. Hormone replacement

Study Group Questions

- What is the normal anatomy and physiology of the urinary system?
- What factors may influence urination?
- What are some common urinary elimination problems, their causes, and patient signs and symptoms?
- How do growth and development influence urinary function and patterns?
- How can urinary drainage be surgically altered, and why would an alteration be necessary?
- What measures may be implemented to prevent infection in the urinary tract?
- How does the nurse assess the patient's urinary function/elimination?
- What noninvasive and invasive procedures may be used to determine urinary function?
- What diagnostic tests are used to determine the characteristics of urine?
- What are the expected characteristics of urine?
- What nursing interventions are appropriate for promoting urination in the health care and home care settings?
- What information should be included in teaching patients/families about promotion of urination and prevention of infection?

Name ____________ Date ________ Instructor's Name ____________

Performance Checklist: Skill 32-1 Inserting a Straight or Indwelling Catheter

	S	U	NP	Comments
Assessment				
1. Assess status of patient and allergy history.	___	___	___	___
2. Review patient's medical record, including physician's or health care provider's order and nurses' notes.	___	___	___	___
3. Assess for previous catheterization.	___	___	___	___
4. Assess patient's knowledge of the purpose of catheterization.	___	___	___	___
Planning				
1. Explain procedure to patient.	___	___	___	___
2. Arrange for extra nursing personnel to assist as necessary.	___	___	___	___
3. Collect appropriate equipment	___	___	___	___
Implementation				
1. Perform hand hygiene.	___	___	___	___
2. Close curtain or door.	___	___	___	___
3. Raise bed to appropriate working height.	___	___	___	___
4. Facing patient, stand on left side of bed if right-handed (on right side if left-handed). Clear bedside table and arrange equipment.	___	___	___	___
5. Raise side rail on opposite side of bed, and put side rail down on working side.	___	___	___	___
6. Place waterproof pad under patient.	___	___	___	___
7. Position patient:				
A. Female Patient				
(1) Assist to dorsal recumbent position (supine with knees flexed). Ask patient to relax thighs so she is able to externally rotate the hip joints.	___	___	___	___
(2) Position female patient in side-lying (Sims') position with upper leg flexed at knee and hip if unable to be supine. Take extra precautions to cover rectal area with drape during procedure to reduce chance of cross-contamination.	___	___	___	___
B. Male Patient				
(1) Assist to supine position. Ensure thighs are slightly abducted.	___	___	___	___

	S	U	NP	Comments
8. Drape patient:				
A. Female Patient				
(1) Drape with bath blanket. Place blanket diamond fashion over patient, with one corner at patient's neck, side corners over each arm and side, and last corner over perineum.	____	____	____	____
B. Male Patient				
(1) Drape upper trunk with bath blanket. Cover lower extremities with bed sheets, exposing only genitalia.	____	____	____	____
9. Wearing disposable gloves, wash perineal area with soap and water as needed; dry and dispose of gloves.	____	____	____	____
10. Position lamp to illuminate perineal area. (When using flashlight, have assistant hold it.)	____	____	____	____
11. Perform hand hygiene. When inserting an indwelling catheter open package containing drainage system; place drainage bag over edge of bottom bed frame and bring drainage tube up between side rail and mattress.	____	____	____	____
12. Open catheterization kit according to directions, keeping bottom of container sterile.	____	____	____	____
13. Place plastic bag that contains kit within reach of work area to use as waterproof bag to dispose of used supplies.	____	____	____	____
14. Apply sterile gloves.	____	____	____	____
15. Organize supplies on sterile field. Open inner sterile package containing catheter. Pour sterile antiseptic solution into correct compartment containing sterile cotton balls. Open lubricant packet. Remove specimen container (lid should be placed loosely on top) and prefilled syringe from collection compartment of tray and set them aside on sterile field if needed.	____	____	____	____

	S	U	NP	Comments
16. Before inserting indwelling catheter, a common practice is to test balloon by injecting fluid from prefilled syringe into balloon port.	_____	_____	_____	__________
17. Lubricate catheter 2.5 to 5 cm (1 to 2 inches) for women and 12.5 to 17.5 cm (5 to 7 inches) for men. NOTE: Some catheter kits will have a plastic sheath over the catheter that must be removed before lubrication. (Optional: Physician may order use of lubricant containing local anesthetic.)	_____	_____	_____	__________
18. Apply sterile drape, keeping gloves sterile:				
A. Female Patient				
(1) Allow top edge of drape to form cuff over both hands. Place drape on bed between patient's thighs. Slip cuffed edge just under buttocks, taking care not to touch contaminated surface with gloves.	_____	_____	_____	__________
(2) Pick up fenestrated sterile drape and allow it to unfold without touching an unsterile object. Apply drape over perineum, exposing labia and being sure not to touch contaminated surface.	_____	_____	_____	__________
B. Male Patient: You will use one of two methods for draping, depending on preference				
(1) First method: Apply drape over thighs and under penis without completely opening fenestrated drape.	_____	_____	_____	__________
(2) Second method: Apply drape over thighs just below penis. Pick up fenestrated sterile drape, allow it to unfold, and drape it over penis with fenestrated slit resting over penis.	_____	_____	_____	__________

	S	U	NP	Comments
19. Place sterile tray and contents on sterile drape between legs. Open specimen container. NOTE: Patient's size and positioning will dictate exact placement.	____	____	____	____
20. Cleanse urethral meatus.				
A. Female Patient				
(1) With nondominant hand, carefully retract labia to fully expose urethral meatus. **Maintain position of nondominant hand throughout procedure.**	____	____	____	____
(2) Holding forceps in sterile dominant hand, pick up cotton ball saturated with antiseptic solution and clean perineal area, wiping front to back from clitoris toward anus. Using a new cotton ball for each area, wipe along the far labial fold, near labial fold, and directly over center of urethral meatus.	____	____	____	____
B. Male Patient				
(1) If patient is not circumcised, retract foreskin with nondominant hand. Grasp penis at shaft just below glans. Retract urethral meatus between thumb and forefinger. **Maintain nondominant hand in this position throughout procedure.**	____	____	____	____
(2) With dominant hand, pick up cotton ball with forceps and clean penis. Move cotton ball in circular motion from urethral meatus down to base of glans. Repeat cleansing three more times, using clean cotton ball each time.	____	____	____	____

	S	U	NP	Comments
21. Pick up catheter with gloved dominant hand 7.5 to 10 cm (3 to 4 inches) from catheter tip. Hold end of catheter loosely coiled in palm of dominant hand. (Optional: may grasp catheter with forceps.) Place distal end of catheter in urine tray receptacle if performing a straight catheterization.	_____	_____	_____	__________
22. Insert catheter.				
A. Female Patient				
(1) Ask patient to bear down gently as if to void and slowly insert catheter through urethral meatus.	_____	_____	_____	__________
(2) Advance catheter a total of 5 to 7.5 cm (2 to 3 inches) in adult **or until urine flows out catheter's end.** When urine appears, advance catheter another 2.5 to 5 cm (1 to 2 inches). Do not force against resistance. Place end of catheter in urine tray receptacle.	_____	_____	_____	__________
(3) Release labia, and hold catheter securely with nondominant hand.	_____	_____	_____	__________
B. Male Patient				
(1) Lift penis to position perpendicular to patient's body, and apply light traction.	_____	_____	_____	__________
(2) Ask patient to bear down as if to void and slowly insert catheter through urethral meatus.	_____	_____	_____	__________
(3) Advance catheter 17.5 to 22.5 cm (7 to 9 inches) in adult or until urine flows out catheter's end. If you initially feel resistance withdraw catheter; do not force it through urethra. When urine appears, advance catheter another 2.5 to 5 cm (1 to 2 inches). **Do not use force to insert a catheter.**	_____	_____	_____	__________

	S	U	NP	Comments
(4) Lower penis and hold catheter securely in nondominant hand. Place end of catheter in urine tray receptacle.	____	____	____	____
(5) Reduce (or reposition) the foreskin.	____	____	____	____
23. Collect urine specimen as needed. Fill specimen cup or jar to desired level (20 to 30 ml) by holding end of catheter in dominant hand over cup.	____	____	____	____
24. Allow bladder to empty fully unless institution policy restricts maximum volume of urine drained with each catheterization (about 800 to 1000 ml).	____	____	____	____
25. Inflate balloon fully per manufacturer's recommendations, and then release catheter with nondominant hand and pull gently to feel resistance.	____	____	____	____
26. Attach end of catheter to collecting tube of drainage system, if necessary. Drainage bag must be below level of bladder; do not place bag on side rails of bed.	____	____	____	____
27. Anchor catheter.				
A. Female Patient				
(1) Secure catheter tubing to inner thigh with strip of nonallergenic tape (commercial multipurpose tube holders with a Velcro strap are available). Allow for slack so movement of thigh does not create tension on catheter.	____	____	____	____
B. Male Patient				
(1) Secure catheter tubing to top of thigh or lower abdomen (with penis directed toward chest. Allow slack in catheter so movement does not create tension on catheter.	____	____	____	____
28. Assist patient to comfortable position. Wash and dry perineal area as needed.	____	____	____	____

	S	U	NP	Comments
29. Remove gloves and dispose of equipment, drapes, and urine in proper receptacles.				
30. Perform hand hygiene.				
Removal of Indwelling Catheter				
31. Palpate bladder.				
32. Before removing an indwelling catheter, check the patient's medical orders to determine if you need a sterile urine specimen.				
33. Explain the procedure to patient.				
34. Place an absorbent, waterproof pad under patient's buttocks.				
35. Perform hand hygiene.				
36. Put on clean disposable gloves.				
37. Remove adhesive tape or velcro tube holder used to pressure and anchor catheter.				
38. Using a sterile syringe fitted with a tip that matches the catheter inflation valve, remove all the instilled fluid in the balloon.				
39. After removing the instilled fluid, gently pull out the catheter while asking the patient to breathe slowly with an open mouth.				
40. After removal of catheter, wrap it in absorbent pad and dispose properly.				
41. Remove any tape residue from abdomen or inner thigh.				
42. Instruct to save urine after removal of catheter and provide measuring device.				
Evaluation				
1. Ask about patient's comfort.				
2. Observe character and amount of urine in drainage system.				
3. Determine that there is no urine leaking from catheter or tubing connections.				
4. Report and record type and size of catheter inserted, amount of fluid used to inflate balloon, characteristics of urine, amount of urine, reasons for catheterization, specimen collection if appropriate, and patient's response to procedure and teaching concepts.				

	S	U	NP	Comments
5. Initiate I&O records.	_____	_____	_____	____________________
6. If catheter is definitely in bladder and no urine is produced within an hour, absence of urine should be reported to physician immediately.	_____	_____	_____	____________________
7. Ensure that times for catheter care are indicated in the care plan. Patients with indwelling catheters receive perineal and catheter care every 8 hours and after bowel movements.	_____	_____	_____	____________________
8. Record in nurses' notes when catheter care was given and condition of urethral meatus.	_____	_____	_____	____________________

Name ____________________ **Date** __________ **Instructor's Name** ________________________

Procedural Guidelines 32-1 Applying a Condom Catheter

	S	U	NP	Comments
1. Check physician or health care provider's order.	____	____	____	____________
2. Perform hand hygiene.	____	____	____	____________
3. Assess urinary elimination patterns, patient's ability to voluntarily urinate, and patient's continence.	____	____	____	____________
4. Assess mental status of patient and explain procedure.	____	____	____	____________
5. Raise bed to working height and raise far upper side rail.	____	____	____	____________
6. Using sheet, drape patient, exposing only the genitalia.	____	____	____	____________
7. Apply disposable gloves; provide perineal care and dry thoroughly.	____	____	____	____________
8. Prepare condom catheter and drainage bag (see manufacturer's directions).	____	____	____	____________
9. Apply gloves and assess condition of penis and scrotum. Provide perineal care.	____	____	____	____________
a. If needed, clip hair at base of penile shaft.	____	____	____	____________
10. Apply skin prep to penile shaft, and allow to dry.	____	____	____	____________
11. Holding penis in nondominant hand, apply condom by rolling smoothly onto penis. NOTE: Leave a space of 2.5 to 5 cm (1 to 2 inches) between tip of penis and end of catheter.	____	____	____	____________
12. Secure condom catheter:				
a. If using elastic adhesive, wrap the strip of adhesive over the condom to secure it in place by using a spiral technique. NOTE: **Never use adhesive tape.**	____	____	____	____________
b. For self-adhesive catheter, follow manufacturer's directions.	____	____	____	____________
13. Attach catheter to large-volume drainage bag or leg bag. Attach large-volume drainage bag to lower bed frame.	____	____	____	____________
14. Make patient comfortable.	____	____	____	____________
15. Observe urinary drainage, drainage tube patency, condition of penis, and tape placement.	____	____	____	____________

33 Bowel Elimination

Case Studies

1. You have arranged with your instructor and the home care agency to visit a 76-year-old female patient. In completing your initial assessment, the patient tells you that she has been having difficulty over the past 2 years in "moving her bowels." She takes you to the bathroom, where she shows you a collection of over-the-counter laxatives and enemas. The patient also tells you that, since the death of her husband, she does not do a lot of cooking, relying on sandwiches and prepared foods.
   a. Based on this information, identify a nursing diagnosis, patient goal(s)/outcomes, and nursing interventions related to bowel elimination.
2. A patient is scheduled to have a colonoscopy performed.
   a. Identify the patient teaching that is provided before the procedure.

Chapter Review

Match the description/definition in Column A with the correct term in Column B.

	Column A	*Column B*
______	1. Propulsion of food through the gastrointestinal (GI) tract	a. Stoma
______	2. Loss of appetite	b. Hemorrhoids
______	3. Artificial opening in the abdominal wall	c. Melena
______	4. Dilated rectal veins	d. Peristalsis
______	5. Blood in the stool	e. Anorexia

Complete the following:

6. Constipation in the older adult is usually the result of:

7. What types of patients should be cautioned against straining during defecation and why?

8. As a result of persistent diarrhea, the patient is at risk for:

9. Provide an example of the effect that fecal incontinence can have on an individual:

10. Identify which of the following factors will interfere with bowel elimination and decrease peristalsis:
    a. Slower esophageal emptying ______
    b. Eating raw vegetables ______
    c. Immobilization ______
    d. Consumption of lean meats ______
    e. Anxiety ______
    f. Emotional depression ______
    g. Abdominal surgery ______
    h. Use of antibiotics ______
    i. Food allergies ______
    j. Parkinson's disease ______
    k. Use of narcotic analgesics ______
    l. Drinking fruit juices ______
    m. Tube feedings ______

11. In taking into account patients' cultural backgrounds, the nurse recognizes that individuals who are ______________ try to avoid exposure of the lower torso.

12. Identify a risk factor for colon cancer:

13. Identify two nursing interventions for a patient who is experiencing:
    a. Constipation:

    b. Diarrhea:

14. Provide an example of how each of the following factors influences bowel elimination:
    a. Positioning:

    b. Pregnancy:

    c. Diagnostic tests:

15. How can the nurse promote comfort for a patient with hemorrhoids?

16. Identify one possible cause for an increase in both the total bilirubin and alkaline phosphatase levels:

17. What is the correct position for an adult patient to receive an enema?

18. An enema that is used to treat patients with hyperkalemia is:

19. For a hypertonic enema:
    a. It works by:

    b. A commonly used over-the-counter hypertonic enema is:

20. The patient receiving tube feedings may experience diarrhea as a result of:

21. Identify what should be included in a focused assessment of a patient's bowel function.

22. What surgical procedures are anticipated for patients with:
    a. Colorectal cancer:

    b. Diverticulitis:

23. Select the correct practices that should be included in the teaching plan for a patient with an ostomy:
    a. Using creams around the peristomal skin _______
    b. Emptying the pouch when it is one-fourth to one-half full _______
    c. Washing the peristomal skin with a detergent soap _______
    d. Applying Kenalog spray for a yeast infection _______
    e. Anticipating a significant amount of bleeding _______
    f. Changing the entire pouching system daily _______
    g. Using the same manufacturer's flange and pouch _______
    h. Cutting the pouch opening 1/16 to 1/8 of an inch larger than the stoma _______
    i. Applying a skin barrier around the stoma _______

24. For the following fecal characteristics, identify whether they are expected or unexpected findings:
    a. Yellow infant's stool

    b. A defecation frequency greater than 3 times per day for an adult

    c. White-colored stool

    d. Tarry stool

    e. Soft, formed stool

    f. 150 mg/day average amount of stool

25. Before giving a patient a bedpan, the nurse should:

26. Select which of the following interventions may be delegated to assistive personnel:
    a. Digital removal of an impaction _______
    b. Enema administration _______
    c. Ostomy pouching _______
27. For an adult patient who will receive an enema, the nurse recognizes that the tube should be inserted __________ inches and the height of the bag for a regular enema should be __________ inches above the anus.

Select the best answer for each of the following questions:

28. The patient expresses a feeling of mild cramping during the administration of a saline enema. The nurse should first:
    1. Discontinue the procedure
    2. Change the salinity of the solution
    3. Lower the bag to slow the infusion
    4. Allow the solution to become cool
29. A patient in a senior day care center is experiencing some constipation. A commonly prescribed medication is a wetting agent or stool softener, such as:
    1. Bisacodyl (Dulcolax)
    2. Phenolphthalein (Ex-Lax)
    3. Magnesium hydroxide (Milk of Magnesia)
    4. Docusate sodium (Colace)
30. The nurse observes the nursing assistant carrying out bowel retraining with a patient in the extended care facility. The nurse identifies that the assistant implements an *incorrect* procedure when:
    1. Allowing the patient adequate time in the bathroom
    2. Taking the patient to the bathroom at regular times throughout the day
    3. Pulling the curtain around the patient while on the commode
    4. Restricting fluids with breakfast and lunch meals
31. For patients that have been prescribed extended bed rest, the prolonged immobility may result in reduced peristalsis and fecal impaction. The nurse is alert to one of the first signs of an impaction when the patient experiences:
    1. Headaches
    2. Abdominal distention
    3. Overflow diarrhea
    4. Abdominal pain with guarding
32. A patient has been admitted to an acute care unit with a diagnosis of biliary disease. When assessing the patient's feces, the nurse expects that they will be:
    1. Bloody
    2. Pus filled
    3. Black and tarry
    4. White or clay colored

33. Upon review of the patient's laboratory results, the nurse notes that the patient is experiencing hypocalcemia. The nurse will plan to implement measures to prevent:
    1. Gastric upset
    2. Malabsorption
    3. Constipation
    4. Fluid secretion
34. The nurse is preparing to administer an enema to a 7-year-old child. When assembling the equipment, the nurse will prepare an enema of:
    1. 150 to 250 ml of fluid
    2. 250 to 350 ml of fluid
    3. 400 to 500 ml of fluid
    4. 500 to 750 ml of fluid
35. The nurse recognizes that the greatest challenge for skin care will be for the patient with a(n):
    1. Ileostomy
    2. Sigmoid colostomy
    3. Descending ostomy
    4. Ileoanal pouch
36. The nurse evaluates that the patient has normal bowel sounds by auscultating all four quadrants and finding:
    1. 4 sounds per minute
    2. 15 sounds per minute
    3. 40 sounds per minute
    4. No bowel sounds after 1 minute
37. The nurse instructs the patient who is taking an iron supplement that his stool may be:
    1. Red and liquid
    2. Pale and frothy
    3. Mucus-filled
    4. Black and tarry
38. The nurse is caring for a patient with a Salem sump tube for gastric decompression. Which of the following actions by the nurse requires correction?
    1. Clamping off the blue lumen or air vent
    2. Using clean technique to insert the tube
    3. Anchoring the tube to the patient's gown
    4. Keeping the nares lubricated
39. The nurse recognizes that the intake of mineral oil to promote bowel elimination interferes with the absorption of:
    1. Vitamin A
    2. Vitamin B_6
    3. Vitamin C
    4. Niacin
40. Further follow-up is required if the patient informs the nurse that he uses:
    1. Fleet enemas
    2. Tap water enemas
    3. Castile soap enemas
    4. Normal saline enemas
41. During a digital removal of a fecal impaction, the nurse notes that the patient has bradycardia. The nurse should:
    1. Provide oxygen
    2. Discontinue the procedure
    3. Turn the patient on the right side
    4. Instruct the patient to take rapid, deep breaths
42. In the teaching plan for a patient who will be having a fecal occult blood test (FOBT), which one of the following foods should be noted for producing a false positive result?
    1. Fish
    2. Pasta
    3. Vitamin B
    4. Whole grain bread

Study Group Questions

- What is the normal anatomy and physiology of the gastrointestinal system?
- How is bowel elimination influenced by the process of growth and development?
- What are some common bowel elimination problems?
- How are continent and incontinent bowel diversions/ostomies different?
- What is included in the nursing assessment of a patient in order to determine bowel elimination status?
- What diagnostic tests may be used to determine the presence of bowel elimination disorders?
- How are the critical thinking and nursing processes applied to situations where patients are experiencing alterations in bowel elimination?

- What nursing interventions may be implemented to promote bowel elimination and comfort for patients in the health promotion, acute care, and restorative care settings?
- What information should be included in the teaching plan for patients/families with regard to promotion and/or restoration of bowel elimination?

Study Chart

Create a study chart to describe Bowel Elimination Problems, *identifying possible causes, signs and symptoms, and nursing interventions for the following: constipation, diarrhea, incontinence, flatulence, hemorrhoids, and bowel obstruction.*

Name ____________________ Date __________ Instructor's Name ____________________

Performance Checklist: Skill 33-1 Administering a Cleansing Enema

	S	U	NP	Comments
Assessment				
1. Assess status of patlient: last bowel movement, normal bowel patterns, hemorrhoids, mobility, external sphincter control, presence of abdominal pain.	____	____	____	____________
2. Assess for presence of increased intracranial pressure, glaucoma, or recent rectal or prostate surgery.	____	____	____	____________
3. Inspect abdomen for distention.	____	____	____	____________
4. Determine patient's level of understanding of purpose of enema.	____	____	____	____________
5. Check patient's medical record to clarify the rationale for the enema.	____	____	____	____________
6. Review physician's or health care provider's order for enema.	____	____	____	____________
Planning				
1. Collect appropriate equipment.	____	____	____	____________
2. Correctly identify patient and explain procedure.	____	____	____	____________
3. Assemble enema bag with appropriate solution and rectal tube.	____	____	____	____________
Implementation				
1. Perform hand hygiene, and apply gloves.	____	____	____	____________
2. Provide privacy by closing curtains around bed or closing door.	____	____	____	____________
3. Raise bed to appropriate working height for nurse; raise side rail on opposite side.	____	____	____	____________
4. Assist patient into left side-lying (Sims') position with right knee flexed. Children may be placed in dorsal recumbent position.	____	____	____	____________
5. Place waterproof pad under hips and buttocks.	____	____	____	____________
6. Cover patient with bath blanket, exposing only rectal area, with anus clearly visible.	____	____	____	____________
7. Separate buttocks and inspect perianal region for abnormalities.	____	____	____	____________

	S	U	NP	Comments
8. Place bedpan or commode in easily accessible position. If patient will be expelling contents in toilet, ensure that toilet is available. (If patient will be repositioning to bathroom to expel enema, place patient's slippers and bathrobe in easily accessible position.)	____	____	____	____
9. Administer enema:				
A. Enema Bag				
(1) Add warmed solution to enema bag (warm tap water as it flows from faucet), place saline container in basin of hot water before adding saline to enema bag, and check temperature of solution by pouring small amount of solution over inner wrist.	____	____	____	____
(2) Raise container, release clamp, and allow solution to flow long enough to fill tubing.	____	____	____	____
(3) Reclamp tubing.	____	____	____	____
(4) Lubricate 6 to 8 cm (3 to 4 inches) of tip of rectal tube with lubricating jelly.	____	____	____	____
(5) Gently separate buttocks and locate anus. Instruct patient to relax by breathing out slowly through mouth.	____	____	____	____
(6) Insert tip of rectal tube slowly by pointing tip in direction of patient's umbilicus. Length of insertion varies:	____	____	____	____
Adult: 7.5 to 10 cm (3 to 4 inches)	____	____	____	____
Child: 5 to 7.5 cm (2 to 3 inches)	____	____	____	____
Infant: 2.5 to 3.75 cm (1 to 1½ inches)	____	____	____	____
(7) Hold tubing in rectum constantly until end of fluid instillation.	____	____	____	____
(8) Open regulating clamp, and allow solution to enter slowly with container at patient's hip level.	____	____	____	____

	S	U	NP	Comments
(9) Raise height of enema container slowly to appropriate level above anus: 30 to 45 cm (12 to 18 inches) for high enema, 30 cm (12 inches) for regular enema, 7.5 cm (3 inches) for low enema. Instillation time varies with volume of solution administered.	____	____	____	____________
(10) Lower container or clamp tubing if patient complains of cramping or if fluid escapes around rectal tube.	____	____	____	____________
(11) Clamp tubing after all solution is instilled.	____	____	____	____________
B. Prepackaged Disposable Container				
(1) Remove plastic cap from rectal tip. Tip is already lubricated, but more jelly can be applied as needed.	____	____	____	____________
(2) Gently separate buttocks and locate rectum. Instruct patient to relax by breathing out slowly through mouth.	____	____	____	____________
(3) Insert tip of bottle gently into rectum toward the umbilicus. Adult: 7.5 to 10 cm (3 to 4 inches) Child: 5 to 7.5 cm (2 to 3 inches) Infant: 2.5 to 3.75 cm (1 to 1½ inches)	____	____	____	____________
(4) Squeeze bottle until all of solution has entered rectum and colon. Instruct patient to retain solution until the urge to defecate occurs, usually 2 to 5 minutes.	____	____	____	____________
10. Place layers of toilet tissue around tube at anus and gently withdraw rectal tube.	____	____	____	____________
11. Explain to patient that feeling of distention is normal, as is some abdominal cramping. Ask patient to retain solution as long as possible while lying quietly in bed. (For infant or young child, gently hold buttocks together for a few minutes.)	____	____	____	____________

	S	U	NP	Comments
12. Discard enema container and tubing in proper receptacle, or rinse out thoroughly with warm soap and water if container is to be reused.	_____	_____	_____	_____
13. Assist patient to bathroom or help position patient on bedpan.	_____	_____	_____	_____
14. Observe character of feces and solution (caution patient against flushing toilet before inspection).	_____	_____	_____	_____
15. Assist patient as needed in washing anal area with warm soap and water (if you administer perineal care, use gloves).	_____	_____	_____	_____
16. Remove and discard gloves, and perform hand hygiene.	_____	_____	_____	_____
Evaluation				
1. Inspect color, consistency, and amount of stool and fluid passed.	_____	_____	_____	_____
2. Assess condition of abdomen; cramping, rigidity, or distention can indicate a serious problem.	_____	_____	_____	_____
3. Record type and volume of enema given and characteristics of results.	_____	_____	_____	_____
4. Record and report patient's tolerance of and responce to procedure.	_____	_____	_____	_____

Name ____________________ **Date** __________ **Instructor's Name** ____________________________

Performance Checklist: Skill 33-2 Inserting and Maintaining a Nasogastric Tube for Gastric Decompression

	S	U	NP	Comments
Assessment				
1. Inspect condition of patient's nasal and oral cavities.	_____	_____	_____	____________________
2. Ask if patient has had history of nasal surgery, and note if deviated nasal septum is present.	_____	_____	_____	____________________
3. Palpate patient's abdomen for distention, pain, and rigidity. Auscultate for bowel sounds.	_____	_____	_____	____________________
4. Assess patient's level of consciousness and ability to follow instructions.	_____	_____	_____	____________________
5. Determine if patient has had an NG tube insertion in the past and which naris was used.	_____	_____	_____	____________________
6. Check medical record for physician's or health care provider's order, type of NG tube to be placed, and whether tube is to be attached to suction or drainage bag.	_____	_____	_____	____________________
Planning				
1. Prepare equipment at the bedside. Have a 4-inch (10-cm) piece of tape ready with one end split in half.	_____	_____	_____	____________________
2. Identify patient, and explain procedure. Let patient know there will be a burning sensation in nasopharynx as tube is passed.	_____	_____	_____	____________________
3. Position patient in high-Fowler's position with pillows behind head and shoulders. Raise bed to a horizontal level comfortable for the nurse.	_____	_____	_____	____________________
Implementation				
1. Perform hand hygiene, and apply disposable gloves.	_____	_____	_____	____________________
2. Place bath towel over patient's chest; give facial tissues to patient. Place emesis basin within reach.	_____	_____	_____	____________________
3. Pull curtain around the bed or close room door.	_____	_____	_____	____________________
4. Stand on patient's right side if right-handed, left side if left-handed.	_____	_____	_____	____________________

	S	U	NP	Comments
5. Instruct patient to relax and breathe normally while occluding one naris. Then repeat this action for other naris. Select nostril with greater airflow.	____	____	____	____________
6. Measure distance to insert tube:				
a. *Traditional method:* Measure distance from tip of nose to earlobe to xiphoid process.	____	____	____	____________
b. *Hanson method:* First mark 50-cm point on tube; then do traditional measurement. Tube insertion should be to midway point between 50 cm (20 inches) and traditional mark.	____	____	____	____________
7. Mark length of tube to be inserted with small piece of tape loosely placed around tube so it can be easily removed.	____	____	____	____________
8. Curve 10 to 15 cm (4 to 6 inches) of end of tube tightly around index finger; then release.	____	____	____	____________
9. Lubricate 7.5 to 10 cm (3 to 4 inches) of end of tube with water-soluble lubricating gel.	____	____	____	____________
10. Alert patient that procedure is to begin.	____	____	____	____________
11. Initially instruct patient to extend neck back against pillow; insert tube slowly through naris with curved end pointing downward.	____	____	____	____________
12. Continue to pass tube along floor of nasal passage, aiming down toward ear. When resistance is felt, apply gentle downward pressure to advance tube (do not force past resistance).	____	____	____	____________
13. If resistance is met, try to rotate the tube and see if it advances. If still resistant, withdraw tube, allow patient to rest, relubricate tube, and insert into other naris.	____	____	____	____________
14. Continue insertion of tube until just past nasopharynx by gently rotating tube toward opposite naris.	____	____	____	____________
a. Once past nasopharynx, stop tube advancement, allow patient to relax, and provide tissues.	____	____	____	____________
b. Explain to patient that next step requires that patient swallow. Give patient glass of water unless contraindicated.	____	____	____	____________

	S	U	NP	Comments
15. With tube just above oropharynx, instruct patient to flex head forward, take a small sip of water, and swallow. Advance tube 2.5 to 5 cm (1 to 2 inches) with each swallow of water. If patient is not allowed fluids, instruct to dry swallow or suck air through straw. Advance tube with each swallow.	____	____	____	____
16. If patient begins to cough, gag, or choke, withdraw slightly and stop tube advancement. Instruct patient to breathe easily and take sips of water.	____	____	____	____
17. If patient continues to cough during insertion, pull tube back slightly.	____	____	____	____
18. If patient continues to gag and cough or complains that the tube feels as though it is coiling in the back of the throat, check back of oropharynx using flashlight and tongue blade. If tube is coiled, withdraw it until the tip is back in the oropharynx. Then reinsert with the patient swallowing.	____	____	____	____
19. After patient relaxes, continue to advance tube with swallowing until tape or mark on tube is reached, which signifies the tube is in the desired distance. Temporarily anchor tube to patient's cheek with a piece of tape until tube placement is verified.	____	____	____	____
20. Verify tube placement: Check agency policy for preferred methods for checking tube placement.	____	____	____	____
a. Ask patient to talk.	____	____	____	____
b. Inspect posterior pharynx for presence of coiled tube.	____	____	____	____
c. Aspirate gently back on syringe to obtain gastric contents, observing color.	____	____	____	____
d. Measure pH of aspirate with color-coded pH paper with range of whole numbers from 1 to 11.	____	____	____	____
e. Have ordered x-ray performed of chest/abdomen.	____	____	____	____

	S	U	NP	Comments
f. If tube is not in stomach, advance another 2.5 to 5 cm (1 to 2 inches) and repeat steps 20a-d to check tube position.	_____	_____	_____	_____
21. Anchoring tube:				
a. After tube is properly inserted and positioned, either clamp end or connect it to drainage bag or suction machine.	_____	_____	_____	_____
b. Tape tube to nose; avoid putting pressure on naris. Cut tape about 5 inches (10 cm), and split halfway.	_____	_____	_____	_____
(1) Before taping tube to nose, apply small amount of tincture of benzoin to lower end of nose and allow to dry (optional). Apply tape to nose, leaving the split end free. Be sure top end of tape over nose is secure.	_____	_____	_____	_____
(2) Carefully wrap two split ends of tape around tube.	_____	_____	_____	_____
(3) Alternative: Apply tube fixation device using shaped adhesive patch.	_____	_____	_____	_____
c. Fasten end of NG tube to patient's gown by looping rubber band around tube in slipknot. Pin rubber band to gown (provides slack for movement).	_____	_____	_____	_____
d. Unless physician orders otherwise, head of bed should be elevated 30 degrees.	_____	_____	_____	_____
e. Explain to patient that sensation of tube should decrease somewhat with time.	_____	_____	_____	_____
f. Remove gloves and perform hand hygiene.	_____	_____	_____	_____
22. Once placement is confirmed:				
a. Place a mark, either a red mark or tape, on the tube to indicate where the tube exits from the nose.	_____	_____	_____	_____
b. Measure the tube length from naris to connector as an alternate method.	_____	_____	_____	_____
c. Document the tube length in the patient record.	_____	_____	_____	_____

	S	U	NP	Comments
23. Tube irrigation:				
a. Perform hand hygiene and apply gloves.	____	____	____	____
b. Check for tube placement in stomach (see step 21). Reconnect NG tube to connecting tube.	____	____	____	____
c. Draw up 30 ml of normal saline into Asepto or catheter-tip syringe.	____	____	____	____
d. Clamp NG tube. Disconnect from connecting tubing, and lay end of connection tubing on towel.	____	____	____	____
e. Insert tip of irrigating syringe into end of NG tube. Remove clamp. Hold syringe with tip pointed at floor, and inject saline slowly and evenly. Do not force solution.	____	____	____	____
f. If resistance occurs, check for kinks in tubing. Turn patient onto left side. Repeated resistance should be reported to surgeon.	____	____	____	____
g. After instilling saline, immediately aspirate or pull back slowly on syringe to withdraw fluid. If amount aspirated is greater than amount instilled, record the difference as output. If amount aspirated is less than amount instilled, record the difference as intake.	____	____	____	____
h. Reconnect NG tube to drainage or suction. (If solution does not return, repeat irrigation.)	____	____	____	____
i. Remove gloves and perform hand hygiene.	____	____	____	____
24. Discontinuation of NG tube:				
a. Verify order to discontinue NG tube.	____	____	____	____
b. Explain procedure to patient, and reassure that removal is less distressing than insertion.	____	____	____	____
c. Perform hand hygiene, and apply disposable gloves.	____	____	____	____
d. Turn off suction and disconnect NG tube from drainage bag or suction. Remove tape or fixation device from bridge of nose and unpin tube from gown.	____	____	____	____

	S	U	NP	Comments
e. Stand on patient's right side if right-handed, left side if left-handed.	____	____	____	____
f. Hand the patient facial tissue; place clean towel across chest. Instruct patient to take and hold a deep breath.	____	____	____	____
g. Clamp or kink tubing securely and then pull tube out steadily and smoothly into towel held in other hand while patient holds breath.	____	____	____	____
h. Measure amount of drainage, and note character of content. Dispose of tube and drainage equipment into proper container.	____	____	____	____
i. Clean nares and provide mouth care.	____	____	____	____
j. Position patient comfortably and explain procedure for drinking fluids, if not contraindicated.	____	____	____	____
25. Clean equipment and return to proper place. Place soiled linen in utility room or proper receptacle.	____	____	____	____
26. Remove gloves and perform hand hygiene.	____	____	____	____
Evaluation				
1. Observe amount and character of contents draining from NG tube. Ask if patient feels nauseated.	____	____	____	____
2. Palpate patient's abdomen periodically, noting any distention, pain, and rigidity and auscultate for the presence of bowel sounds. Turn off suction while auscultating.	____	____	____	____
3. Inspect condition of nares and nose.	____	____	____	____
4. Observe position of tubing.	____	____	____	____
5. Ask if patient feels sore throat or irritation in pharynx.	____	____	____	____
6. Record length, size, and type of gastric tube inserted and naris used, patient's tolerance to procedure, confirmation of tube placement, character of gastric contents, pH value, whether the tube is clamped or connected to drainage or to suction, and the amount of suction supplied.	____	____	____	____

	S	U	NP	Comments
7. Record difference between amount of normal saline instilled and amount of gastric aspirate removed on intake and output (I&O) sheet. Record in nurses' notes or flow sheet amount and character of contents draining from NG tube every shift.	_____	_____	_____	_____
8. Report any unexpected outcomes.	_____	_____	_____	_____

Name ____________ Date ________ Instructor's Name ____________

Performance Checklist: Skill 33-3 Pouching an Ostomy

	S	U	NP	Comments
Assessment				
1. Perform hand hygiene, and put on clean gloves. Auscultate for bowel sounds.	____	____	____	____________
2. Observe skin barrier and pouch for leakage and length of time in place.	____	____	____	____________
3. Observe stoma for color, swelling, trauma, and healing. Assess type of stoma.	____	____	____	____________
4. Observe abdominal contour and abdominal incision (if present).	____	____	____	____________
5. Observe effluent from stoma, and keep a record of intake and output. Ask patient about skin tenderness.	____	____	____	____________
6. When assessing skin for irritation, check that pouching system is not leaking.	____	____	____	____________
7. To minimize skin irritation avoid unnecessary changing of pouching system.	____	____	____	____________
8. Assess abdomen for best type of pouching system to use.	____	____	____	____________
9. Assess the patient's self-care ability to determine the best type of pouching system to use.	____	____	____	____________
10. Remove used pouch and skin barrier gently by pushing skin away from barrier. After skin barrier and pouch removal, assess skin around stoma, noting scars, folds, skin breakdown, and peristomal suture line if present.	____	____	____	____________
11. Remove gloves, and perform hand hygiene.	____	____	____	____________
12. Determine patient's emotional response and knowledge and understanding of an ostomy and its care.	____	____	____	____________
Planning				
1. Explain procedure to patient; encourage patient's interaction and questions.	____	____	____	____________
2. Assemble equipment, and close room curtains or door.	____	____	____	____________

	S	U	NP	Comments
Implementation				
1. Position patient either standing or supine, and drape. If seated, position patient either on or in front of toilet.	_____	_____	_____	__________
2. Perform hand hygiene, and apply disposable gloves.	_____	_____	_____	__________
3. Place towel or disposable waterproof barrier under patient.	_____	_____	_____	__________
4. Cleanse peristomal skin gently with warm tap water using gauze pads or clean washcloth; do not scrub skin. Dry completely by patting skin with gauze or towel.	_____	_____	_____	__________
5. Measure stoma for correct size of pouching system needed using the manufacturer's measuring guide.	_____	_____	_____	__________
6. Select appropriate pouch for patient based on patient assessment. With a custom cut-to-fit pouch, use an ostomy guide to cut opening on the pouch 1/16 to 1/8 inch larger than stoma before removing backing. Prepare pouch by removing backing from barrier and adhesive. With ileostomy, apply thin circle of barrier paste around opening in pouch; allow to dry.	_____	_____	_____	__________
7. Apply skin barrier and pouch. If creases next to stoma occur, use barrier paste to fill in; let dry 1 to 2 minutes.				
A. For One-Piece Pouching System				
(1) Use skin sealant wipes on skin directly under adhesive skin barrier or pouch; allow to dry. Press adhesive backing of pouch and/or skin barrier smoothly against skin, starting from the bottom and working up and around sides.	_____	_____	_____	__________
(2) Hold pouch by barrier, center over stoma, and press down gently on barrier; bottom of pouch should point toward patient's knees.	_____	_____	_____	__________
(3) Maintain gentle finger pressure around barrier for 1 to 2 minutes.	_____	_____	_____	__________

	S	U	NP	Comments
B. If Using Two-Piece Pouching System				
(1) Apply barrier-paste flange (barrier with adhesive) as in steps above for one-piece system. Snap on pouch and maintain finger pressure.	____	____	____	____________
C. For both pouching systems, gently tug on pouch in a downward direction.	____	____	____	____________
8. Gently press on pectin or karaya flange.	____	____	____	____________
9. Although many ostomy pouches are odor-proof, some nurses and patients like to add a small amount of ostomy deodorant into pouch. Do not use "home remedies," which can harm stoma, to control ostomy odor. Do not make a hole in pouch to release flatus.	____	____	____	____________
10. Fold bottom of drainable open-ended pouches up once, and close using a closure device such as a clamp (or follow manufacturer's instructions for closure).	____	____	____	____________
11. Properly dispose of old pouch and soiled equipment. Some patients will also request you to spray the room with air freshener.	____	____	____	____________
12. Remove gloves, and perform hand hygiene.	____	____	____	____________

Evaluation

	S	U	NP	Comments
1. Ask if patient feels discomfort around stoma.	____	____	____	____________
2. Note appearance of stoma around skin and existing incision (if present) while pouch is removed and skin is cleansed. Reinspect condition of skin barrier and adhesive.	____	____	____	____________
3. Auscultate bowel sounds, and observe characteristics of stool.	____	____	____	____________
4. Observe patient's nonverbal behaviors as pouch is applied. Ask if patient has any questions about pouching.	____	____	____	____________
5. Document type of pouch and skin barrier applied.	____	____	____	____________

	S	U	NP	Comments
6. Record amount and appearance of stool, texture, condition of peristomal skin, and sutures.	____	____	____	____________
7. Record and report any of the following to the charge nurse and/or physician:				
a. Abnormal appearance of stoma, suture line, peristomal skin, character of output, abdominal tenderness or distention, and absence of bowel sounds.	____	____	____	____________
b. No flatus in 24 to 36 hours and no stool by third day.	____	____	____	____________
8. Record patient's level of participation and need for teaching.	____	____	____	____________

Name ____________________ Date __________ Instructor's Name __________________________

Procedural Guidelines 33-1 Measuring Fecal Occult Blood

	S	U	NP	Comments
1. Explain purpose of test and ways patient will assist. Some patients collect own specimen, if possible.	_____	_____	_____	_____
2. Perform hand hygiene.	_____	_____	_____	_____
3. Apply clean, disposable gloves.	_____	_____	_____	_____
4. Use tip of wooden applicator to obtain a small portion of uncontaminated stool specimen. Be sure specimen is free of toilet paper.	_____	_____	_____	_____
5. Perform hemoccult slide test:				
a. Open flap of slide and, using a wooden applicator, thinly smear stool in first box of the guaiac paper. Apply a second fecal specimen from a different portion of the stool to slide's second box.	_____	_____	_____	_____
b. Close slide cover and turn the packet over to reverse side. Open cardboard flap and apply two drops of developing solution on each box of guaiac paper. A blue color indicates a positive guaiac, or presence of fecal occult blood.	_____	_____	_____	_____
c. Observe the color of the guaiac paper after 30 to 60 seconds.	_____	_____	_____	_____
d. Dispose of test slide in proper receptacle.	_____	_____	_____	_____
6. Wrap wooden applicator in paper towel, remove gloves, and discard in proper receptacle.	_____	_____	_____	_____
7. Perform hand hygiene.	_____	_____	_____	_____
8. Record results of test; note any unusual fecal characteristics.	_____	_____	_____	_____

Name ____________ Date ________ Instructor's Name ____________

Procedural Guidelines 33-2 Assisting Patient On and Off a Bedpan

	S	U	NP	Comments
1. Assess the patient's level of mobility, strength, ability to help, and presence of any condition (e.g., orthopedic injury) that interferes with the use of a bedpan.	____	____	____	____________
2. Explain to the patient the technique you will use for turning and positioning.	____	____	____	____________
3. Offer the bedpan at a time that coincides with the duodenocolic or mass peristaltic reflex.	____	____	____	____________
4. Perform hand hygiene, and apply disposable gloves.	____	____	____	____________
5. Close the room curtain for privacy.	____	____	____	____________
6. If using a metal bedpan, hold it under warm running water for a couple of minutes, and then dry.	____	____	____	____________
7. Raise the bed to a comfortable working height and be sure patient is positioned high in bed with head elevated 30 degrees (unless contraindicated). Raise the side rail opposite the side where you are standing.	____	____	____	____________
8. Fold back top linen to patient's knees.	____	____	____	____________
9. Assist with positioning: Instruct patient to bend knees and place weight on heels. Place your hand, palm up, under patient's sacrum, resting elbow on mattress. Then have patient lift hips while you slip bedpan into place with other hand.	____	____	____	____________
10. Dependent patient: Lower head of bed flat and have patient roll onto side opposite nurse. Apply powder lightly to lower back and buttocks (optional). Place bedpan firmly against buttocks and push down into mattress with open rim toward patient's feet. Keeping one hand against bedpan, place other hand around patient's forehip. Ask patient to roll onto pan, flat on bed. With patient positioned comfortably, raise head of bed 30 degrees.	____	____	____	____________

	S	U	NP	Comments
11. Place rolled towel under lumbar curve of patient's back.	____	____	____	____________
12. Place call light and toilet tissue within patient's reach, and keep side rails up as needed.	____	____	____	____________
13. Remove bedpan as patient lifts hips up or as patient carefully rolls off pan and to side. Hold pan firmly as patient moves.	____	____	____	____________
14. Assist in cleansing anal area. Wipe from pubic area toward anus. Replace top covers.	____	____	____	____________
15. If you collect a specimen or intake and output, do not dispose of tissue in bedpan.	____	____	____	____________
16. Have patient wash and dry hands.	____	____	____	____________
17. Empty pan's contents, dispose of gloves, and perform hand hygiene.	____	____	____	____________
18. Inspect stool for color, amount, consistency, odor, or presence of abnormal substances.	____	____	____	____________

Name ____________________ Date __________ Instructor's Name ________________________

Procedural Guidelines 33-3 Digital Removal of Stool

	S	U	NP	Comments
1. Obtain patient's baseline vital signs and level of comfort, observe for abdominal distention, and auscultate for bowel sounds before the procedure.	____	____	____	____________
2. Explain the procedure, and help the patient to lie on the left side in Sims' position with knees flexed and back toward you.	____	____	____	____________
3. Perform hand hygiene.	____	____	____	____________
4. Drape the trunk and lower extremities with a bath blanket, and place a waterproof pad under the buttocks. Keep a bedpan next to the patient.	____	____	____	____________
5. Apply disposable gloves, and lubricate the index finger of dominant hand with anesthetic lubricating jelly.	____	____	____	____________
6. Instruct the patient to take slow, deep breaths. Gradually and gently insert the index finger into the rectum and advance the finger slowly along the rectal wall toward the umbilicus.	____	____	____	____________
7. Gently loosen the fecal mass by massaging around it. Work the finger into the hardened mass.	____	____	____	____________
8. Work the feces downward toward the end of the rectum. Remove small pieces at a time and discard into bedpan.	____	____	____	____________
9. Periodically reassess the patient's heart rate and look for signs of fatigue. Stop the procedure if the heart rate drops significantly or the rhythm changes.	____	____	____	____________
10. Continue to clear rectum of feces, and allow the patient to rest at intervals.	____	____	____	____________
11. After completion, wash and dry the buttocks and anal area.	____	____	____	____________
12. Remove bedpan; inspect feces for color and consistency. Dispose of feces. Remove gloves by turning them inside out; then discard.	____	____	____	____________
13. Assist patient to toilet or clean bedpan if urge to defecate develops.	____	____	____	____________

	S	U	NP	Comments
14. Perform hand hygiene. Record results of procedure by describing fecal characteristics and amount.	_____	_____	_____	_____
15. Follow procedure with enemas or cathartics as ordered by physician.	_____	_____	_____	_____
16. Reassess patient's vital signs and level of comfort, observe status of abdominal distention, and auscultate bowel sounds.	_____	_____	_____	_____

Immobility 34

Case Study

1. Your patient, Mrs. B., has just come to the rehabilitation facility. She has been immobilized with a spinal cord injury from an automobile accident. You are aware of the physical hazards of immobility, but Mrs. B.'s withdrawn behavior is your concern now.

a. What can you do to prevent the possible psychological and emotional effects of Mrs. B.'s period of immobility?

Chapter Review

Match the descriptions/definitions in Column A with the correct term in Column B.

	Column A	Column B
______	1. Characterized by bone resorption	a. Renal calculi
______	2. Temporary decrease in blood supply to an organ or tissue	b. Diuresis
		c. Hypostatic pneumonia
______	3. Capacity to maneuver around freely	d. Mobility
______	4. Permanent plantar flexion	e. Ischemia
______	5. Lung inflammation from stasis or pooling of secretions	f. Atelectasis
		g. Thrombus
______	6. Increased urine excretion	h. Activities of daily living
______	7. Collapse of alveoli	i. Disuse osteoporosis
______	8. Bathing, dressing, eating	j. Footdrop
______	9. Calcium stones in the kidney	k. Orthostatic hypotension
______	10. Accumulation of platelets, fibrin, clotting factors, and cellular elements attached to the interior wall of an artery or vein	

Complete the following:

11. The objectives or advantages of bed rest are:

12. Identify all of the following pathophysiological changes that occur with immobility:
    a. Increased basal metabolic rate ______
    b. Decreased gastrointestinal motility ______
    c. Orthostatic hypotension ______
    d. Increased appetite ______
    e. Increased oxygen availability ______
    f. Hypercalcemia ______
    g. Increased lung expansion ______
    h. Decreased cardiac output ______
    i. Increased dependent edema ______
    j. Decreased stressors ______
    k. Increased urinary stasis ______
    l. Decreased passive behaviors ______
    m. Increased sensory overload ______

13. An example of a fluid and electrolyte imbalance that may occur with prolonged immobility is:

14. An example of a common behavioral change that may be observed in the immobilized patient is:

15. The nurse anticipates that the patient on prolonged bed rest will have a heart rate that is ______________________ beats per minute

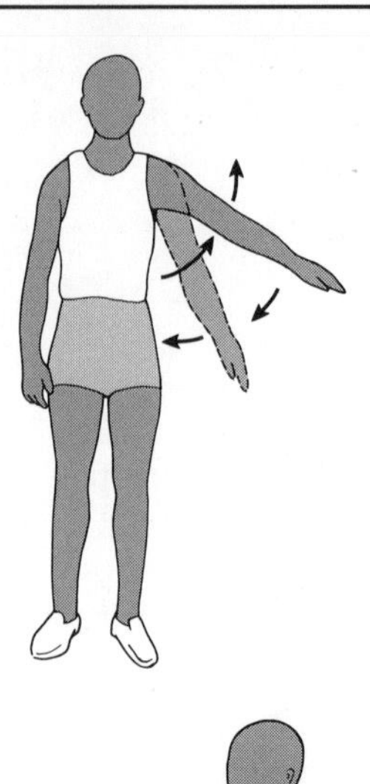

16. Virchow's triad is related to __________, and the three associated problems are:

17. With an immobilized child, the nurse's focus is on:

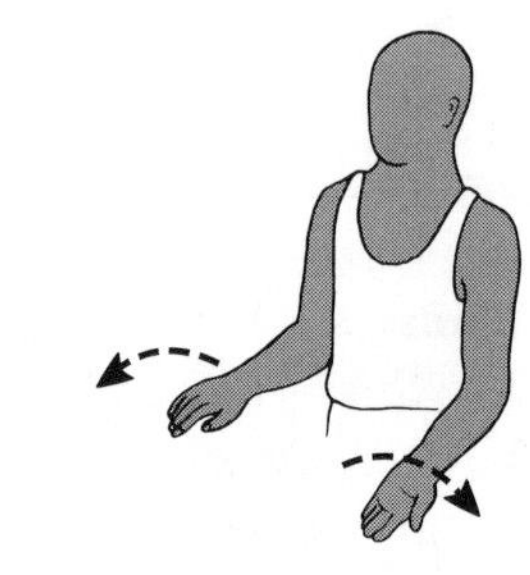

18. An important concept when working with patients who are immobilized is to maintain the patient's autonomy. The nurse can accomplish this by:

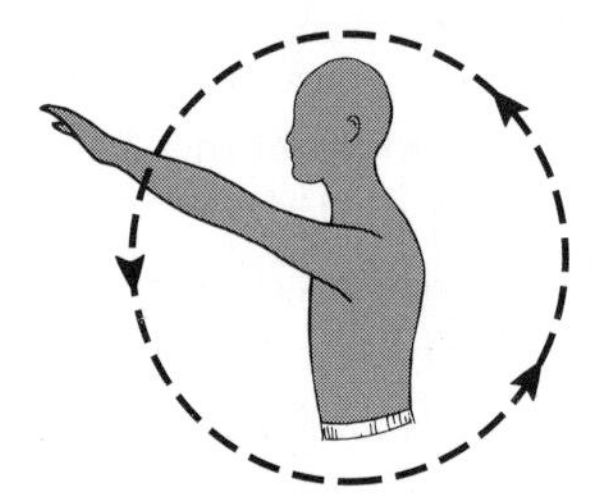

19. Identify at least one major change that may occur in the cardiovascular system as a result of immobility, and a nursing intervention to prevent or treat the change:

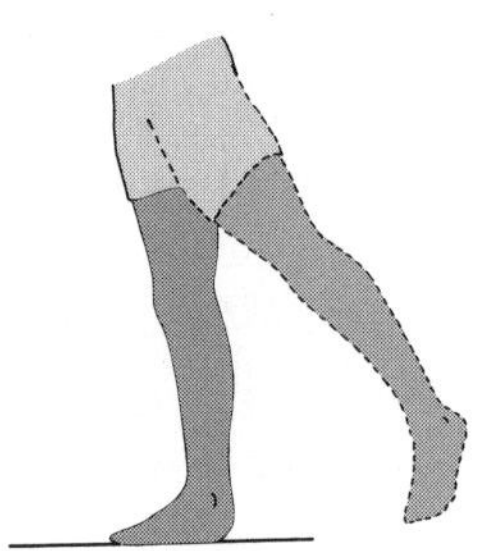

20. Identify at least one potential respiratory complication of immobility, and the nursing intervention to prevent or treat the complication:

21. What areas are included in a focused assessment of patient mobility?

22. Identify for each of the following illustrations what joint range of motion (JROM) exercise is being performed:

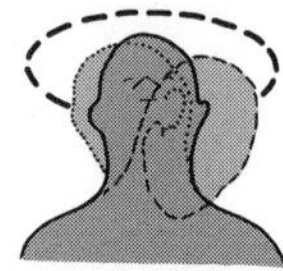

23. To evaluate muscle atrophy, the nurse should:

24. Where should the nurse check for edema in the immobilized patient?

25. For the immobilized patient, identify the usual frequency of assessment for the following:
    a. Respiratory status:

    b. Anorexia:

    c. Urinary elimination:

    d. Intake and output:

26. Specific joint range of motion (JROM) exercises to prevent thrombophlebitis include:

27. For the patient who will have antiembolic stockings:
    a. The contraindications for their use are:

    b. They are removed:

    c. The nurse makes sure that the stockings are NOT:

28. For a sequential compression device, select all of the following that are correct:
    a. The back of the patient's ankle and knee are aligned with markings on the sleeve. _______
    b. A hand's width is left between the sleeve and the patient's skin. _______
    c. The sleeve and device are removed once daily. _______
    d. The unit is observed through one complete cycle after application. _______

29. A medication that is used to reduce the risk of thrombophlebitis is:

    It is usually given every ________ hours by the ____________________ route.

30. The immobilized patient is experiencing shortness of breath and chest pain and the nurse suspects a pulmonary emboli. Independent or nurse-initiated actions that should be taken immediately include:
    a. Administering heparin _______
    b. Placing the patient in high-Fowler's position _______
    c. Drawing arterial blood gases _______
    d. Administering fluids _______
    e. Checking the patient's oxygen saturation _______

31. Identify at least one change that may occur in the following systems as a result of immobility, and a nursing intervention to prevent or treat the problem:
    a. Integumentary:

    b. Gastrointestinal:

    c. Urinary:

    d. Musculoskeletal:

Select the best answer for each of the following questions:

32. The patient has been prescribed prolonged bed rest following a cerebral vascular accident (stroke). During assessment, the nurse is alert to the presence of:
    1. An increased blood pressure reading
    2. Warmth to the calf area
    3. Increased muscle mass

4. An increased hemoglobin level

33. An older adult patient had a fractured hip repaired 2 days ago. The patient is having more difficulty than expected in moving around, and the nurse is concerned about possible respiratory complications. In assessing the patient for possible atelectasis, the nurse expects to find:
    1. A decreased respiratory rate
    2. Wheezing on inspiration
    3. Asymmetrical breath sounds
    4. Rubbing sounds during inspiration and expiration
34. For a patient who has been placed in a spica (full body) cast, the nurse remains alert to possible changes in the cardiovascular system as a result of immobility. The nurse may find that the patient has:
    1. Hypertension
    2. Tachycardia
    3. Hypervolemia
    4. An increased cardiac output
35. A possible complication for the patient who has been prescribed prolonged bed rest is thrombus formation. For the nurse to assess the presence of this serious problem, the nurse should:
    1. Attempt to elicit Chvostek's sign
    2. Palpate the temperature of the feet
    3. Measure the patient's calf and thigh diameters
    4. Observe for hair loss and skin turgor in the lower legs
36. The patient has been prescribed extended bed rest following abdominal surgery. The patient now has an order to be out of bed. The nurse should first:
    1. Assess respiratory function
    2. Obtain the patient's blood pressure measurement
    3. Ask if the patient feels light-headed
    4. Assist the patient to the edge of the bed
37. The patient has been placed in skeletal traction and will be immobilized for an extended period of time. The nurse recognizes that there is a need to prevent respiratory complications and intervenes by:
    1. Suctioning the airway every hour
    2. Changing the patient's position every 4 to 8 hours
    3. Using oxygen and nebulizer treatments regularly
    4. Encouraging deep breathing and coughing every hour
38. Patients who are immobilized in health care facilities require that their psychosocial needs be met along with their physiological needs. The nurse recognizes the patient's psychosocial needs when telling the patient the following:
    1. "The staff will limit your visitors so that you will not be bothered."
    2. "We will help you get dressed so you look more like yourself."
    3. "We can discuss the routine to see if there are any changes that we can make with you."
    4. "A roommate can sometimes be a real bother and very distracting. We can move you to a private room."
39. A patient is transferred to the rehabilitation facility from the medical center following a CVA (cerebral vascular accident/stroke). The CVA resulted in severe right-sided paralysis, and the patient is very limited in mobility. To prevent the complication of external hip rotation for this patient, the nurse uses a:
    1. Footboard
    2. Bed board
    3. Trapeze bar
    4. Trochanter roll
40. The patient who has deep vein thrombosis is at risk for:
    1. Atelectasis
    2. Pulmonary emboli
    3. Orthostatic hypotension
    4. Hypostatic pneumonia
41. The equipment that is used on the bed to assist the patient to raise up the trunk is a:
    1. Sandbag
    2. Bed board
    3. Trapeze bar
    4. Wedge pillow

42. For exercise, which of the following is appropriate for the immobilized older adult?
    1. Gradual, extended warm-ups
    2. Rapid transitions and movements
    3. Sustained isometric exercises of at least a minute
    4. Slowing of exercise rate in the presence of angina or breathlessness
43. The nurse is instructing the patient on joint range of motion (JROM) and performance of shoulder abduction. The nurse correctly instructs the patient to:
    1. Raise the arm straight forward
    2. Move the arm in a full circle
    3. Move the arm until the thumb is turned inward and toward the back
    4. Raise the arm to the side to a position above the head
44. The nurse is instructing the patient on joint range of motion (JROM) and performance of forearm supination. The nurse correctly instructs the patient to:
    1. Move the palm toward the inner aspect of the forearm
    2. Turn the lower arm and hand so the palm is up
    3. Straighten the elbow by lowering the hand
    4. Touch the thumb to each finger of the hand
45. The patient is being instructed to perform dorsiflexion of the foot. The nurse observes the patient's ability to:
    1. Turn the foot and leg toward the other leg
    2. Move the foot so the toes point upward
    3. Turn the sole of the foot medially
    4. Straighten and spread the toes of the foot

Study Group Questions

- What are the basic concepts of mobility?
- What is immobility?
- How is bed rest used therapeutically?
- What physiological changes may occur throughout the body as a result of immobility?
- What psychosocial and developmental changes may occur as a result of immobility?
- What assessments should be made by the nurse to determine the effect of immobility on the patient?
- What nursing interventions should be implemented to prevent or treat the effects of immobility?

Name ____________ Date ________ Instructor's Name ____________

Procedural Guidelines 34-1 Applying Antiembolic Elastic Stockings

	S	U	NP	Comments
1. Assess patient for risk factors in Virchow's triad.	___	___	___	___
2. Observe for signs, symptoms, and conditions that might contraindicate use of elastic stockings.	___	___	___	___
3. Assess and document the condition of patient's skin and circulation to the legs.	___	___	___	___
4. Obtain physician's or health care provider's order.	___	___	___	___
5. Assess patient's or caregiver's understanding of use and application of elastic stockings.	___	___	___	___
6. Assess the condition of the patient's skin and circulation to the leg and foot.	___	___	___	___
7. Use tape measure to measure patient's legs to determine proper stocking size.	___	___	___	___
8. Explain procedure and reasons for applying stockings.	___	___	___	___
9. Perform hand hygiene. Provide hygiene to patient's lower extremities as needed.	___	___	___	___
10. Position patient in supine position.	___	___	___	___
11. Apply stockings:				
a. Turn elastic stocking inside out up to the heel. Place one hand into stocking, holding heel. Pull top of stocking with other hand inside out over foot of stocking.	___	___	___	___
b. Place patient's toes into foot of elastic stocking, making sure that stocking is smooth.	___	___	___	___
c. Slide remaining portion of stocking over patient's foot, being sure that the toes are covered. Make sure the foot fits into the toe and heel position of the stocking.	___	___	___	___
d. Slide top of stocking up over patient's calf until stocking is completely extended. Be sure sock is smooth and no ridges or wrinkles are present, particularly behind the knee.	___	___	___	___
e. Instruct patient not to roll socks partially down.	___	___	___	___

	S	U	NP	Comments
12. Reposition patient to position of comfort, and perform hand hygiene.	_____	_____	_____	__________
13. Remove stockings at least once per shift.	_____	_____	_____	__________
14. Inspect stockings for wrinkles or constriction.	_____	_____	_____	__________
15. Inspect elastic stockings to determine that there are no wrinkles, rolls, or binding.	_____	_____	_____	__________
16. Observe circulatory status of lower extremities. Observe color, temperature, and condition of skin. Palpate pedal pulses.	_____	_____	_____	__________
17. Observe patient's response to wearing the antiembolic stockings.	_____	_____	_____	__________
18. Observe patient or caregiver apply stockings.	_____	_____	_____	__________
19. Record date and time of stocking application and stocking length and size.	_____	_____	_____	__________
20. Record condition of skin and circulatory assessment.	_____	_____	_____	__________
21. Report changes indicating a decline in circulation.	_____	_____	_____	__________

Name ____________________ Date __________ Instructor's Name ________________________

Procedural Guideline 34-2 Application of Sequential Compression Devices (SCD)

	S	U	NP	Comments
1. Assess patient's need for sequential compression stockings.	____	____	____	____________
2. Obtain baseline assessment data about the status of circulation, pulses, and skin integrity on patient's lower extremities before initiating sequential compression stockings.	____	____	____	____________
3. Perform hand hygiene. Provide hygiene to lower extremities, as needed.	____	____	____	____________
4. Assemble and prepare equipment.	____	____	____	____________
5. Arrange SCD sleeve under the patient's leg according to the leg position indicated on the inner lining of the sleeve.	____	____	____	____________
a. Back of patient's ankle should align with the ankle marking on inner lining of the sleeve.	____	____	____	____________
b. Position back of knee with the popliteal opening.	____	____	____	____________
6. Wrap SCD sleeve securely around patient's leg.	____	____	____	____________
7. Verify fit of SCD sleeves by placing two fingers between patient's leg and sleeve.	____	____	____	____________
8. Attach SCD sleeve's connector to plug on mechanical unit. Arrows on compressor line up with arrows on plug from mechanical unit.	____	____	____	____________
9. Turn mechanical unit on. Green light indicates unit is functioning.	____	____	____	____________
10. Observe functioning of unit for one complete cycle.	____	____	____	____________
11. Reposition patient for comfort and perform hand hygiene.	____	____	____	____________
12. Remove compression stockings at least once per shift.	____	____	____	____________
13. Monitor skin integrity and circulation to patient's lower extremities as ordered or as recommended by SCD manufacturer.	____	____	____	____________

Skin Integrity and Wound Care 35

Case Study

1. You are a student nurse assigned to provide care to a patient in an extended care facility. While assisting the patient from the bed to the shower chair, you notice reddened areas on her sacral region, and on both elbows and heels. The skin on these areas is intact, but the redness does not go away.
   a. Identify a nursing diagnosis, patient goal/outcomes, and nursing interventions related to this patient's assessment data.

Chapter Review

Match the description/definition in Column A with the correct term in Column B.

	Column A	Column B
_______	1. Localized collection of blood under the tissues	a. Cachexia
_______	2. Separation of wound layers with protrusion of visceral organs	b. Approximate
_______	3. Wound edges come together	c. Abrasion
_______	4. Superficial loss of dermis	d. Laceration
_______	5. Pressure exerted against the skin when the patient is moved	e. Dehiscence
_______	6. General ill health and malnutrition, with weakness and emaciation	f. Fistula
_______	7. Removal of devitalized tissue	g. Maceration
_______	8. Torn, jagged damage to dermis and epidermis	h. Hematoma
_______	9. Separation of skin and tissue layers	i. Evisceration
_______	10. Abnormal passage between two body organs, or between an organ and the outside of the body	j. Debridement
		k. Shearing force

Complete the following:

11. Mark the areas on the body that are common sites for pressure ulcer development.

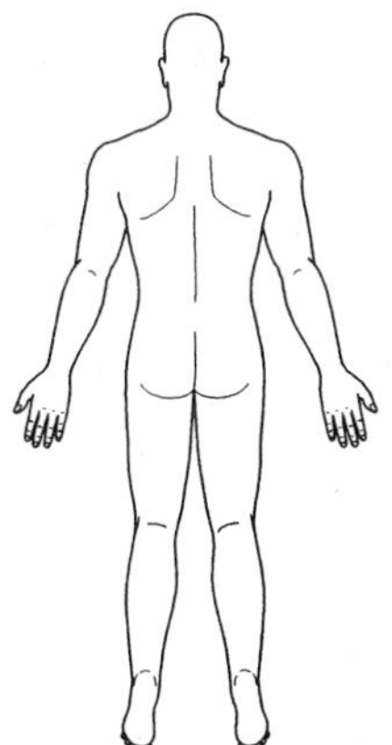

12. Identify the following stages of pressure ulcer development:
    a.

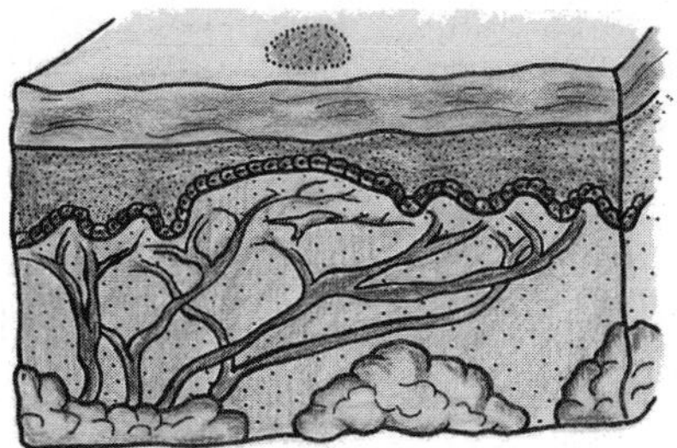

b.

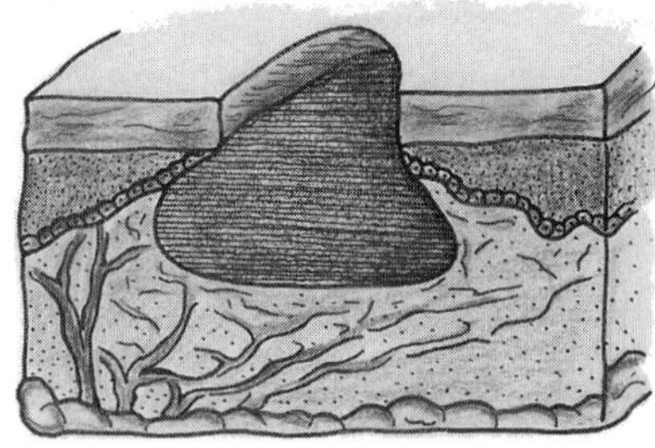

13. Provide an example of a contributing factor for pressure ulcer formation:

14. Patients in which age-groups are at the highest risk for both pressure ulcer development and sensitivity to heat and cold applications:

15. The major change in the older adult's skin that contributes to pressure ulcer development is:

16. Identify the following related to wound healing:
    a. A clean surgical wound with little tissue loss heals by:

    b. A severe laceration or chronic wound heals by:

17. Identify if the following statements are true or false:
    a. Wounds that are kept moist for several days heal faster than those that are kept dry.
    True _____ False _____
    b. Reddened areas that are noted on the patient's skin should be massaged.
    True _____ False _____
    c. Use of a foam ring or donut is effective for pressure reduction for the patient sitting out of bed.
    True _____ False _____

18. Identify a complication of wound healing that is assessed by the nurse in the following examples:
    a. Separation of the layers of the skin with serosanguineous drainage noted:

    b. Bluish swelling or mass at the site:

    c. Fever, general malaise, and increased WBC count:

    d. Green, odorous local drainage:

    e. Decreased blood pressure, increased pulse rate, increased respirations:

    f. Visceral organs protruding through abdominal wall:

    g. Wound edges swollen, painful, with redness extending from the edges outward:

19. Identify the methods or indicators that are used for assessing darkly pigmented skin:
    a. Lighting source:

b. Unexpected consistency:
c. Unexpected change in color:

20. Identify an example of how each of the following factors influences wound healing:
   a. Age:
   b. Obesity:
   c. Diabetes:
   d. Immunosuppression:

21. Match each of the following types of wound drainage with their correct description:

Drainage	*Description*
a. Serous	1. Pale, more watery, with plasma and red blood cells
b. Sanguineous	2. Thick, yellow, green, or brown with organisms and white blood cells
c. Serosanguineous	3. Clear, watery plasma
d. Purulent	4. Fresh bleeding

22. Provide at least one nursing intervention that should be implemented to prevent pressure ulcer formation specifically related to:
   a. Pressure reduction:
   b. Skin care:

23. Arrange the steps for obtaining an aerobic wound culture in order from 1 to 5:
   a. Return the swab to the culture tube.
   b. Apply pressure to express fluid from wound onto swab.
   c. Moisten swab with normal saline.
   d. Swab wound in a 1 × 1 cm area.
   e. Cleanse the wound and allow to dry.

24. The nurse investigates if the patient has had a tetanus toxoid injection within the past year if the patient has a(n):

25. Identify how the nurse determines whether a wound is healing:

26. A patient who is sitting out of bed in a chair and requires assistance to move around should be limited to _____ hours sitting and should be repositioned every _____ hour(s).

27. The nurse can reduce friction or shear by:

28. Nursing care of an abrasion or laceration includes:

29. For use of a wound vacuum-assisted closure (V.A.C.) ®System:
    a. The purpose of the Wound V.A.C. is to:
    b. The tube is attached to:
    c. The dressing that is used for this system is:
    d. The transparent dressing should:

30. For wound irrigation, identify the following that are considered as safe guidelines:
    a. Syringe size:
    b. Needle gauge:
    c. psi:
    d. During an irrigation, the nurse notes sanguineous return. The nurse should:

31. Identify what is pictured in the following illustrations:

    a.

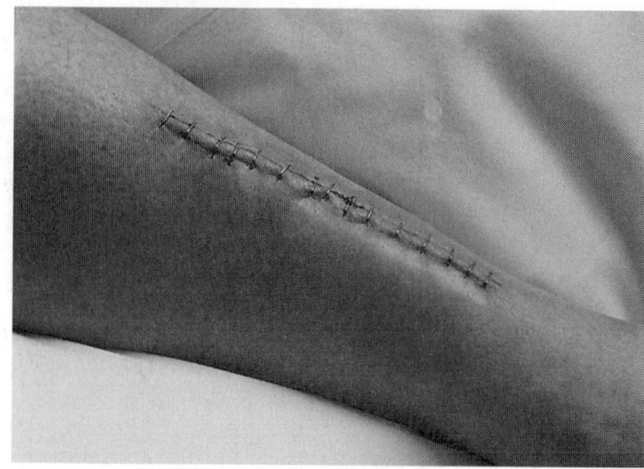

    b.

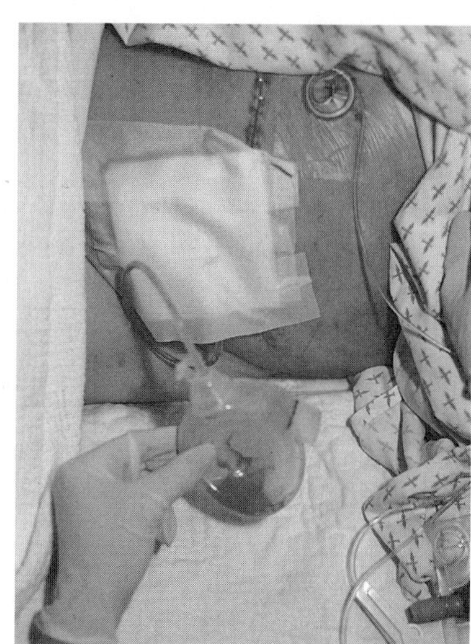

32. Select all of the following that are correct nursing interventions for elastic bandages:
    a. Placing the body part to be bandaged in anatomical position _______
    b. Applying a bandage to an extremity from proximal to distal _______

c. Positioning pins or knots toward the wound _______
d. Overlapping turns by one half to two thirds the width of the bandage _______
e. Assessing circulation once daily _______

33. Identify the steps in caring for a traumatic wound:

34. Specify whether the following effects are a result of heat (H) or cold (C) therapy:
a. Vasoconstriction _______
b. Decreased blood viscosity _______
c. Increased tissue metabolism _______
d. Decreased muscle tension _______
e. Increased capillary permeability _______

35. Provide an instance where the application of heat is contraindicated: _______
Provide an instance where the application of cold is contraindicated: _______

36. The usual duration of time for the application of heat or cold is: _______

37. Select all of the following that are correct for the application of heat or cold:
a. Provide a timer or clock so the patient may help time the application _______
b. Allow the patient to adjust the temperature setting _______
c. Do not place the patient in a position that prevents movement away from the temperature source _______
d. Maintain the temperature as hot or cold as the patient is able to tolerate _______
e. Apply a heating pad or cold pack directly to the skin _______
f. Add hotter solution to a soak to maintain temperature while the patient remains immersed _______
g. Keep the rest of the patient draped or covered while receiving treatment _______

38. Using the Braden scale, what is this patient's risk for pressure ulcer development?

		Score
Sensory	Very Limited	_____
Moisture	Occasionally	_____
Activity	Chairfast	_____
Mobility	Very Limited	_____
Nutrition	Probably Inadequate	_____
Friction/ Shear	Potential Problem	_____
	Total Score	_____
	Patient Risk	_____

Select the best answer for each of the following questions:

39. To avoid pressure ulcer development for an immobilized patient at home, the nurse recommends a surface to use on the bed. A surface type that is low-cost and easy to use in the home is a(n):
1. Foam overlay surface
2. Air overlay surface
3. Air fluidized surface
4. Low air loss surface

40. For the patient in the extended care facility who has a nursing diagnosis of *Impaired physical mobility,* the nurse will implement:
1. Massage of reddened skin areas
2. Movement of the patient in the chair every 2 hours
3. Maintenance of low-Fowler's position while in bed (30 degrees or lower)
4. Placement of plastic absorptive pads directly beneath the patient

41. The patient has experienced a traumatic injury that will require applications of heat. The nurse implements the treatment based on the principle that:
1. Long exposures help the patient develop tolerance to the procedure
2. The foot and the palm of the hand are the most sensitive to temperature
3. Patient response is best to minor temperature adjustments
4. Patients are more tolerant to temperature changes over a large body surface area

42. A severely overweight patient has returned to the unit after having major abdominal surgery. When the nurse enters the room, it is evident that the patient has moved or coughed and the wound has eviscerated. The nurse should immediately:
    1. Assess vital signs
    2. Contact the physician
    3. Apply light pressure on the exposed organs
    4. Place sterile towels soaked in saline over the area
43. A patient with a knife protruding from his upper leg is brought into the emergency department. The nurse is waiting for the physician to arrive when a newly hired nurse comes to assist. The nurse delegates the new staff member to do all of the following as soon as possible **except:**
    1. Assess vital signs
    2. Remove the knife to cleanse the wound
    3. Wrap a bandage around the knife and injured site
    4. Apply pressure to the surrounding area to stop bleeding
44. The nurse is assessing the patient's wound and notices that it has very minimal tissue loss and drainage. There are a number of dressings that may be used according to the protocol on the unit. The nurse selects:
    1. Gauze
    2. Alginate
    3. Wound V.A.C.
    4. Transparent film
45. The nurse is completing an assessment of the patient's skin integrity and identifies that an area is a full-thickness wound with damage to the subcutaneous tissue. The nurse identifies this stage of ulcer formation as:
    1. Stage I
    2. Stage II
    3. Stage III
    4. Stage IV
46. The patient has a large wound to the sacral area that requires irrigation. The nurse explains to the patient that irrigation will be performed to:
    1. Decrease scar formation
    2. Decrease wound drainage
    3. Remove debris from the wound
    4. Improve circulation in the wound
47. The nurse is working with an older adult patient in the extended care facility. While turning the patient, the nurse notices that there is a reddened area on the patient's coccyx. The nurse implements skin care that includes:
    1. Soaking the area with normal saline
    2. Cleaning the area with mild soap, drying, and applying a protective moisturizer
    3. Washing the area with an astringent and painting it with povidone-iodine solution
    4. Applying a dilute solution of hydrogen peroxide and water and using a heat lamp to dry the area
48. A patient has a wound to the left lower extremity that has minimal exudates and collagen formation. The nurse identifies the healing phase of this wound as:
    1. Primary intention
    2. Proliferative phase
    3. Secondary intention
    4. Inflammatory phase
49. Following neurosurgery, the nurse assesses the patient's bandage and finds that there is thin, clear drainage coming from the operative site. The nurse describes this drainage to the surgeon as:
    1. Serous
    2. Purulent
    3. Sanguineous
    4. Serosanguineous
50. The patient has a surgical wound on the right upper aspect of the chest that requires cleansing. The nurse implements aseptic technique by:
    1. Cleaning the wound twice and discarding the swab
    2. Moving from the outer region of the wound toward the center
    3. Using an antiseptic solution followed by a normal saline rinse
    4. Starting at the drainage site and moving outward with circular motions
51. The nurse is working in a physician's office and is asked by one of the patients when heat or cold should be applied.

In providing an example, the nurse identifies that cold therapy should be applied for the patient with:
1. A newly fractured ankle
2. Menstrual cramping
3. An infected wound
4. Degenerative joint disease

52. The patient will require the application of a binder to provide support to the abdomen. When applying the binder, the nurse uses the principle that:
1. The binder should be kept loose for patient comfort
2. The patient should be sitting or standing when it is applied
3. The patient must maintain adequate ventilatory capacity
4. The binder replaces the need for underlying bandages or dressings

53. The nurse is aware that malnutrition places a patient at a greater risk for tissue damage. The patient with the greatest risk is the individual who:
1. Experienced a 7% weight loss over 4 months
2. Is between 45 and 60 years of age
3. Has an albumin level of 3 mg/dl
4. Has a transferrin level of 120 mg/dl

54. The agent that is most effective and safest for cleaning a granular wound is:
1. Acetic acid
2. Normal saline
3. Povidone-iodine
4. Hydrogen peroxide

55. The nurse is working with a patient who has a stage III, clean ulcer with significant exudate. The nurse anticipates that which one of the following dressings will be used:
1. Composite film dressing
2. Transparent dressing
3. Calcium alginate dressing
4. Hydrogel dressing

56. For the patient's optimal nutritional intake that will promote formation of new blood vessels and collagen synthesis, the nurse plans to teach the patient to include a sufficient intake of:
1. Fats
2. Proteins
3. Carbohydrates
4. Fat-soluble vitamins

Study Group Questions

- What are pressure ulcers and what contributes to their development?
- Where are pressure ulcers most likely to develop?
- What are the stages of pressure ulcer development?
- What are the classifications of wounds?
- How do wounds heal?
- What are the possible complications of wound healing?
- How do pressure ulcers affect health care costs?
- What tools may be used to predict patients' risks for pressure ulcer development?
- What should be included in the nursing assessment of patients to determine their risk for pressure ulcer development?
- How are wounds managed in both emergency and nonemergency health care settings?
- What types of drainage may be seen in wounds?
- How are wound cultures obtained?
- How can the nurse prevent pressure ulcer development?
- What nursing interventions may be implemented to treat pressure ulcers and wounds?
- What are the procedures for dressing changes and wound care?
- What criteria are used in the selection of dressings and sutures or staples?
- What are the principles involved in heat and cold therapy, including patient safety?
- What information should be included in patient/family teaching for prevention and treatment of pressure ulcers, wound care, and use of heat and cold therapy?

Name ____________________ Date __________ Instructor's Name ________________________

Performance Checklist: Skill 35-1 Assessment of Patient for Pressure Ulcer: Risk and Skin Assessment

	S	U	NP	Comments
Assessment				
1. Close room door or bedside curtains.	____	____	____	____________________
2. Identify patient's risk for pressure ulcer formation using the Braden scale; assign a score for each of the subscales.	____	____	____	____________________
3. Obtain the risk score and evaluate based upon patient's overall condition.	____	____	____	____________________
4. Conduct a systematic skin assessment of bony prominences. Wear examination gloves when applying pressure to reddened areas.	____	____	____	____________________
5. Assess the following potential areas of skin breakdown ears and nares, lips, tube sites, orthopedic and positioning devices.	____	____	____	____________________
6. Assess all skin surfaces for tissue damage or loss.	____	____	____	____________________
Implementation				
1. If any of the risk factors receive low scores on the risk assessment tool, consider one or more interventions.	____	____	____	____________________
2. Assist patient when changing positions during the assessment.	____	____	____	____________________
3. When you note a reddened area, inspect for erythema, pallor, or mottling.	____	____	____	____________________
4. Remove gloves, perform hand hygiene, and reposition patient.	____	____	____	____________________
Evaluation				
1. Evaluate patient's skin regularly.	____	____	____	____________________
2. Compare current risk score with previous scores.	____	____	____	____________________
3. Record risk score and frequency of risk assessment.	____	____	____	____________________
4. Record appearance of skin, especially pressure points.	____	____	____	____________________
5. Describe positioning and turning schedule.	____	____	____	____________________
6. Describe preventative skin interventions.	____	____	____	____________________
7. Report changes in skin care protocol.	____	____	____	____________________
8. Document consultation from skin/wound care specialists.	____	____	____	____________________

Name ____________________ Date __________ Instructor's Name ____________________

Performance Checklist: Skill 35-2 Treating Pressure Ulcers

	S	U	NP	Comments
Assessment				
1. Assess the patient's comfort level and need for pain medication.	____	____	____	____________
2. Determine if patient has allergies to topical agents.	____	____	____	____________
3. Review the order for topical agent or dressing.	____	____	____	____________
4. Assess each of the patient's pressure ulcer(s) and surrounding skin to determine ulcer characteristics.	____	____	____	____________
5. Assess the type of tissue in the wound bed. Chart the approximate amount of each tissue found in the wound bed.	____	____	____	____________
6. Assess need for revisions to therapy during each dressing change.	____	____	____	____________
a. Note color, temperature, edema, moisture, and condition of skin around the ulcer. Modify the assessment technique based on the patient's individual skin color.	____	____	____	____________
b. Measure the wound's length and width per agency policy.	____	____	____	____________
c. Measure the depth of the pressure ulcer using a sterile cotton-tipped applicator or other device that will allow measurement of wound depth. Place the applicator *gently* into the pressure ulcer until it touches the bottom. Mark the place on the applicator where it reaches the top of the wound, and then remove the applicator from the ulcer. Measure the distance from the tip of the applicator to the mark using a measuring tape or ruler to determine the depth of the pressure ulcer.	____	____	____	____________
d. Measure depth of undermining tissue. Use a cotton-tipped applicator, and gently probe under skin edges.	____	____	____	____________
7. Remove gloves, discard appropriately, and perform hand hygiene.	____	____	____	____________

	S	U	NP	Comments
Planning				
1. Explain procedure to patient and family.	____	____	____	____________
2. Prepare the following necessary equipment and supplies:	____	____	____	____________
a. Washbasin, warm water, soap, washcloth, and bath towel	____	____	____	____________
b. Normal saline or other wound-cleansing agent in sterile solution container	____	____	____	____________
c. Prescribed topical agent	____	____	____	____________
d. Appropriate dressing	____	____	____	____________
Implementation				
1. Close room door or bedside curtains. Perform hand hygiene, and apply gloves. Open sterile packages and topical solution containers. (Goggles and moisture-proof cover gown should be worn if indicated.)	____	____	____	____________
2. Remove bed linen and patient's gown to expose ulcer and surrounding skin. Keep remaining body parts draped.	____	____	____	____________
3. Gently wash skin surrounding ulcer with warm water and soap.	____	____	____	____________
4. Rinse area thoroughly with water.	____	____	____	____________
5. Gently dry skin thoroughly by patting lightly with towel.	____	____	____	____________
6. Perform hand hygiene and change gloves.	____	____	____	____________
7. Cleanse ulcer thoroughly with normal saline or prescribed wound-cleansing agent.	____	____	____	____________
8. Use whirlpool treatments if needed to assist with wound debridement. Keep the wound directly away from the water jets.	____	____	____	____________
9. Apply topical agents, if prescribed.				
a. Enzymes:				
(1) Using a wooden tongue blade, apply a small amount of enzyme debridement ointment directly to the necrotic areas on the base of pressure ulcer. Avoid getting the enzyme on the surrounding skin. Do not apply enzyme to surrounding skin.	____	____	____	____________

	S	U	NP	Comments
(2) Place gauze dressing directly over ulcer, and tape it in place. Follow specific manufacturer's recommendation for type of dressing material to use to cover a pressure ulcer when using enzymatic agent.	_____	_____	_____	_____
(3) If using an antibiotic solution, apply per order and cover with gauze pad.	_____	_____	_____	_____
b. Hydrogel agents:				
(1) Cover surface of ulcer with hydrogel using applicator or gloved hand.	_____	_____	_____	_____
(2) Apply a secondary dressing, such as dry gauze, hydrocolloid, or transparent dressing, over gel to completely cover ulcer.	_____	_____	_____	_____
c. Calcium alginates:				
(1) Pack wound with alginate using applicator or gloved hand.	_____	_____	_____	_____
(2) Apply a secondary dressing, such as dry gauze, foam, or hydrocolloid, over alginate.	_____	_____	_____	_____
10. Reposition patient comfortably off pressure ulcer.	_____	_____	_____	_____
11. Remove gloves, and dispose of soiled supplies. Perform hand hygiene.	_____	_____	_____	_____
Evaluation				
1. Observe skin surrounding ulcer for inflammation, edema, and tenderness.	_____	_____	_____	_____
2. Inspect dressings and exposed ulcers, observing for drainage, foul odor, and tissue necrosis. Monitor patient for signs and symptoms of infection, including fever and elevated white blood cell (WBC) count.	_____	_____	_____	_____
3. Compare subsequent ulcer measurements.	_____	_____	_____	_____
4. Use one of the scales designed to measure wound healing.	_____	_____	_____	_____
5. Record appearance of ulcer in patient's record.	_____	_____	_____	_____
6. Describe the type of topical agent used, dressing applied, and patient's response.	_____	_____	_____	_____
7. Report any deterioration in ulcer appearance.	_____	_____	_____	_____

Name ____________________ **Date** __________ **Instructor's Name** __________________________

Performance Checklist: Skill 35-3 Applying Dressings: Dry or Wet-to-Dry and Transparent

	S	U	NP	Comments
Assessment				
1. Assess size of wound to be dressed.	____	____	____	____________
2. Assess location of wound.				
3. Ask patient to rate pain using a scale of 0 to 10.	____	____	____	____________
4. Assess patient's knowledge of purpose of dressing change.	____	____	____	____________
5. Assess need and readiness for patient or family member to participate in dressing wound.	____	____	____	____________
6. Review medical orders for dressing change procedure.	____	____	____	____________
7. Identify patients with risk factors for wound-healing problems.	____	____	____	____________
Planning				
1. Explain procedure to patient.	____	____	____	____________
2. Position patient to allow access to area to be dressed.	____	____	____	____________
3. Plan dressing change to occur 30 minutes following administration of analgesic.	____	____	____	____________
Implementation				
1. Close room or cubicle curtains. Perform hand hygiene. Apply gown, goggles, and mask if risk of spray exists.	____	____	____	____________
2. Position patient comfortably and drape to expose only wound site. Instruct patient not to touch wound or sterile supplies.	____	____	____	____________
3. Place disposable bag within reach of work area. Fold top of bag to make cuff. Put on clean disposable gloves.	____	____	____	____________
4. Remove tape: pull parallel to skin, toward dressing, and hold down uninjured skin. If tape over hairy areas, remove in the direction of hair growth. Remove remaining adhesive from skin.	____	____	____	____________

	S	U	NP	Comments
5. With clean-gloved hand or forceps, remove dressings. Carefully remove outer secondary dressing first, and then remove inner primary dressing that is in contact with the wound bed. If drains are present, slowly and carefully remove dressings one layer at a time. Keep soiled undersurface from patient's sight.	_____	_____	_____	_____
6. Inspect wound for color, edema, drains, exudate, and integrity. Observe appearance of drainage on dressing. Assess for odor. Gently palpate the wound edges for drainage, bogginess, or patient report of increased pain. Measure wound size.	_____	_____	_____	_____
7. Describe the appearance of the wound and any indicators of wound healing to the patient.	_____	_____	_____	_____
8. Dispose of soiled dressings in disposable bag. Remove gloves by pulling them inside out. Dispose of gloves in bag. Perform hand hygiene.	_____	_____	_____	_____
9. Open sterile dressing tray or individually wrapped sterile supplies. Place on bedside table.	_____	_____	_____	_____
10. Open prescribed cleansing solution and pour over sterile gauze.	_____	_____	_____	_____
11. Put on gloves, clean or sterile depending on institution policy.	_____	_____	_____	_____
12. Cleanse wound:				
a. Use separate swab for each cleansing stroke, or spray wound surface.	_____	_____	_____	_____
b. Clean from least contaminated area to most contaminated.	_____	_____	_____	_____
c. Cleanse around the drain (if present), using circular stroke starting near drain and moving outward and away from the insertion site.	_____	_____	_____	_____
13. Use dry gauze to blot in same manner as in step 12 to dry wound.	_____	_____	_____	_____
14. Apply antiseptic ointment if ordered, using same technique as for cleansing.	_____	_____	_____	_____

	S	U	NP	Comments
15. Apply dressings to incision or wound site:	_____	_____	_____	_____
a. **Dry Dressing**				
(1) Apply loose woven gauze as contact layer.	_____	_____	_____	_____
(2) Cut 4 × 4 gauze flat to fit around drain if present or use precut split gauze.	_____	_____	_____	_____
(3) Apply additional layers of gauze as needed.	_____	_____	_____	_____
(4) Apply thicker woven pad (e.g., abdominal dressing or large woven pad).	_____	_____	_____	_____
b. **Wet-to-Dry Dressing**				
(1) Place fine mesh gauze in container of sterile solution.	_____	_____	_____	_____
(2) Wring out excess fluid and apply moist fluffed woven-mesh gauze or packing strip directly onto wound surface without having the gauze touch the surrounding skin.	_____	_____	_____	_____
(3) Make sure any dead space from sinus tracts, undermining, or tunneling is loosely packed with gauze.	_____	_____	_____	_____
(4) Apply dry sterile gauze over wet gauze.	_____	_____	_____	_____
(5) Cover the packed wound with a secondary dressing such as an ABD pad, abdominal dressing, or large woven pad.	_____	_____	_____	_____
c. **Transparent Dressing**				
(1) Apply dressing according to manufacturer's direction. Do not stretch film during application. Avoid wrinkles in film.	_____	_____	_____	_____
16. Secure dressing with roll gauze, tape, Montgomery ties or straps, or binder.	_____	_____	_____	_____
17. Remove gloves and gown if worn, and dispose of them in bag. Dispose of all supplies. Remove goggles if worn.	_____	_____	_____	_____
18. Assist patient to comfortable position.	_____	_____	_____	_____
19. Perform hand hygiene.	_____	_____	_____	_____

	S	U	NP	Comments
Evaluation				
1. Inspect condition of wound and presence of any drainage.	_____	_____	_____	____________________
2. Ask if patient had pain during procedure.	_____	_____	_____	____________________
3. Inspect condition of dressing at least every shift.	_____	_____	_____	____________________
4. Ask patient to describe steps and techniques of dressing change.	_____	_____	_____	____________________
5. Record appearance of wound; color, presence, and characteristics of exudate; change in wound characteristics (especially drainage amount); type and amount of dressings applied; and tolerance of patient to dressing change.	_____	_____	_____	____________________
6. Report unexpected appearance of wound drainage or accidental removal of drain, bright red bleeding, or evidence of wound dehiscence or evisceration.	_____	_____	_____	____________________
7. Write your initials, date, and time of dressing change on a piece of tape in ink (not marker) and place on dressing.	_____	_____	_____	____________________

Name ____________________ Date __________ Instructor's Name ____________________

Performance Checklist: Skill 35-4 Wound Vacuum Assisted Closure

	S	U	NP	Comments
Assessment				
1. Assess location, appearance, and size of wound to be dressed.	____	____	____	____________
2. Review physician's or health care provider's orders for frequency of dressing change, type of foam to use, and amount of negative pressure to be used.	____	____	____	____________
3. Assess patient's level of comfort using a scale of 0 to 10.	____	____	____	____________
4. Assess patient's and family member's knowledge of purpose of dressing.	____	____	____	____________
Planning				
1. Collect appropriate equipment.	____	____	____	____________
2. Explain procedure to patient.	____	____	____	____________
3. Position patient to allow access to dressing site.	____	____	____	____________
Implementation				
1. Close room door or cubicle curtains.	____	____	____	____________
2. Position patient, expose wound site, and cover patient.	____	____	____	____________
3. Cuff top of disposable waterproof bag, and place within reach of work area.	____	____	____	____________
4. Perform hand hygiene, and put on clean disposable gloves. If risk of spray exists, apply protective gown, goggles, and mask.	____	____	____	____________
5. Push therapy on/off button on V.A.C.®	____	____	____	____________
6. Raise the tubing connectors above the level of the V.A.C.® System, and disconnect tubes from each other to drain fluids into canister. Before lowering, tighten clamp on canister tube.	____	____	____	____________
7. With dressing tube unclamped, introduce 10 to 30 ml of normal saline, if ordered, into tubing to soak underneath foam. Let set for 15 to 30 minutes.	____	____	____	____________
8. Gently stretch transparent film horizontally, and slowly pull up from the skin.	____	____	____	____________
9. Remove old V.A.C.® dressing, observing appearance and drainage on dressing. Use caution to remove dressing around drains. Dispose of soiled dressings in waterproof bag. Remove gloves by pulling	____	____	____	____________

	S	U	NP	Comments
them inside out, and dispose of them in waterproof bag. Avoid having patient see old dressing because the site of wound drainage may be upsetting to the patient. Perform hand hygiene.				
10. Apply sterile or clean gloves. Irrigate the wound with normal saline or other solution ordered by the physician. Gently blot to dry.	_____	_____	_____	____________________
11. Measure wound as ordered: at baseline, first dressing change, weekly, and discharge from therapy. Remove and discard gloves. Perform hand hygiene.	_____	_____	_____	____________________
12. Depending on the type of wound, apply sterile or new clean gloves.	_____	_____	_____	____________________
13. Select appropriate foam dressing depending on wound type and stage of healing. Use sterile scissors to cut foam to exact wound size, making sure to fit the size and shape of the wound, including tunnels and undermined areas.	_____	_____	_____	____________________
14. Gently place foam in wound, making sure that the foam is in contact with entire wound (base, margins, and tunneled and undermined areas)	_____	_____	_____	____________________
15. Apply tubing to foam in the wound.	_____	_____	_____	____________________
16. Apply skin protectant, such as skin prep or Stomahesive wafer, to skin around the wound.	_____	_____	_____	____________________
17. Apply V.A.C.® transparent dressing, covering the V.A.C.® foam and 3 to 5 cm of surrounding healthy tissue. Make sure transparent dressing is wrinkle-free. Secure tubing to transparent film, aligning drainage hole to ensure an occlusive seal. Be careful not to apply tension to drape and tubing.	_____	_____	_____	____________________
18. Secure tubing several centimeters away from the dressing.	_____	_____	_____	____________________
19. After the wound is completely covered, connect the tubing from the dressing to the tubing from the canister and V.A.C.® System.				
a. Remove canister from sterile packaging and push into V.A.C.® System until a click is heard. **An alarm will sound if the canister is not properly engaged.**	_____	_____	_____	____________________

	S	U	NP	Comments
b. Connect the dressing tubing to the canister tubing. Make sure both clamps are open.	_____	_____	_____	__________________________
c. Place V.A.C. unit on a level surface or hang from the foot of the bed. **The V.A.C.® System will sound an alarm and deactivate therapy if the unit is tilted beyond 45 degrees.**	_____	_____	_____	__________________________
d. Press green power button and set pressure as ordered.	_____	_____	_____	__________________________
20. Discard soiled dressing change materials properly. Perform hand hygiene.	_____	_____	_____	__________________________
21. Inspect V.A.C.® System to verify that negative pressure is achieved.				
a. Verify that display screen reads THERAPY ON.	_____	_____	_____	__________________________
b. Be sure clamps are open and tubing is patent.	_____	_____	_____	__________________________
c. Identify air leaks by listening with stethoscope or by moving hand around edges of wound while applying light pressure.	_____	_____	_____	__________________________
d. If a leak is present, use strips of transparent film to patch areas around the edges of the wound.	_____	_____	_____	__________________________
22. Assist patient to a comfortable position.	_____	_____	_____	__________________________
Evaluation				
1. Inspect condition of wound on ongoing basis; note drainage and odor.	_____	_____	_____	__________________________
2. Ask patient to rate pain using a scale of 0 to 10.	_____	_____	_____	__________________________
3. Verify airtight dressing seal and correct negative pressure setting.	_____	_____	_____	__________________________
4. Observe patient's or family member's ability to perform dressing change.	_____	_____	_____	__________________________
5. Record wound appearance, color and characteristics of any drainage, presence of wound healing, and patient tolerance to procedure. Record date and time of new dressing on the dressing as per agency policy.	_____	_____	_____	__________________________
6. Report any brisk, bright red bleeding; evidence of poor wound healing; evisceration or dehiscence; and possible wound infection.	_____	_____	_____	__________________________

Name ____________________ Date __________ Instructor's Name ________________________

Performance Checklist: Skill 35-5 Performing Wound Irrigation

	S	U	NP	Comments
Assessment				
1. Review physician's or health care provider's order for irrigation of open wound and type of solution to be used.	____	____	____	____________
2. Assess recently recording of signs and symptoms assessments related to patient's open wound:	____	____	____	____________
a. Extent of impairment of skin integrity, including size of wound	____	____	____	____________
b. Elevation of body temperature	____	____	____	____________
c. Drainage from wound (amount, color, and consistency) Amount can be measured by part of dressing saturated or in terms of quantity.	____	____	____	____________
d. Odor	____	____	____	____________
e. Wound color	____	____	____	____________
f. Consistency of drainage	____	____	____	____________
g. Culture report	____	____	____	____________
h. Stage of healing of the patient's wound	____	____	____	____________
i. Dressing: dry and clean, evidence of bleeding, profuse drainage	____	____	____	____________
3. Assess comfort level or pain on a scale of 0 to 10, and identify symptoms of anxiety.	____	____	____	____________
4. Assess patient for history of allergies to antiseptics, tapes, or dressing material.	____	____	____	____________
Planning				
1. Explain procedure of wound irrigation and cleansing.	____	____	____	____________
2. Administer prescribed anesthetic 30 to 45 minutes before starting wound irrigation procedure.	____	____	____	____________
3. Position patient.				
a. Position patient comfortably to permit gravitational flow of irrigating solution through wound and into collection receptable.	____	____	____	____________
b. Position patient so that wound is vertical to collection basin.	____	____	____	____________
c. Place padding or extra towels.	____	____	____	____________
d. Expose wound only.	____	____	____	____________

	S	U	NP	Comments
Implementation				
1. Perform hand hygiene.	_____	_____	_____	_____
2. Form cuff on waterproof bag, and place it near bed.	_____	_____	_____	_____
3. Close room door or bed curtains.	_____	_____	_____	_____
4. Apply gown and goggles if needed.	_____	_____	_____	_____
5. Apply clean gloves, remove soiled dressing, and discard dressing in waterproof bag. Discard gloves.	_____	_____	_____	_____
6. Prepare equipment; open sterile supplies.	_____	_____	_____	_____
7. Apply sterile gloves.	_____	_____	_____	_____
8. To irrigate wound with wide opening:				
a. Fill 35-ml syringe with irrigation solution.	_____	_____	_____	_____
b. Attach 19-gauge needle or angiographic catheter.	_____	_____	_____	_____
c. Hold syringe tip 2.5 cm (1 inch) above upper end of wound and over area being cleansed.	_____	_____	_____	_____
d. Using continuous pressure, flush wound; repeat steps 9a through 8c until solution draining into basin is clear.	_____	_____	_____	_____
9. To irrigate deep wound with minimal pressure:				
a. Attach soft angiographic catheter to piston syringe filled with irrigation solution.	_____	_____	_____	_____
b. Lubricate tip of catheter with irrigating solution and gently insert tip of catheter.	_____	_____	_____	_____
c. Using slow, continuous pressure, flush wound.	_____	_____	_____	_____
d. Refill syringe, and repeat until solution draining into basin is clear.	_____	_____	_____	_____
10. When indicated, obtain cultures after cleansing with nonbacteriostatic saline.	_____	_____	_____	_____
11. Dry wound edges with gauze; dry patient if shower or whirlpool is used.	_____	_____	_____	_____
12. Apply appropriate dressing.	_____	_____	_____	_____
13. Remove gloves, mask, goggles, and gown.	_____	_____	_____	_____
14. Assist patient to comfortable position.	_____	_____	_____	_____
15. Dispose of equipment and soiled supplies, and perform hand hygiene.	_____	_____	_____	_____

	S	U	NP	Comments
Evaluation				
1. Observe type of tissue in wound bed.	_____	_____	_____	_____
2. Inspect dressing periodically.	_____	_____	_____	_____
3. Evaluate skin integrity.	_____	_____	_____	_____
4. Observe patient for signs of discomfort.	_____	_____	_____	_____
5. Observe for presence of retained irrigant.	_____	_____	_____	_____
6. Record wound irrigation and patient response on progress notes.	_____	_____	_____	_____
7. Immediately report to attending physician any evidence of fresh bleeding, sharp increase in pain, retention of irrigant, or signs of shock.	_____	_____	_____	_____

Name ____________________ Date __________ Instructor's Name ____________________

Procedural Guidelines 35-1 Applying Abdominal or Breast Binders

	S	U	NP	Comments
1. Observe patient with need for support of thorax or abdomen. Observe ability to breathe deeply and cough effectively.	____	____	____	____________
2. Review medical record if medical prescription for particular binder is necessary and evaluate reasons for application.	____	____	____	____________
3. Inspect skin for actual or potential alterations in integrity. Observe for irritation, abrasion, skin surfaces that rub against each other, or allergic response to adhesive tape used to secure dressing.	____	____	____	____________
4. Inspect any surgical dressing.	____	____	____	____________
5. Assess patient's comfort level using analog scale of 0 to 10 (see Chapter 30) and noting any objective signs and symptoms.	____	____	____	____________
6. Gather necessary data regarding size of patient and appropriate binder.	____	____	____	____________
7. Explain procedure to patient.	____	____	____	____________
8. Perform hand hygiene, and apply gloves (if likely to contact wound drainage).	____	____	____	____________
9. Close curtains or room door.	____	____	____	____________
10. Apply binder.				
a. Abdominal binder:				
(1) Position patient in supine position with head slightly elevated and knees slightly flexed.	____	____	____	____________
(2) Fanfold far side of binder toward midline of binder.	____	____	____	____________
(3) Instruct and assist patient in rolling away from you toward raised side rail while firmly supporting abdominal incision and dressing with hands.	____	____	____	____________
(4) Place fanfolded ends of binder under patient.	____	____	____	____________
(5) Instruct or assist patient in rolling over folded ends toward you.	____	____	____	____________
(6) Unfold and stretch ends out smoothly on far side of bed.	____	____	____	____________

	S	U	NP	Comments
(7) Instruct patient to roll back into supine position.	_____	_____	_____	_____
(8) Adjust binder so that supine patient is centered over binder using symphysis pubis and costal margins as lower and upper landmarks, respectively.	_____	_____	_____	_____
(9) Close binder. Pull one end of binder over center of patient's abdomen. While maintaining tension on that end of binder, pull opposite end of binder over center and secure with Velcro closure tabs, metal fasteners, or horizontally placed safety pins.	_____	_____	_____	_____
(10) Assess patient's comfort level.	_____	_____	_____	_____
(11) Adjust binder as necessary.	_____	_____	_____	_____
b. Breast binder:				
(1) Assist patient in placing arms through binder's armholes.	_____	_____	_____	_____
(2) Assist patient to supine position in bed.	_____	_____	_____	_____
(3) Pad area under breasts if necessary.	_____	_____	_____	_____
(4) Using Velcro closure tabs or horizontally placed safety pins, secure binder at nipple level first. Continue closure process above and then below nipple line until entire binder is closed.	_____	_____	_____	_____
(5) Make appropriate adjustments, including individualizing fit of shoulder straps and pinning waistline darts to reduce binder size.	_____	_____	_____	_____
(6) Instruct and observe skill development in self-care related to reapplying breast binder.	_____	_____	_____	_____
11. Remove gloves, and perform hand hygiene.	_____	_____	_____	_____
12. Observe site for skin integrity, circulation, and characteristics of the wound.	_____	_____	_____	_____

	S	U	NP	Comments
13. Assess comfort level of patient using analog scale of 0 to 10 and noting any objective signs and symptoms.	_____	_____	_____	_____________________
14. Assess patient's ability to ventilate properly, including deep breathing and coughing.	_____	_____	_____	_____________________

Name ____________________ Date __________ Instructor's Name ____________________

Procedural Guidelines 35-2 Applying Elastic Bandages

	S	U	NP	Comments
1. Review patient's medical record and order for application of elastic bandage.	_____	_____	_____	____________________
2. Inspect areas to be bandaged for				
a. Intact skin	_____	_____	_____	____________________
b. Abrasions	_____	_____	_____	____________________
c. Draining wounds	_____	_____	_____	____________________
d. Skin discoloration	_____	_____	_____	____________________
3. Note circulation to the area requiring an elastic bandage.				
a. Palpate skin, noting temperature, color.	_____	_____	_____	____________________
b. Palpate pulse, noting pulse quality.	_____	_____	_____	____________________
c. Observe extremity for edema or dehydration.	_____	_____	_____	____________________
4. Determine level of function of affected extremity.	_____	_____	_____	____________________
5. Assess level of pain severity to area (scale 9 to 10).	_____	_____	_____	____________________
6. Explain procedure to patient.	_____	_____	_____	____________________
7. Perform hand hygiene, and apply gloves, if indicated.	_____	_____	_____	____________________
8. Close curtains or room door.	_____	_____	_____	____________________
9. Hold roll of elastic bandage in dominant hand, and use other hand to tightly hold the beginning of bandage at distal body part.	_____	_____	_____	____________________
10. Apply bandage from distal point toward proximal boundary, stretching the bandage slightly, using a variety of bandage turns to cover various body shapes. Prevent uneven bandage tension or circulatory impairment by overlapping turns by one-half to two-thirds width of bandage roll. NOTE: Be sure bandage is smooth (without creases).	_____	_____	_____	____________________
11. Secure each roll with clip or tape before applying additional roll(s).	_____	_____	_____	____________________
12. When finished with application, secure last elastic roll with clip, adhesive tape, or mesh to prevent wrap from becoming dislodged and thus decreasing extremity support.	_____	_____	_____	____________________
13. Remove gloves, and perform hand hygiene.	_____	_____	_____	____________________

	S	U	NP	Comments
14. Evaluate circulation to bandaged area every 4 hours.				
a. Palpate distal pulse.	_____	_____	_____	____________________
b. Palpate skin, noting temperature every 4 hours.	_____	_____	_____	____________________
c. Observe skin color.	_____	_____	_____	____________________
15. Determine patient's level of comfort, using analog scale of 0 to 10 and noting any objective signs and symptoms.	_____	_____	_____	____________________
16. Observe for changes from baseline assessment in level of extremity function.	_____	_____	_____	____________________

Sensory Alterations 36

Case Studies

1. You are making a home visit to a patient with diabetes mellitus who is losing his eyesight (diabetic retinopathy).
   a. What interventions may be implemented with the patient to assist in maintaining adequate sensory stimulation and personal safety?

2. You have been assigned to care for a patient in the intensive care unit (ICU).
   a. What sensory alterations may this patient experience, and how can you prevent their occurrence?

Chapter Review

Complete the following:

1. Identify other terms for the following:
   a. Sight: _______
   b. Hearing: _______
   c. Taste: _______
   d. Smell: _______
   e. Touch: _______
   f. Position sense: _______
2. Identify one of the major diseases that can lead to visual impairment:
3. Identify at least one factor that can lead to each of the following:
   a. Sensory deprivation:
   b. Sensory overload:
4. Provide the correct term for the following:
   a. A buildup of ear wax in the external auditory canal:
   b. Hearing loss associated with aging:
   c. Opacity of the lens resulting in blurred vision:
   d. Decreased salivary production/dry mouth:
   e. Intermittent hearing loss, vertigo, tinnitus, and pressure in the ears:
5. Identify how the following factors may influence sensory function:
   a. Age—older adulthood:
   b. Medications:
   c. Smoking:
   d. Environment:

6. Identify a way that the nurse can evaluate the patient's vision and hearing during routine interactions or care:

7. A common cause of blindness in children is:

Identify an area that should be included when teaching parents about eyesight safety:

8. A common cause of hearing impairment in children is:

9. Identify a way that the nurse can modify sensory stimulation in the health care environment:

10. The nurse may communicate with a hearing-impaired patient by:

11. Provide an example of a drug that may cause ototoxicity in patients:

12. Identify how the nurse may assist patients with the following deficits to adapt their home environments for safety:
   a. Hearing deficit:

   b. Diminished sense of smell:

   c. Diminished sense of touch:

13. Identify a nursing diagnosis that may be formulated for a patient with a sensory deficit:

14. Provide an example of a general screening that is conducted to determine visual and/or auditory deficits:

15. Select all of the following that are appropriate in promoting sensory stimulation in the home environment:
   a. Reducing glare by using sheer curtains on windows _______
   b. Using pale colors on surfaces _______
   c. Serving bland foods with similar textures _______
   d. Using a pocket magnifier _______
   e. Introducing fragrant flowers _______
   f. Playing recorded music with high-frequency sound _______

Select the best answer for each of the following questions:

16. An expected outcome for a patient with an auditory deficit should include:
   1. Minimizing use of affected sense(s)
   2. Preventing additional sensory losses
   3. Promoting the patient's acceptance of dependency
   4. Controlling the environment to reduce sensory stimuli
17. The nurse is working with patients at the senior day care center and recognizes that changes in sensory status may influence the older adult's eating patterns. For patients who are experiencing changes in their dietary intake, the nurse will assess for:
   1. Presbycusis
   2. Xerostomia
   3. Vestibular ataxia
   4. Peripheral neuropathy
18. Parents arrive at the pediatric clinic with their 1½-year-old child. The parents ask the nurse if there are signs that may indicate that the child is not able to hear

well. The nurse explains to the parents that they should be alert to the child:
1. Awakening to loud noises
2. Responding reflexively to sounds
3. Having delayed speech development
4. Remaining calm when unfamiliar people approach

19. The nurse is assessing the patient for a potential gustatory impairment. This may be indicated if the patient has a(n):
1. Weight loss
2. Blank look or stare
3. Increased sensitivity to odors
4. Period of excessive clumsiness or dizziness

20. A patient has come to the local walk-in emergency center with flu-like symptoms. After seeing the physician, the patient shows the nurse the prescriptions the physician has written. The patient should be informed that ototoxicity may occur with the administration of:
1. Vitamin C
2. Acetaminophen
3. Erythromycin
4. Cough suppressant with codeine

21. A responsive patient has had eye surgery, and patches have been temporarily placed on both eyes for protection. The evening meal has arrived, and the nurse will be assisting the patient. In this circumstance, the nurse should:
1. Feed the patient the entire meal
2. Encourage family members to feed the patient
3. Allow the patient to be totally independent and feed himself
4. Orient the patient to the locations of the foods on the plate and provide the utensils

22. Following a CVA (cerebral vascular accident/stroke), the patient is found to have receptive aphasia. The nurse may assist this patient with communication by:
1. Obtaining a referral for a speech therapist
2. Using a system of simple gestures and repeated behaviors
3. Providing the patient with a letter chart to use to answer questions
4. Offering the patient a notepad and pen to write down questions and concerns

23. A mother is bringing in her newborn for his first physical examination. She expresses concern because during her pregnancy she may have been exposed to an infectious disease, and the baby's hearing could be affected. The nurse inquires if the patient was exposed to:
1. Rubella
2. Pneumonia
3. Excessive oxygen
4. A urinary tract infection

24. For a patient with a hearing deficit, the best way for the nurse to communicate is to:
1. Approach the patient from the side
2. Use visible facial expressions
3. Shout or speak very loudly to the patient
4. Repeat the entire conversation if it is not totally understood

Study Group Questions

- What are the human senses and their functions?
- What factors influence sensory function?
- What are some common sensory alterations?
- What types of patients are at risk for developing sensory alterations?
- How should the nurse assess a patient's sensory function?
- What behaviors or changes in lifestyle patterns or socialization may indicate a sensory alteration?
- How can the nurse promote sensory function and prevent injury and isolation in the health promotion and acute and restorative care settings?
- What screening processes are used to determine the presence of sensory alterations?
- How may the family/significant others be involved in the care of the patient with a sensory alteration?
- What information should be included in patient/family teaching for promotion of sensory function and prevention of injury?

37 Surgical Patient

Case Studies

1. Your patient is scheduled to have extensive abdominal surgery with a large, midline incision.
   a. How can you assist this patient to promote respiratory function postoperatively?
2. A patient is having outpatient surgery.
   a. How may preoperative teaching be conducted?
3. While completing the preoperative checklist, the nurse discovers that the patient's temperature is 101° F.
   a. What should the nurse do?
4. Your patient insists that his good luck medallion must go with him everywhere, even to surgery.
   a. What should you do?

Chapter Review

Match the description/definition in Column A with the correct term in Column B.

	Column A	Column B
________	1. Performed on the basis of the patient's choice; not essential for health	a. Palliative surgery
________	2. Involves extensive reconstruction or alteration in body parts; poses risks to well-being	b. Transplant surgery
________	3. Relieves or reduces intensity of disease symptoms; will not produce cure	c. Major surgery
________	4. Must be done immediately to save life or preserve function of body part	d. Ablative surgery
________	5. Surgical exploration that allows physician to confirm medical status; may involve removal of body tissue for analysis	e. Cosmetic surgery
________	6. Performed to improve personal appearance	f. Emergency surgery
________	7. Amputation or removal of diseased body part	g. Elective surgery
________	8. Performed to replace malfunctioning organs or structures	h. Diagnostic surgery

Complete the following:

9. The patient who smokes cigarettes is at a greater risk for:

   Postoperative care for this patient will require more aggressive:

10. Identify a medical condition that may increase the patient's surgical risk:

11. Identify an example of how changes in each of the following body systems place the older adult patient at risk during surgery:
    a. Cardiovascular:

b. Pulmonary:

c. Renal:

d. Neurological:

12. Obesity places a patient at greater risk for surgery as a result of:

13. Identify a consideration for surgical patients who are taking the following medications:
    a. Insulin:

    b. Antibiotics:

    c. NSAIDs:

14. Provide two examples of information that is usually included in preoperative teaching:

15. Identify a routine screening test that may be ordered for a patient preoperatively:

16. Identify the commonly used types of preoperative medications:

17. Identify two nursing diagnoses that may be formulated for a patient who will be having his or her first surgery:

18. The patient is going to receive general anesthesia for the surgical procedure. Specify the general NPO criteria for the following:
    a. No food or fluids _____ hours before surgery
    b. No meat or fried foods _____ hours before surgery

19. Identify the adverse effects associated with the following types of anesthesia:
    a. General anesthesia:

    b. Regional anesthesia:

    c. Local anesthesia:

    d. Conscious sedation:

20. Select all of the following preoperative interventions that are appropriate:
    a. Completing bowel preparation before GI surgery _______
    b. Shaving the surgical site with a razor _______
    c. Providing antimicrobial soap for bathing _______
    d. Removing the patient's wig _______
    e. Leaving artificial fingernails intact _______
    f. Removing a hearing aid when the patient gets to the OR _______

21. In the presurgical care unit (PSCU), verification is done to determine:

22. Identify which of the following tasks are responsibilities of the circulating nurse (C) or scrub nurse (S):
    a. Completion of preoperative assessments/verification _______
    b. Application of sterile drapes _______
    c. Establishment of the intraoperative plan of care _______

d. Calculation of blood loss and urinary output _______
e. Provision of sterile equipment for the surgeon _______
f. Documentation of the procedure _______
g. Maintenance of the sterile field _______

23. For the following, identify a nursing intervention for intraoperative patient care:
  a. Prevention of injury:
  b. Maintenance of patient's body temperature:
  c. Prevention of infection:

24. Identify a specific nursing intervention to prevent the following postoperative complications:
  a. Pulmonary stasis:
  b. Venous stasis:
  c. Wound infection:

25. Select the assessment findings for a patient in the postanesthesia care unit (PACU) that signify the patient is qualified to be discharged from the unit:
  a. Oxygen saturation 96% _______
  b. Rales on auscultation _______
  c. Pulse rate 110 beats per minute _______
  d. Bilateral peripheral pulses _______
  e. Abdominal distention _______
  f. Response to verbal stimuli _______
  g. Sluggish hand grasp and pupillary response _______
  h. Quarter-size sanguineous spot maintained on incisional dressing _______
  i. 30 ml/hour urinary output _______

26. The nurse is aware that the patient should void within _____ hours after surgery.

27. Following general anesthesia, postoperative oral intake usually begins with an order for _______________________ (diet).

28. With regard to postoperative wound healing and care, select all of the following statements that are correct:
  a. The surgical dressing is changed after the patient leaves the PACU. _______
  b. Any visible drainage on the surgical dressing should be marked. _______
  c. The patient who has an order for an oral analgesic should be medicated 20 minutes before an uncomfortable dressing change. _______
  d. Redness, warmth, and edema should be expected at the incision site. _______
  e. Wound drainage should be measured once a day. _______
  f. The patient should be draped during a dressing change to minimize exposure. _______

29. The patient in the illustration is demonstrating the use of a(n):

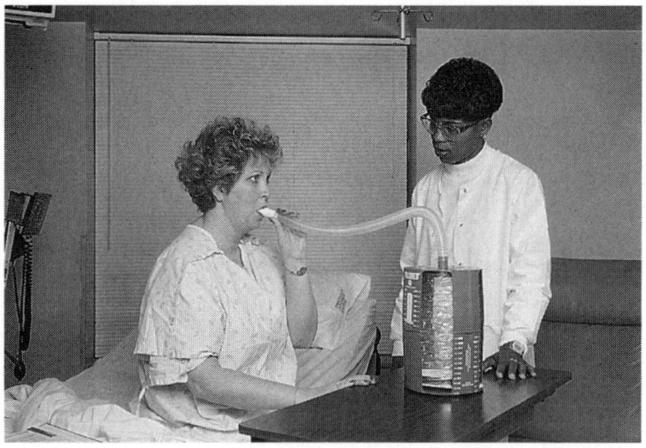

Select the best answer for each of the following questions:

30. The nurse is starting the preparations for the patient who is having surgery tomorrow morning. The nurse prepares to have the consent form completed. The nurse recognizes that informed consent:
    1. Is valid if the patient is disoriented
    2. Is signed by the patient after the administration of preoperative medications
    3. Indicates that the patient is aware of the procedure and its possible complications
    4. Requires that the nurse provide information about the surgery before the consent can by signed
31. The patient is brought to PACU after surgery. The nurse is assessing the patient and is alert to the indication of a postoperative hemorrhage if the patient exhibits:
    1. Restlessness
    2. Warm, dry skin
    3. A slow, steady pulse rate
    4. A decreased respiratory rate
32. The nurse is checking the vital signs of the patient who had major surgery yesterday. The nurse discovers that the patient's temperature is slightly elevated. This finding is usually indicative of:
    1. A postoperative wound infection
    2. An allergic response to latex
    3. A response to the anesthesia
    4. Extensive neural damage
33. The nurse is completing the preoperative checklist for a female patient who will be having surgery. The nurse determines that the surgeon and anesthesiologist should be informed of which of the patient's laboratory results?
    1. Hemoglobin level—10 g/dl
    2. Potassium level—4.2 mEq/L
    3. Platelet count—210,000/mm^3
    4. Prothrombin time (PT)—11 seconds
34. The patient has received a spinal anesthetic during the surgical procedure. The nurse is alert to possible complications of the anesthetic and is assessing the patient for a:
    1. Rash
    2. Headache
    3. Nephrotoxic response
    4. Hyperthermic response
35. The patient is being evaluated for transfer from the PACU to the patient's unit. The nurse determines that the patient will be approved for transfer if the patient exhibits:
    1. Increased wound drainage
    2. Pulse oximetry of 95%
    3. Respirations of 30 breaths per minute
    4. Nonpalpable peripheral pulses
36. The patient is scheduled to have abdominal surgery later this morning. At 9:00 AM, while completing the preoperative checklist, the nurse recognizes the need to contact the surgeon immediately. The nurse has identified that the patient:
    1. Received an enema at 6:00 AM
    2. Admitted to recent substance abuse
    3. Ate a hamburger last evening at 6:00 PM
    4. Has bowel sounds in all four quadrants of the abdomen
37. The patient is being positioned in the PACU after surgery. Unless contraindicated, the nurse should place the patient:
    1. Prone
    2. In high Fowler's
    3. Supine with arms across the chest
    4. On the side with the face turned downward
38. When the patient first arrives at PACU, there are general nursing measures that are implemented. The nurse will:
    1. Provide oral fluids
    2. Allow the patient to sleep
    3. Provide a warm blanket
    4. Remove the urinary catheter
39. The nurse is visiting the patient who had surgery 9 hours ago. The nurse asks if the patient has voided, and the patient

responds negatively. At this time, the nurse:
1. Provides more oral fluids
2. Inserts an IV and administers fluids
3. Obtains an order for urinary catheterization
4. Recognizes that this is a normal outcome

40. During a patient assessment in the PACU, the nurse finds that the patient's operative site is swollen and appears tight. The nurse suspects:
    1. Infection
    2. Hemorrhage
    3. Lymphedema
    4. Subcutaneous emphysema
41. An immediate postoperative priority in providing nursing care for the patient is:
    1. Airway patency
    2. Relief of pain
    3. Sufficient circulation to the extremities
    4. Prevention of wound infection
42. A 54-year-old patient is scheduled to have a gastric resection. The nurse informs the surgeon preoperatively of the patient's history of:
    1. A tonsillectomy at age 10
    2. Employment as a telephone repair person
    3. Smoking two packs of cigarettes per day
    4. Taking acetaminophen for minor body aches
43. The patient has been taking Coumadin (warfarin) at home. The patient is going to be admitted for a surgical procedure, and the nurse anticipates that this prescribed medication will be:
    1. Administered as usual
    2. Increased in dose immediately before the procedure
    3. Reduced in dose by half immediately before the procedure
    4. Discontinued at least 2 days before the procedure
44. During the intraoperative phase, the nurse's responsibility is reflected in the statement:
    1. "I think that the patient requires more information about the procedure and its consequences."
    2. "There seems to be a missing sponge, so a recount must be done to see that all of the sponges were removed."
    3. "The patient has signed the request. I will prepare the medications and then get the record completed."
    4. "The patient appears reactive and stable. Dressing to wound is dry and intact. Analgesic administered per order."
45. The nurse is assisting the patient with postoperative exercises. The patient tells the nurse, "Blowing into this thing (incentive spirometer) is a waste of time." The nurse explains to the patient that the specific purpose of this therapy is to:
    1. Stimulate the cough reflex
    2. Promote lung expansion
    3. Increase pulmonary circulation
    4. Directly remove excess secretions from the respiratory tract
46. The patient is scheduled for surgery, and the nurse is completing the final areas of the preoperative checklist. After administering the preoperative medications, the nurse should:
    1. Assist the patient to void
    2. Obtain the informed consent
    3. Prepare the skin at the surgical site
    4. Place the side rails up on the bed or stretcher
47. At the ambulatory surgery center, a patient is having surgery using general anesthesia. The nurse will expect this patient to:
    1. Ambulate immediately after being admitted to the recovery area
    2. Meet all of the identified criteria in order to be discharged home
    3. Remain in the phase I recovery area longer than a hospitalized patient
    4. Receive large amounts of oral fluids immediately upon entering the recovery area
48. The nurse is preparing a patient for surgery and recognizes that the greatest risk of bleeding is for the patient with:
    1. Diabetes mellitus

2. Emphysema
3. Thrombocytopenia
4. Immunodeficiency syndrome

49. The patient has a nasogastric tube in place following surgery and complains to the nurse of nausea. The nurse should:
   1. Remove the NG tube
   2. Provide oral fluids
   3. Move the patient side to side
   4. Irrigate the tube with normal saline

Study Group Questions

- How are surgeries classified?
- What are some surgical risk factors and why do they increase the patient's risk?
- How does the incision site influence a patient's recovery?
- How may prior surgical experiences influence the patient's expectations of surgery?
- What general information should be included in preoperative teaching?
- What is the purpose of the preoperative exercises that are explained and demonstrated to patients?
- What preoperative assessments should be made by the nurse?
- What are some common preoperative diagnostic tests that may be ordered for the patient?
- What nursing interventions are implemented in the preoperative care of patients?
- How does the nurse prepare and assist the patient in the acute care setting on the day of surgery?
- What are the roles of nurses in the operating room and in the recovery setting?
- What interventions are implemented to maintain patient safety and well-being in the operating room and postanesthesia care area?
- What nursing care is critical in the immediate postoperative stage?
- What are the similarities and differences between preanesthesia and postanesthesia care for patients in the acute care and ambulatory surgery settings?
- What general information should be included in postoperative teaching for patients/families in the acute care and ambulatory surgery settings?
- How may the family/significant others be involved in the patient's perioperative experience?

Study Chart

Create a study chart on Surgical Risk Factors, *identifying how age, nutritional status, obesity, immunocompetence, fluid/electrolyte balance, and pregnancy may affect the patient's perioperative experience.*

Name ____________________ **Date** __________ **Instructor's Name** __________________________

Performance Checklist: Skill 37-1 Teaching Postoperative Exercises

	S	U	NP	Comments
Assessment				
1. Assess patient's risk for postoperative respiratory complications.	_____	_____	_____	__________________________
2. Auscultate lungs.				
3. Assess patient's ability to cough and deep breathe by having patient take a deep breath and observing movement of shoulders, chest wall, and abdomen. Measure chest excursion during a deep breath. Ask patient to cough after taking a deep breath.	_____	_____	_____	__________________________
3. Assess patient's risk for postoperative thrombus formation. Observe for a positive Homans' sign by monitoring calf pain when dorsiflexing the patient's foot with the knee flexed. Observe for calf pain, redness, swelling, or vein distention, usually unilaterally.	_____	_____	_____	__________________________
4. Assess patient's ability to move independently while in bed.	_____	_____	_____	__________________________
5. Assess patient's willingness and capability to learn exercises.	_____	_____	_____	__________________________
6. Assess family members' or significant others' willingness to learn and to support patient postoperatively.	_____	_____	_____	__________________________
7. Assess patient's medical orders preoperatively and postoperatively.	_____	_____	_____	__________________________
Planning				
1. Prepare equipment.	_____	_____	_____	__________________________
2. Plan teaching sessions.	_____	_____	_____	__________________________
3. Explain importance of exercises.	_____	_____	_____	__________________________
4. Prepare room for teaching.	_____	_____	_____	__________________________
Implementation				
1. Teach importance of postoperative exercises to recovery and physiological benefits.	_____	_____	_____	__________________________
A. Diaphragmatic Breathing				
(1) Assist patient to a comfortable sitting or standing position with knees flexed. If patient chooses to sit, raise the head of bed to semi-Fowler's or Fowler's position, assist to side of bed or to upright position in chair.	_____	_____	_____	__________________________

	S	U	NP	Comments
(2) Stand or sit, facing patient.	_____	_____	_____	_____
(3) Instruct patient to place palms of hands across from each other, down, and along lower borders of anterior rib cage; place tips of third fingers lightly together. Demonstrate for patient.	_____	_____	_____	_____
(4) Have patient take slow, deep breaths, inhaling through nose and pushing abdomen against hands. Tell patient to feel middle fingers separate as patient inhales. Explain that patient will feel normal downward movement of diaphragm during inspiration.	_____	_____	_____	_____
(5) Explain that abdominal organs descend and chest wall expands. Demonstrate for patient.	_____	_____	_____	_____
(6) Instruct patient to avoid using chest and shoulders while inhaling.	_____	_____	_____	_____
(7) Have patient hold a slow, deep breath; hold for count of three; and then slowly exhale through mouth as if blowing out a candle (pursed lips). Tell patient middle fingertips will touch as chest wall contracts.	_____	_____	_____	_____
(8) Repeat breathing exercise 3 to 5 times.	_____	_____	_____	_____
(9) Have patient practice exercise. Instruct patient to take 10 slow, deep breaths every hour while awake.	_____	_____	_____	_____
B. Incentive Spirometry				
(1) Perform hand hygiene.	_____	_____	_____	_____
(2) Instruct patient to assume semi-Fowler's or high-Fowler's position.	_____	_____	_____	_____
(3) Indicate on the device the volume level to be obtained with each inhalation.	_____	_____	_____	_____
(4) Have patient demonstrate how to place mouthpiece so that lips completely cover mouthpiece.	_____	_____	_____	_____

	S	U	NP	Comments
(5) Instruct patient to inhale slowly and maintain constant flow through unit. When maximal inspiration is reached, patient should hold breath for 2 to 3 seconds and then exhale slowly. Number of breaths should not exceed 10 to 12 per minute.	____	____	____	__________
(6) Instruct patient to breathe normally for short period.	____	____	____	__________
(7) Have patient repeat maneuver until goals are achieved.	____	____	____	__________
(8) Perform hand hygiene.	____	____	____	__________
C. Positive Expiratory Pressure therapy and "huff" coughing				
(1) Perform hand hygiene.	____	____	____	__________
(2) Set positive expiratory pressure (PEP) device for setting ordered.	____	____	____	__________
(3) Instruct patient to assume semi-Fowler's or high-Fowler's position, and place nose clip on patient's nose.	____	____	____	__________
(4) Have patient place lips around mouthpiece. Patient should take a full breath and then exhale 2 or 3 times longer than inhalation. Pattern should be repeated for 10 to 20 breaths.	____	____	____	__________
(5) Remove device from mouth, and have patient take a slow, deep breath and hold for 3 seconds.	____	____	____	__________
(6) Instruct patient to exhale in quick, short, forced "huffs."	____	____	____	__________
D. Controlled Coughing				
(1) Explain importance of maintaining an upright position.	____	____	____	__________
(2) If surgical incision is to be either abdominal or thoracic, teach patient to place pillow or bath blanket over incisional area and place hands over pillow to splint incision. During breathing and coughing exercises, press gently against incisional area for splitting or support.	____	____	____	__________

	S	U	NP	Comments
(3) Demonstrate coughing. Take two slow, deep breaths, inhaling through nose and exhaling through mouth.				
(4) Inhale deeply a third time, and hold breath to count of three. Cough fully for two or three consecutive coughs without inhaling between coughs. (Tell patient to push all air out of lungs.)				
(5) Caution patient against just clearing throat instead of coughing. Explain that coughing will not cause injury to incision.				
(6) Instruct patient to continue to practice coughing exercises, splinting imaginary incision. Instruct the patient to cough 2 or 3 times while awake.				
(7) Instruct patient to examine sputum for consistency, odor, amount, and color changes.				
E. Turning				
(1) Instruct patient to assume supine position and move toward left side of bed by bending knees and pressing heels against the mattress to raise and move buttocks.				
(2) Instruct patient to place the right hand over incisional area to splint it.				
(3) Instruct patient to keep right leg straight and flex left knee up.				
(4) Have patient grab right side rail with left hand, pull toward right, and roll onto right side.				
(5) Instruct patient to turn every 2 hours while awake.				
F. Leg Exercises				
(1) Have patient assume supine position in bed. Demonstrate leg exercises by performing passive range-of-motion exercises and simultaneously explaining exercise.				
(2) Rotate each ankle in complete circle. Instruct patient to draw imaginary circles with big toe. Repeat 5 times.				

	S	U	NP	Comments
(3) Alternate dorsiflexion and plantar flexion of both feet. Direct patient to feel calf muscles contract and relax alternately.	____	____	____	____
(4) Perform quadriceps stretching by tightening thigh muscle and bringing knee down toward mattress, then relaxing. Repeat 5 times.	____	____	____	____
(5) Have patient alternately raise each leg up from bed surface, keeping legs straight, and then have patient bend leg at hip and knee. Repeat 5 times.	____	____	____	____
2. Have patient continue to practice exercises at least every 2 hours while awake. Instruct patient to coordinate turning and leg exercises with diaphragmatic breathing, incentive spirometry, and coughing exercises.	____	____	____	____
Evaluation				
1. Observe patient performing exercises independently.	____	____	____	____
2. Observe family members' or significant others' ability to coach patient.	____	____	____	____
3. Record which exercises have been demonstrated to patient and whether patient can perform exercises independently.	____	____	____	____
4. Record physical assessment findings.	____	____	____	____
5. Report any problems patient has in practicing exercises to nurse assigned to patient on next shift.	____	____	____	____

Answers to Case Study Questions and Chapter Reviews

CHAPTER 1: Health and Wellness

Case Study

a. This is an individual entering her middle adult years who is experiencing stress in her personal and professional life. She is being called upon by her employer and her child to meet their expectations, and she believes that this does not allow her the time to meet her health needs. The symptoms of gastrointestinal distress may be a response to the pressures in her life.

b. Initially the nurse may spend time with this patient to discuss the patient's personal feelings and needs. The patient may benefit from instruction in stress reduction and relaxation techniques, along with a review of time management. The nurse may investigate with her if there are support people at work and in the neighborhood to assist her in keeping up with her busy schedule. This individual also may be assisted in making an appointment for medical follow-up to determine her current health status.

Chapter Review

1. e
2. d
3. g
4. c
5. b
6. f
7. False
8. a. External variable
   b. External variable
   c. Internal variable
   d. External variable
   e. Internal variable
9. Positive health behaviors include immunizations, adequate sleep, exercise, and good nutrition.
10. Negative health behaviors include smoking, substance abuse, poor diet, and refusal to take medication or follow a treatment regimen.
11. 2
12. 3
13. 1
14. 2
15. 1
16. 3
17. 2
18. 4
19. 3
20. 1
21. 3

CHAPTER 2: The Health Care Delivery System

Case Studies

1. a. You may tell the neighbor that managed care is a type of program in which the health needs of the patient are funneled through to one party—the case manager. The design of this program is to control the cost of health care services while maintaining quality. Specific guidelines are in place for the type of services covered, length of hospital stay, and access to specialty care. An HMO (health maintenance organization) is a type of managed care program in which the focus is on primary care. A comprehensive number of services usually are provided; the services can be found in one location or in different facilities that are specified by the organization.

b. You could review the HMO book with your neighbor to clarify some of the terms and conditions of the coverage, which may be confusing for someone without any experience with the health care delivery system. If there are specific questions, the neighbor could be referred to an information telephone number for the program.

2. a. This individual should be eligible for benefits as a veteran and may be referred to the Department of Veterans Affairs to receive further information.

b. He could be admitted to a military or Veterans Administration hospital for ongoing treatment.

3. a. This patient could benefit from the services of a hospice organization for either home care and/or inpatient care, depending on the program.

Chapter Review

1.	f	4.	g	7.	d
2.	i	5.	a	8.	c
3.	b	6.	h	9.	Hospice

10. Discharge planning should begin the moment the patient enters the health care agency; the planning assists in the transition of the patient's care from one environment to the other (such as from the hospital to the home). The patient's ongoing needs are anticipated and identified, and necessary services/resources are coordinated before the patient's discharge.
11. Developments in technology influence many aspects of health care delivery. New types of equipment for patient monitoring, computerization, and electronic communication and record-keeping systems create a need for further education on the part of the health care provider.
12.

a.	Primary	g.	Primary
b.	Tertiary	k.	Secondary
c.	Restorative	h.	Preventive
d.	Restorative	i.	Secondary
e.	Continuing	j.	Continuing
f.	Preventive	l.	Restorative

13. The role of the case manager is to coordinate efforts of all the disciplines to achieve the most efficient and appropriate plan of care for the patient. The focus of case management is on discharge planning.
14. Vulnerable populations include children and women, older adults, and the mentally ill and homeless.
15. Patients who require subacute care are termed outliers because of their increased length of hospital stay and greater need for ongoing care.
16. Access to health care options are found in selections a and e.

17.	3	21.	2	25.	3
18.	2	22.	3	26.	1
19.	1	23.	4	27.	3
20.	4	24.	1	28.	2

CHAPTER 3: Community-Based Nursing Practice

Case Study

a. There are a variety of physiological, psychological, and sociocultural problems that the older adult may have, including:

   Physiological—heart disease, hypertension, arthritis, stroke (cerebral vascular accident), diabetes, sensory impairments (failing eyesight and hearing), cognitive impairments (Alzheimer's disease), cancer, malnutrition

   Psychological—depression, anxiety, substance abuse, dependence, other altered coping abilities, loss

   Sociocultural—finances, housing, separation from family

b. The nurse should investigate what is already available for older adults. This information should be available at the local municipal building/center, library, and/or health department. If not already available, the nurse should look into the possibility of working with the local government, health department, and other members of the community to offer such services as the following: senior day care; community activities (e.g., day trips and exercise groups) and transportation; health screenings; nutritional programs; in-person and telephone support groups; advice regarding security, financial and housing concerns; and reduced or no-cost home maintenance assistance. Older adults should be encouraged, whenever possible, to become involved in activites that provide mutual satisfaction and stimulation, such as school programs where they can read to elementary school children or consultation to businesses in their area of expertise.

Chapter Review

1. Challenges for community-based nursing practice include increased sexually transmitted diseases, pollution, new life-threatening diseases, and under-immunization of infants.

2. People who live in poverty are more likely to live in dangerous environments, work in high-risk jobs, have less nutritious diets, and experience multiple stressors.
3. Mentally ill patients in the community are at a greater risk for abuse, assault, and injury.
4. The role of the nurse in community-based practice is:
   a. Case manager
   b. Patient advocate
   c. Counselor
   d. Educator/teacher
5. Public policy to improve health includes legislation for seat belt use, smoking restrictions, and immunizations.
6. Nurse specialists in community or public health are educated at the graduate level.
7. High-risk or vulnerable populations include the homeless, substance abusers, victims of domestic violence, the mentally ill, older adults, women and children.

8.	a. False	9. 3	12. 2
	b. False	10. 4	
	c. True	11. 1	

CHAPTER 4: Legal Principles in Nursing

Case Studies

1. A patient who does not appear to understand a procedure should not sign a consent form. The physician will need to be contacted to provide the information to the patient. The nurse's role in this situation is to witness the signing of the consent form only if the patient demonstrates an understanding of the procedure. Because the nurse will not be performing the procedure, it is not his or her responsibility to describe what will or will not be done during the surgery.

2. a. Any question of a written order should be clarified with the prescriber. You should not depend on the "guess" of another colleague, even if it is a supervisor.
   b. If the medication is administered according to the charge nurse's belief, and the order is not correct, then you are accountable for the result.

3. In an emergency situation, treatment may be provided to an individual without obtaining consent. If there is sufficient opportunity to obtain consent, then the divorced parent who has legal custody of the child will need to be contacted.

4. You will need to investigate your state's statutes to determine what information is required to be reported for a colleague in a suspected substance abuse situation. In many states, the nurse is held accountable if he or she is knowledgeable about an impaired practitioner but does not report the situation to the Board of Nursing. For most instances, the situation is not acted on immediately; it is investigated further by the appropriate authorities.

Chapter Review

1. j	5. e	9. c
2. f	6. b	10. g
3. a	7. i	
4. k	8. d	

11. The nurse may avoid being liable by following the standards of care, providing competent care, communicating with other health care providers, documenting fully, and developing an empathetic rapport with patients.
12. Standards of care are defined in Nurse Practice Acts by Boards of Nursing, state and federal hospital licensing laws, professional and specialty organizations, and agency policies and procedures.
13. Informed consent requires the following:
    - A competent adult individual
    - Consent given voluntarily
    - Options for care understood
    - Opportunity provided for questions
    - A physician/patient relationship in which risks and alternatives are explained
    - Nurse witnessing of the patient's signature
14. True
15. Professional negligence is termed malpractice.
16. The Good Samaritan laws offer legal immunity.
17. Verbal or telephone orders should be signed within 24 hours.

18. The two standards for determination of death are cardiopulmonary and whole brain.
19. Proof of negligence requires:
    - The nurse owed a duty to the patient
    - The nurse did not carry out the duty or breached the duty
    - The patient was injured
    - The patient's injury was caused by the nurse's failure to carry out that duty
20. The coroner is notified if the patient's death is unforeseen or sudden or if the patient was not seen by a physician within 36 hours of death.
21. Advance directives act to specify decisions regarding life-saving treatment and to designate a power of attorney.
22. Health care workers are required to report attempted suicide, rape, gunshot wounds, unsafe or impaired professional practice, child abuse, and certain communicable diseases.

23. 2
24. 3
25. 4
26. 3
27. 1
28. 2
29. 1
30. 4
31. 1
32. 4

CHAPTER 5: Ethics

Case Study

a. **Step 1**. Is this an ethical dilemma?
Review of scientific data does not resolve Mr. R.'s situation, his question is perplexing, and your response and his action will have a profound relevance for human concern.
Step 2. Gather all the information relevant to the case.
Mr. R. is a 42-year-old man with severe multiple sclerosis who is unable to perform the simplest activities of daily living. He appears to be aware of his situation and is seeking an alternative to his present lifestyle. You are his home care nurse and are aware of the patient's situation.
Step 3. Examine and determine one's own values on the issues.
Use of the values' clarification process may assist you in determining your beliefs about assisted suicide and the quality and sanctity of life.
Step 4. State the problem clearly.
Mr. R. has an interest in being "helped to die," and he has involved you in a possible dilemma by asking you to assist him in getting more information about this method.
Step 5. Consider possible courses of action.
You may or may not be able to assist the patient in his actual pursuit of an assisted suicide because of your beliefs. In addition, the legal view on assisted suicide varies from state to state and will need to be investigated before any action is taken by you or the home care agency. A discussion with your supervisor and colleagues may assist in determining a course of action. (You will want to inform the patient that you will be sharing this information with other members of the health team.) If Mr. R. is intent on finding out about, and possibly pursuing, an assisted suicide, his family members (if available) may become involved.
Step 6. Negotiate the outcome.
Communication with the patient may determine whether there are other alternatives to the patient's plan. Work with the patient to consider all of the possibilities, but respect the patient's wish even if it is to pursue assisted suicide.
Step 7. Evaluate the action.
The actions taken by the nurse and other members of the home care agency should be documented. Recognize that satisfaction with the outcome by both the patient and the nurse may not be possible. There are no right or wrong answers to ethical questions. Evaluation is based on the effectiveness of working through the problem to a reasonable solution.

b. The nurse in this situation should be the patient's advocate. The first step is to determine if the patient is truly intent on pursuing this alternative measure. If he really is interested, then the nurse may assist him in a number of ways. Information on assisted suicide may be obtained directly or indirectly for the patient. The nurse may not be able to become involved but can be supportive of the patient's decision to investigate the procedure. There are legal and ethical considerations that may inhibit the nurse from having *any* involvement, in which case Mr. R. should be referred to others who may support him in his actions.

Chapter Review

1. f
2. g
3. i
4. b
5. c
6. a
7. e
8. d
9. j
10. Access to a patient's medical record requires the patient's consent.
11. The nursing shortage is influenced by the number of students and the age of practicing nurses.
12. End-of-life issues include "do not resuscitate" (DNR) orders, assisted suicide/euthanasia, living wills, and maintenance or removal of life-sustaining measures.
13. a. Deontology
    b. Feminist ethics
    c. Utilitarianism
    d. Ethics of care
14. a. *Cost containment:* Not having enough staff or equipment with monetary cutbacks, having limitations on coverage and benefits, providing restricted hours and services
    b. *Cultural sensitivity:* Accepting a patient's refusal of treatment (e.g., Christian Scientist's beliefs), recognizing the need for special diets or concern for the body of the deceased
15. 4
16. 4
17. 4
18. 3
19. 1
20. 4
21. 1

CHAPTER 6: Critical Thinking and Nursing Judgment

Case Study

a. The nurse may choose to return to the office to obtain supplies and then make a later visit to this patient. This option is possible if the nurse has other patients to visit or if there is work to be done at the office. This option will, however, take time away from the nurse and extend visiting hours. The nurse may choose to purchase necessary items from a local pharmacy, but the nurse may not have the necessary funds or be able to be reimbursed for this purchase. It may be most appropriate for the nurse to investigate what alternative resources are available in the patient's home, such as clean cloths, boiled water, salt, and tongs (all used with patient permission).

b. The nurse should determine what resources the patient has in the home, including running water, waste disposal, and methods for heating and refrigeration. In addition, a financial screening may be needed if indicated for the determination of available funds and/or insurance coverage for supplies and equipment.

Chapter Review

1. e
2. d
3. b
4. c
5. a
6. Examples of critical thinking throughout the nursing process:
   a. *Assessment:* collecting and analyzing data
   b. *Nursing diagnosis:* identifying the appropriate patient problems
   c. *Planning:* establishing expected outcomes, prioritizing, collaborating, and delegating
   d. *Implementation:* performing nursing interventions safely
   e. *Evaluation:* determining achievement of outcomes, reassessing as indicated
7. The levels of critical thinking are:
   a. Basic
   b. Complex
   c. Commitment
8. Examples of critical thinking attitudes:
   a. Confidence
   b. Thinking independently
   c. Discipline
   d. Creativity
   e. Integrity
9. 4
10. 3
11. 1
12. 3
13. 3
14. 4
15. 2
16. 1
17. 4
18. 1
19. 2

CHAPTER 7: Nursing Process

Case Studies

1. a. The nurse should obtain additional data about Mr. B.'s medical history and current health status. Mr. B. may be seeing a physician or other primary care provider and have medication prescribed for hypertension.

b. A community health fair allows for general screening of large numbers of people, but it usually does not offer opportunity or space for privacy to complete health histories or physical assessments. Individuals demonstrating alterations from expected norms, such as Mr. B., are referred to clinics, personal physicians, or other health care delivery agencies, as appropriate.

2. a. The relevant assessment data obtained from Mr. B. include:
- Being newly diagnosed with hypertension
- Having a new prescription of an antihypertensive medication
- Demonstrating insecurity about the medication regimen
- Relating his father's death at age 54 from a heart attack

b. Nursing diagnoses for Mr. B. may include:
- *Knowledge deficit related to unfamiliarity with the diagnosis and treatment of hypertension*
- *Knowledge deficit related to newly prescribed medication* (as manifested by his verbalization of uncertainty as to how and when to take his medications)
- *Fear related to possible repeat of father's medical history and early death*

3. a. Sample diagnoses, goals, and outcomes for Mr. B:

b. Nursing interventions may include:

Nursing Diagnoses	*Goals*	*Expected Outcome*
Knowledge deficit related to newly prescribed medication (as manifested by his verbalization of uncertainty as to how and when to take his medications).	Mr. B. will recognize the purpose of the hypertensive medication and prepare an administration schedule by the end of the clinic visit.	Mr. B. will restate the use of the antihypertensive medication and scheduling of administration during the visit.
Fear related to possible repeat of father's medical history and early death (as manifested by verbalization of concern over similar family history).	Mr. B. will demonstrate effective coping mechanisms within the next month. Mr. B. will identify a reduction or elimination of feelings of fear.	Mr. B. will discuss his concerns about his father's medical history and early death during this visit. Mr. B. will acknowledge his fear of repeating this history during his visits.
Knowledge deficit related to unfamiliarity with diagnosis of hypertension.	Mr. B. will make specific lifestyle alterations and participate in the treatment regimen.	Mr. B. will identify the etiology and therapeutic regimen for hypertension after the next two clinic visits.

Knowledge deficit	*Fear*
• Assess Mr. B.'s willingness and readiness to learn about his diagnosis and medication regimen • Identify and present appropriate information about hypertension and the medication regimen counseling, as indicated • Establish an environment and strategy for teaching Mr. B. that are conducive to learning • Provide effective learning materials, including pamphlets, videos, photos, and charts, for example	• Assess the degree of Mr. B.'s fear • Observe nonverbal and verbal responses • Listen to Mr. B.'s concerns and feelings • Provide information on coping mechanisms to assist in reducing his level of fear • Offer referral to a support program/counseling, as indicated

4. a. For his hypertension to be controlled, Mr. B. will need to take his medication on a regular basis. The nurse should focus on the implementation method of teaching. Counseling also may be involved, especially if Mr. B. is experiencing other difficulties at work or home that are interfering with his ability to manage his therapeutic regimen. Emphasis may be placed on Mr. B. taking his medication along with a daily routine, such as with meals or after bathing.

b. The nurse will need to look at the original goals, outcomes, and nursing interventions to determine what alterations may be necessary. The strategies for providing the information on Mr. B.'s diagnosis and medication may not have been appropriate. In addition, the patient's fear about his father's medical history may have been blocking his ability to focus and/or influencing his degree of motivation to participate in the therapeutic plan.

5. a. Mr. B. appears to be achieving most of his goals. He states that he is exercising regularly and trying to use the relaxation techniques when he feels stressed. Mr. B. also is expressing his method of coping with his father's medical history.

b. Areas for reassessment may include Mr. B.'s actual medication schedule (because his blood pressure is still slightly elevated) to determine that it is within the prescribed regimen. Determination also may be made to see if Mr. B. may benefit from additional exercise (per review with the physician), and a review of his relaxation techniques may be conducted.

Chapter Review

1. k
2. g
3. j
4. d
5. e
6. f
7. b
8. h
9. i
10. a
11. The three phases of the interview are the orientation phase, working phase, and termination phase.
12. a. *Knowledge deficit related to the need for postoperative care at home*
    Goal: Perform, or obtain assistance in performing, postoperative care at home
    Expected outcome:
    - State the purpose and procedure for postoperative care
    - Demonstrate postoperative care before discharge

    Nursing intervention:
    - Provide appropriate materials for patient review of postoperative care before surgery

- Review and demonstrate the postoperative care to patient after surgery
- Observe the patient's independent performance of postoperative care before discharge

b. *Alteration in elimination: constipation related to lack of physical activity*
Goal:
- Reestablish normal pattern of elimination
- Participate in specified daily physical activity, to tolerance

Expected outcome:
- Ambulate in hallway 3 times each day
- Perform active range-of-motion exercises twice each day

Nursing intervention:
- Instruct and assist patient in performance of physical activity
- Observe tolerance to physical activity
- Assess elimination pattern daily
- Promote additional measures to improve elimination, such as the intake of fluids and fiber

13. a. Psychomotor
 b. Interpersonal
 c. Interpersonal
 d. Psychomotor
 e. Cognitive
14. Before implementing standing orders, the nurse should determine the accuracy and appropriateness of the standing orders for the patient. In addition, the nurse should have the knowledge and competency necessary to carry out each order safely.
15. Possible nursing diagnoses are:
 a. *Diarrhea*
 b. *Activity intolerance*
16. The steps of the implementation phase of the nursing process are as follows: reassess, review/revise the care plan, organize resources and care delivery, and anticipate and prevent complications.
17. If a new patient need is identified, the nurse should modify the care plan.
18. Specific procedures are termed a protocol for care.
19. Indirect nursing interventions include the following: delegation, environmental safety, infection control, documentation, and collaboration.
20. Activities a, c, d, and g can usually be delegated.
21. Examples of how patient outcomes may be improved are:
 a. Erythema will be reduced in area by 2 inches within 2 days
 b. Pulse rate will be within the patient's baseline of 60 to 70 beats per minute following medication administration
 c. Patient will have a daily increase of 50 to 100 calories at each meal until ideal weight is achieved

22.	4	29.	4	36.	2
23.	1	30.	1	37.	3
24.	1	31.	2	38.	4
25.	2	32.	2	39.	3
26.	3	33.	1	40.	2
27.	4	34.	4	41.	4
28.	4	35.	4		

CHAPTER 8: Documentation and Reporting

Case Studies

1. a. A transfer report should include the following information:
- Patient's name and age, name of primary physician, and medical diagnosis
- Summary of medical progress up to the time of transfer
- Current physiological and psychological status
- Current nursing diagnoses/plan of care
- Critical assessments to be completed shortly after transfer
- Any special equipment needed

 b. More specifically, the primary nurse may want to know about the surgical procedure, how it was tolerated by the patient, how the patient responded to the anesthesia, and observations made and treatments completed in the PACU.

2. a. Sample SOAP documentation for Mrs. Q:

S—Patient states she is having intense pain in her right hip area and does not want to move because of the pain.
O—Patient is grimacing and moaning in pain.
A—There is an alteration in comfort related to new surgical incision to right hip.
P—Reduce or eliminate discomfort by administering analgesic medication as ordered and assisting patient to more comfortable position.

Sample DAR documentation for Mrs. Q:
D—Patient is grimacing and moaning in pain. States that she is having intense pain to right hip and does not want to move because it "really hurts." Dressing is dry and intact.
A—Patient assisted to more comfortable position, with leg supported. Analgesic administered per order.
R—Patient expressed reduction in discomfort to tolerable level.

Chapter Review

1. d
2. e
3. a
4. b
5. c
6. a. Draw a single line through the error, write the word *error* above the line, initial or sign the error, and complete the correct notation.
   b. Use only objective descriptions of the patient and use quotes for patient comments.
   c. Use complete, concise descriptions of patient interactions.
   d. Draw a single line through the error, write the word *error* above the line, initial or sign the error, and complete the correct notation.
   e. Use consecutive lines for charting and do not leave margins. Draw lines through unused space and sign your name at the end of the notation.
   f. Only include factual information in the notation.
   g. Identify that the physician was called to clarify an order for the patient.
   h. Have the other caregiver document the information, unless the individual calls with additional information. Document that the information was provided by another individual.
   i. Record pertinent information throughout the shift, signing each entry.
7. False
8. Standards are set by the Joint Commission on Accreditation of Healthcare Organizations (JCAHO)
9. a. Communication: for continuity of care and accurate patient status
   b. Financial: for reimbursement, DRGs, insurance audits
   c. Educational: for teaching nursing and medical students
   d. Research: for statistical data and patient responses
   e. Auditing/Monitoring: for JCAHO standards, incidence of patient falls, pain management
10. Malpractice issues related to documenting include the following: failure to document, verbal orders, charting in advance of care, timing of events, incorrect data, and failure to report.
11. Documentation should be completed immediately after patient care.
12. Subjective statements by the patient should be quoted and may be supported with objective findings.
13. Student nurses should sign their names, followed by either SN or NS and the school affiliation.
14. Both notations are vague and should include more specific information. For example:
    a. Consumed 8 ounces of hot cereal, 6 ounces of orange juice, and an 8-ounce cup of coffee for breakfast.
    b. Voided 200 ml of clear amber urine.
15. Documentation for patient teaching on insulin self-injection should include the verbal and written information provided to the patient, demonstration provided, observation of patient's ability to perform the skill, and patient responses to the activity.

16. Discharge summaries should include the following: procedures that should be peformed and the instructions given, medications prescribed and precautions, signs and symptoms of complications, names and phone numbers of health care providers, names of community resources, follow-up requirements, actual time of discharge, transportation used, and name of person accompanying the discharged patient.
17. Home care documentation is also completed for financial reimbursement.
18. The process of completing narrative notes only when abnormalities exist is part of "charting by exception."

19.	3	23.	4	27.	4
20.	4	24.	4	28.	2
21.	3	25.	4	29.	1
22.	3	26.	2		

CHAPTER 9: Communication

Case Study

a. The following techniques may be effective for an older individual with a moderate hearing impairment:
    - Reducing background noise
    - Checking and cleaning a hearing aid
    - Speaking slowly and clearly
    - Using a low-pitched rather than high-pitched voice
    - Avoiding shouting at the patient
    - Using short, simple sentences
    - Facing the patient to allow for lip reading
    - Not covering the mouth while talking
    - Talking toward the unaffected ear
    - Using facial expressions and gestures

b. The following techniques may be effective for individuals who do not speak English:
    - Speaking in a normal tone of voice
    - Establishing signals or methods of nonverbal communication
    - Obtaining an interpreter familiar with the language and culture
    - Allowing time for communication to take place
    - Developing a communication board, pictures, or cards for common requests
    - Having a dictionary available for reference

c. The following techniques may be effective for an individual who is blind:
    - Announcing yourself when entering the room
    - Communicating verbally before touching the patient
    - Orienting the patient to the environment
    - Explaining the procedure in advance
    - Having the patient handle the equipment, as appropriate
    - Informing the patient when you are done and will be leaving the room

d. The following techniques may be effective for an individual of another culture who is experiencing an invasive procedure for the first time:
    - Explaining the procedure in advance, using an interpreter if necessary
    - Recognizing possible discomfort with exposure and maintaining privacy
    - Staying with the patient to provide emotional support

Chapter Review

1.	c	5.	e	9.	b
2.	h	6.	j	10.	a
3.	g	7.	f		
4.	i	8.	d		

11. a. Intrapersonal level
    b. Interpersonal level
    c. Public level
12. a. Public zone
    b. Social zone
    c. Intimate zone
    d. Social zone
    e. Intimate zone
    f. Public zone
    g. Personal zone
13. Appropriate communication techniques for the older adult with impaired communication include selections a, c, and d.
14. a. Courtesy is not being used. The patient should be called by his or her name, such as Mrs. Jones or Mr. Brown.

b. Courtesy is not being used. The patient should be identified by name, not by room number or diagnosis.
c. Confidentiality is not being applied. The patient should not be discussed outside of the immediate patient area where anyone not involved in the patient's care may overhear the conversation.
d. Availability is not being applied. The nurse should spend time with the patient or identify to the patient when he or she will return to be with the patient.
e. Avoidance of medical jargon is not being considered. The nurse should explain to the patient, in understandable terms, what to expect of the procedure.

15. Examples of ways in which the nurse could enhance communication with the patient include:
    a. "How do you feel today?"
    b. "Do you take any medications at home?" or "What types of medication do you take at home?"
    c. "Have you noticed any areas of swelling around your arms or legs?"
    d. "Do you have any questions about the procedure that will be done today?" or "Has the physician explained the procedure to you?"
16. The communication strategies being used are:
    a. Using silence
    b. Attentive listening
    c. Encouraging conversation
    d. Clarifying
    e. Focusing
17. To assist the patient who has an aphasia, the nurse may:
    - Use simple gestures and statements
    - Provide visual cues, such as pictures or flash cards
    - Listen and observe attentively
    - Allow time for responses, either verbal or nonverbal
    - Have call bells within easy reach
    - Encourage the patient to interact as much as possible
18. Positive responses include answers c and d.
19. Considering the patient's culture, assigning a female nurse to the female Amish patient is appropriate. Selection a is inappropriate.
20. The acronym SOLER is:
    S—Sit facing the patient
    O—Offer an open posture
    L—Lean toward the patient
    E—Establish and maintain intermittent eye contact
    R—Relax

21. 3
22. 2
23. 4
24. 1
25. 4
26. 1
27. 3
28. 3
29. 3
30. 1
31. 4
32. 3
33. 4
34. 1
35. 3
36. 1
37. 4

CHAPTER 10: Patient Education

Case Study

a. Ms. T. has no prior knowledge about her diagnosis or prescribed medication. She also has a prior family history of coronary disease, with her father dying of a heart attack at 54 years of age.
b. Sample teaching plan for Ms. T.:

Learning Need	*Resources*	*Objectives*	*Teaching Strategies*
Knowledge deficit related to newly diagnosed hypertension and antihypertensive medication therapy	Educational media: Video and audio programs on hypertension, written materials on the diagnosis and the medication, information from the physician and other health	Ms. T. will be able to: Describe the diagnosis, etiology, treatment, and complications; describe the actions, side effects, and time of administration for the antihypertensive;	Provide Ms. T. with available educational media and written information on hypertension and antihypertensive medications; use

Continued

Learning Need	*Resources*	*Objectives*	*Teaching Strategies*
	care providers, (e.g., dietitian), nurse's knowledge of diagnosis and treatment regimen	identify when to contact the physician if complications or problems occur; independently monitor and record her blood pressure daily and as necessary; develop a meal plan for a week that incorporates the therapeutic diet	illustrations to explain the functions of the heart and circulatory system and the effects of hypertension; demonstrate the technique for monitoring blood pressure, and have the patient and/or significant other return to demonstrate the procedure; involve significant others in the educational program

Chapter Review

1. d
3. f
5. b
2. c
4. a
6. True
7. Examples of health maintenance and promotion topics include selections a, d, and f.
8. Specific teaching methods that may be implemented for an infant include maintaining consistency in routines (bathing, feeding), holding the child firmly while smiling and speaking softly, and having the infant touch different textures.
9. The presence of pain, anxiety, and distractions may make it difficult for the learner to concentrate.
10. The nurse should consider the following factors when selecting an environment for teaching: privacy, room temperature, lighting, noise, ventilation, furniture, and space.
11. Written materials are generally at the fifth grade level.
12. Teaching sessions should last about 20 to 30 minutes, with critical information being taught first.
13. For the diagnosis *Noncompliance with medication regimen related to insufficient knowledge of purpose and actions*, possible goals/outcomes and nursing interventions include:

    Goals/outcomes:
    - Verbalize purpose and actions of medication regimen
    - Take medications as prescribed

    Nursing interventions:
    - Provide information about prescribed medications, including purpose and actions—give patient written information about medications and their use; use visual aids as necessary to reinforce the material
    - Allow opportunity for patient to express concerns and ask questions
14. The domains of learning are:
    a. Psychomotor
    b. Affective
    c. Cognitive
    d. Affective
    e. Psychomotor
    f. Cognitive
15. Recommendations for instructional techniques are:
    a. Lecture, group discussion
    b. Demonstration and return demonstration
    c. Demonstration and role-playing
16. Explaining in advance is preparatory instruction.

17. Almost 50% of adults in the United States have difficulty reading and understanding health information.

18. 4	22. 3	26. 4
19. 4	23. 2	27. 1
20. 3	24. 1	28. 4
21. 4	25. 2	

CHAPTER 11: Infection Control

Case Studies

1. The nurse should implement the following measures to prevent a urinary tract infection:
   - Provide personal hygiene, perineal care
   - Use aseptic technique when manipulating the catheter and drainage equipment
   - Keep the drainage bag unobstructed and below the level of the bladder
   - Provide ample fluids, within patient's limitations
2. To prevent a wound infection, the nurse should:
   - Maintain sterile technique during dressing changes
   - Use medical asepsis in all interactions with the patient
   - Instruct the patient in hand washing/asepsis
   - Dispose of contaminated materials appropriately and promptly
   - Assist in keeping the patient and environment clean and dry
   - Limit the number of caregivers working with the patient
   - Provide optimum nutrition and fluids, within patient's limitations
   - Administer antibiotics, if prescribed

Chapter Review

1. k	5. b	9. a
2. f	6. g	10. e
3. j	7. d	11. l
4. c	8. h	12. m

13. Clean technique is demonstrated in options a and d. Sterile technique is required for options b, c, and e.
14. Examples of outcomes for this patient are the following: Wound will decrease in diameter by 1 cm in 2 days; wound will be free of signs of infection, including edema and drainage.
15. Immunizations are available for selections a, b, c, and f.
16. The nurse should discard the package with the tear and obtain a new one.
17. Nursing interventions include:
    a. Control or eliminate the infectious agent—clean, disinfect, and sterilize contaminated objects
    b. Control or eliminate the reservoir—remove sources of body fluids, drainage (dressings), or solutions that harbor microorganisms; discard disposable articles contaminated with infectious material
    c. Control the portals of exit—avoid talking, sneezing, or coughing directly over a wound or sterile dressing field; teach patient to protect others; and handle all body fluids carefully (hand hygiene and use of gloves)
    d. Control the transmission—disinfect equipment, provide a personal set of equipment for patients, do not shake linens or allow them to come in contact with the uniform, and perform hand hygiene
    e. Susceptible host—hygienic care, adequate nutritional and fluid intake
18. a. White blood cell count—elevated in an acute infection, decreased in viral/overwhelming infections
    b. Erythrocyte sedimentation rate—elevated with infectious processes
    c. Iron level—decreased in chronic infections
    d. Neutrophils—elevated with acute, supportive infections; decreased with overwhelming bacterial infections
    e. Basophils—remain normal during infections
19. The major cause of health-care–associated infections is inadequate hand hygiene.
20. A patient's gastrointestinal defenses are altered by the administration of antacids and beta-blockers.
21. Appropriate techniques for isolation precautions include selections b, d, and f.

22. Handling of biohazardous waste includes "red" bagging for incineration or special handling.
23. The order for application of PPE is mask, gown, and then gloves.
24. The first items removed when leaving the isolation room are the gloves.
25. Appropriate asepsis is demonstrated in selections b, c, f, and h.
26. For the nursing diagnosis *Impaired skin integrity, related to 2 inch diameter pressure ulcer on sacrum*, possible patient outcomes and nursing interventions include:

    Patient goals/outcomes:
    - Sacral ulcer will reduce in size by 1 inch (within time frame)
    - Skin will remain intact over remainder of body surfaces
    - Sacral ulcer will remain free of infection

    Nursing interventions:
    - Provide wound care as prescribed using aseptic technique
    - Assess condition of ulcer
    - Provide skin care—keep clean and dry, and apply moisturizers as needed
    - Turn and position patient every hour
    - Assess wound for presence of infection, and obtain culture if indicated
    - Provide for patient's nutritional and fluid needs
27. c, first; b, second and third; a, last

28.	1	33.	2	38.	1
29.	1	34.	4	39.	4
30.	3	35.	4	40.	4
31.	4	36.	3		
32.	4	37.	4		

CHAPTER 12: Vital Signs

Case Studies

1. a. Generally, an individual who has a blood pressure reading of above 120-139/80-89 mm Hg on repeated assessments should be referred for medical follow-up. An average of two or more systolic readings above 140 mm Hg and diastolic readings above 90 mm Hg are usually indicative of hypertension.

b. Additional information should be noted such as the arm used and the position (e.g., sitting, standing, lying down) of the patient during the measurement, previous blood pressure readings, known medical problems, and any medical care being received and medications being taken by the patient.

2. The patient's pulse rate and blood pressure reading may be obtained in the lower extremities. The pulses available include the femoral, popliteal, posterior tibial, and dorsalis pedis. The blood pressure is assessed by placing the thigh-sized cuff over the posterior aspect of the middle thigh region while the patient is in the prone position. The popliteal artery is used for palpation and auscultation of the blood pressure. Measurement in the lower extremities may be 10 to 40 mm Hg higher in the systolic reading than that of the upper extremities.

3. a. A febrile patient may exhibit the following signs and symptoms:
- Increased body temperature
- Flushed, dry, warm skin
- Chills
- Feeling of malaise
- Tachycardia

b. Nursing interventions for febrile patients may include:
- Assessment of vital signs, especially temperature
- Observation of patient response, including skin color and temperature, and chills
- Promotion of patient comfort, responding to chills, thirst
- Collection of appropriate specimens, such as blood cultures
- Promotion of rest and reduction of activities that increase heat production
- Promotion of heat loss by removing coverings and keeping the patient dry
- Provision of care to meet increased metabolic demands, including oxygen, nutrition, and fluid requirements
- Monitoring of ongoing status

4. If the pulse oximeter does not appear to be working, there may be problems with light transmission or a reduction of the patient's arterial pulsations. The site for measurement should be checked to determine that it is clean, warm, and dry; not directly near another light source; and receiving adequate circulation. The patient also may need to be reminded to limit excessive motion of the extremity that is being used for measurement.

Chapter Review

1. g
2. l
3. h
4. k
5. f
6. j
7. a
8. d
9. i
10. e
11. c
12. b
13. n
14. m
15. a. (97° F – 32) × 5/9 = 36° C
    b. 9/5 × (38.4° C + 32) = 101.1° F
    c. 38.9° C
    d. 102.9° F
    e. The nurse is alerted to temperature alterations of above 100.4° F or below 96.8° F on an oral Fahrenheit thermometer, and measurements above 38° C or below 36° C on an oral centigrade scale. Rectal temperature readings may be 0.9° F or 0.5° C higher than oral measurements, with axillary readings ranging this same number of degrees lower than oral temperatures.
16. The pulses should be palpated as follows:

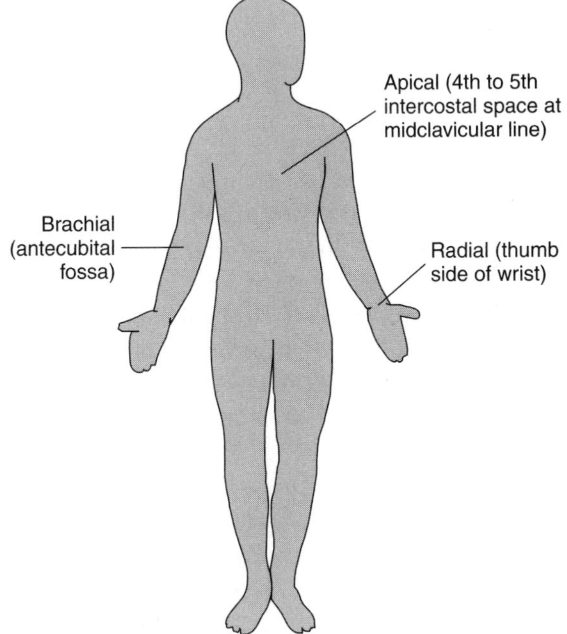

17. a. Aneroid scale:

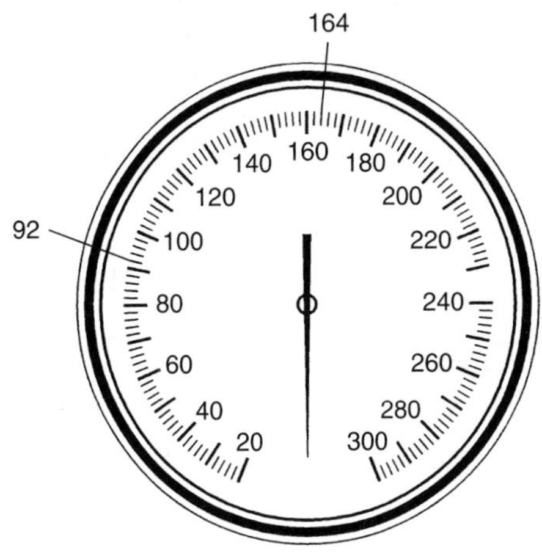

    b. Mercury scale:

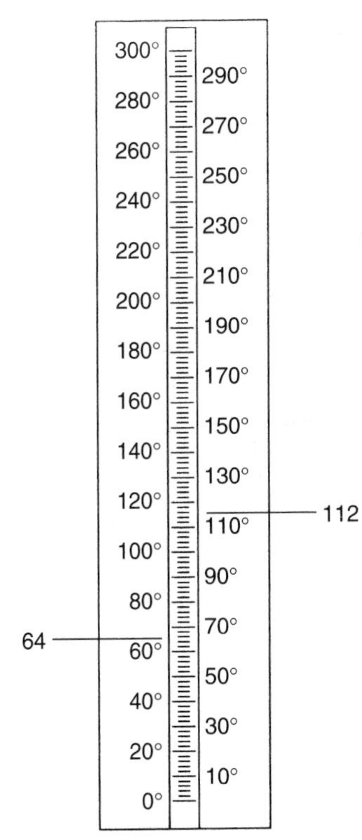

18. False
19. Interventions to reduce body temperature by:
    a. Conduction—ice packs, tepid baths
    b. Convection—fans
20. The thermometer of choice for a patient in isolation is a disposable chemical dot thermometer.

21. The blood pressure measurement should be taken in the lower extremities for a patient with bilateral arm casts, and the popliteal artery should be used.
22. For a patient who has had a right mastectomy, the left arm or lower extremities should be used for blood pressure measurement.
23. Vital signs are usually recorded on a graphic or flow sheet.
24. Decreasing hemoglobin levels will increase the respiratory rate.
25. A pulse oximeter may be applied to the earlobe, finger, toe, or bridge of the nose.
26. The expected SpO_2 level is above 90%.
27. The correct techniques for blood pressure measurement include options a, c, e, and f.
28. The difference between the radial and apical pulses is the pulse deficit.
29. The difference between the systolic and diastolic blood pressure measurements is the pulse pressure.

30.	1	39.	3	48.	1
31.	3	40.	1	49.	4
32.	3	41.	4	50.	2
33.	2	42.	2	51.	1
34.	4	43.	2	52.	4
35.	1	44.	3	53.	2
36.	4	45.	1	54.	1
37.	1	46.	4		
38.	1	47.	3		

CHAPTER 13: Health Assessment and Physical Examination

Case Study

For the 4-year-old boy, you are aware that the experience may be new and frightening. You can show the child the assessment procedures on a doll or model, while giving simple, understandable information, and he may handle equipment that will be used (as appropriate). The exam should be conducted in a comfortable environment, with time allowed for the child to play. The child may be called by his first name, and he may be asked assessment questions that he will understand.

For the 16-year-old female, the nurse may begin the health assessment with the parent(s) in the room with the patient. There should be time, however, when the patient is by herself with the nurse to discuss concerns. The adolescent female should be asked if she wants a parent present during the physical assessment, but the option is provided for the patient to not be accompanied. Procedures and findings should be explained to both the parent(s) and the patient.

The older Hispanic woman may have responses to the exam that are influenced by her culture. She will need to be informed and prepared for the breast and pelvic assessments, with consideration given to her privacy. This patient may desire another female to be present during the examination or to conduct the physical. Care should be taken to determine that this patient understands the information and instruction provided by an examiner who may speak only English. An interpreter may be obtained if the patient is conversant in Spanish. The environment should be warm and comfortable. Ample time should be allowed for the patient to answer questions and assume necessary positions for the exam.

For each of the patients, opportunity should be provided to use the bathroom before, during, and following the examination.

Chapter Review

1.	f	5.	h	9.	e
2.	c	6.	g	10.	i
3.	b	7.	d		
4.	a	8.	j		

11. The five skills used in physical assessment include:
    - Inspection—use of vision and hearing to detect characteristics of body parts and functions
    - Palpation—use of the hands to touch body parts to determine temperature, texture, position, and movement
    - Percussion—striking the body surface with the finger to produce a vibration and elicit sounds
    - Auscultation—listening to sounds created in the body organs (use of stethoscope)

- Olfaction—use of smell to determine the presence of characteristic odors

12. The positions for the physical examination are:
Sitting, supine, dorsal recumbent, lithotomy, Sims', prone, lateral recumbent, and knee-chest
13. The pulses being palpated are:
    a. Ulnar
    b. Posterior tibial
    c. Femoral
    d. Brachial
    e. Dorsalis pedis
14. The skin lesions are:
    a. Papule
    b. Ulcer
    c. Macule
    d. Atrophy
    e. Wheal
15. The PMI is located in the left anterior chest wall, at approximately the fourth to fifth intercostal space, at the midclavicular line.

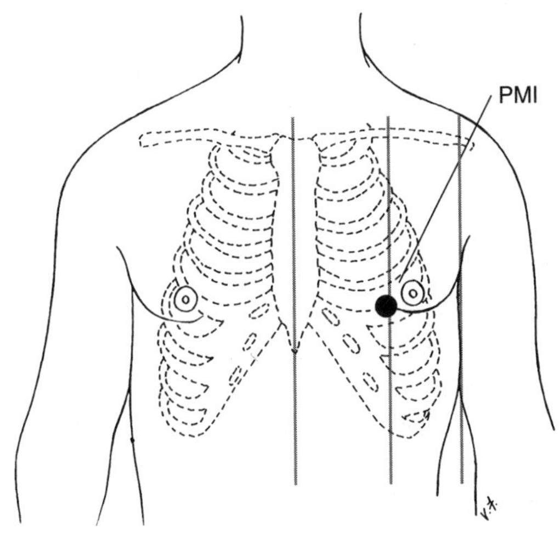

16. The following are findings that may indicate abuse:
    a. Child sexual abuse
    Physical findings:
        - Genital discharge, bleeding, pain, itching
        - Difficulty sitting or walking
        - Foreign bodies in genital tract or rectum

    Behavioral findings:
        - Problems eating or sleeping
        - Fear of certain people or places
        - Regressive or acting-out behavior
        - Preoccupation with own genitals

    b. Domestic abuse
    Physical findings:
        - Injuries and trauma inconsistent with reported cause
        - Multiple injuries, burns, bites
        - Old and new fractures

    Behavioral findings:
        - Eating or sleeping disorders
        - Anxiety, panic attacks
        - Low self-esteem
        - Depression, sense of helplessness
        - Attempted suicide

    c. Older adult abuse
    Physical findings:
        - Injuries and trauma inconsistent with reported cause
        - Bruises, hematomas, burns, fractures
        - Prolonged interval between injury and treatment

    Behavioral findings:
        - Dependent on caregiver
        - Physically and/or cognitively impaired
        - Combative, belligerent
17. Abdominal assessment:

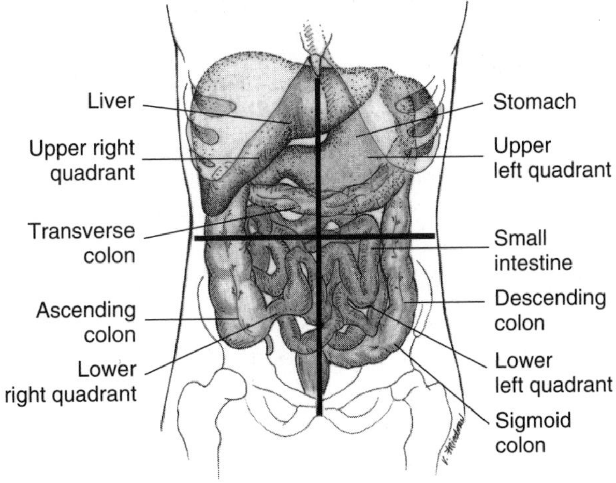

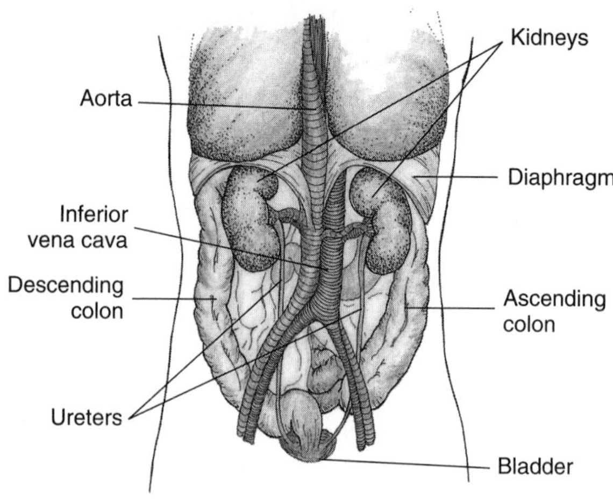

18.

a.	Expected	v.	Unexpected
b.	Unexpected	w.	Expected
c.	Expected	x.	Unexpected
d.	Expected	y.	Unexpected
e.	Unexpected	z.	Unexpected
f.	Unexpected	aa.	Expected
g.	Expected	bb.	Unexpected
h.	Unexpected	cc.	Expected
i.	Unexpected	dd.	Unexpected
j.	Expected	ee.	Expected
k.	Expected	ff.	Unexpected
l.	Expected	gg.	Expected
m.	Unexpected	hh.	Unexpected
n.	Unexpected	ii.	Expected
o.	Unexpected	jj.	Expected
p.	Expected	kk.	Expected
q.	Expected	ll.	Expected
r.	Unexpected	mm.	Unexpected
s.	Expected	nn.	Expected
t.	Expected	oo.	Unexpected
u.	Expected	pp.	Expected

19. The nurse examines the area of discomfort last (b).
20. High-pitched sounds are best heard with the diaphragm of a stethoscope (a).
21. The nurse pulls the ear up and back (a).
22. The patient is placed in lithotomy position, if possible.
23. The patient is placed in the dorsal recumbent position.
24. In the CAGE questionnaire, the 'A' stands for: "Have people Annoyed you by criticizing your substance abuse?"
25. A weight gain of 5 lb or 2.2 kg/day indicates fluid retention.
26. The correct examination techniques are answers a, d, and e.
27. True
28. The correct techniques are c and d.
29. The patient is given a grade of 3 and a F (fair) on the Lovett scale.
30. Tests for colorectal cancer include fecal immunochemical test (FIT), fecal occult blood test (FOBT), colonoscopy, and barium enema.
31. Positions for cardiac assessment include answers b, d, and e.

32.	4	41.	4	50.	1
33.	2	42.	3	51.	4
34.	1	43.	1	52.	1
35.	2	44.	1	53.	2
36.	1	45.	4	54.	3
37.	4	46.	1	55.	3
38.	1	47.	4	56.	1
39.	4	48.	1	57.	1
40.	3	49.	1	58.	4

CHAPTER 14: Administering Medications

Case Studies

1. To assist this patient to maintain the medication regimen at home, you may create a large, colorful, easy-to-read schedule, chart, or calendar that the patient can use to check when medications have been taken. The patient's medications also may be arranged, by time of administration, in a commercially available or homemade container so that the patient also may be able to determine if the medications were taken as prescribed. (Some commercial devices will "beep" when it is time for medications to be taken.)

2. If the prescriber's handwriting is illegible, it is unsafe to make assumptions about the medication order. To avoid errors, you should contact the prescriber as soon as possible and clarify the medication orders.

3. A patient without an identification band should not receive medications. To verify the identity of the patient, find another nurse or health care worker who is familiar with the patient. On verifying the name of the patient, obtain and provide the identification band for the patient. Asking the patient his or her name assists in verification but may be inaccurate if the patient is not aware or oriented to the surroundings.

4. When administering an injection to a child, you need to be very careful to avoid injuring or severely agitating the child. An appropriate, well-developed muscle site should be selected. You also may need to have someone else assist in holding or distracting the child by talking. The injection should be given quickly and accurately. An anesthetic ointment may be applied to the site before the injection to decrease the amount of discomfort. Children should not be told that they are receiving a "shot" or that it will not hurt. A sleeping child should be awakened before being given an injection.
5. This discrepancy in the narcotic count should be reported immediately to the nurse in charge. Usually an attempt is made to determine if the missing dose can be accounted for by checking with all of the other staff members. If the missing medication cannot be tracked down, the discrepancy will need to be documented on the computerized or written record. The agency's protocol for this situation then should be followed in relation to where and how the documentation is forwarded.
6. For the patient who requires an antipyretic but is experiencing nausea and vomiting, the nurse should contact the prescriber and have the medication order changed to a rectal suppository. For patients who have difficulty tolerating oral medications, the nurse should investigate alternative forms of the medication.

Chapter Review

1. i	5. c	9. b
2. j	6. e	10. h
3. k	7. m	11. d
4. g	8. f	12. a

13. Federal and state legislation, state nurse practice acts, and agency policies and procedures control or regulate the nurse's administration of medications.
14. Strategies to prevent errors with look-alike medications include the following: ordering medications by the generic name, including the diagnosis on the prescription, repeating verbal orders back to the prescriber, discussing the medications with the patient, reinforcing instructions with the patient, advising patients to check medication labels, and having the patient report any changes in the medication's appearance.
15. Factors influencing the actions of medications:
    a. Dietary factors—drug and nutrient interactions can alter a drug's action or the effect of the nutrient; proper drug metabolism relies on good nutrition
    b. Physiological variables—age, sex, weight, nutritional status, disease states
    c. Environmental conditions—stress, exposure to heat/cold, comfort of the setting
16. The routes for parenteral administration include intramuscular, intradermal, subcutaneous, and intravenous.
17. The components that are missing in the orders are:
    a. Dosage
    b. Route
    c. Time for administration
    d. Route
18. The rights are right drug, right dose, right patient, right route, right time, and right documentation.
19. The correct sequence for mixing two insulins in the same syringe is: g, d, h, i, a, e, f, c, b.
20. The forms of medication are:
    a. Capsule
    b. Suppository
    c. Tincture
    d. Elixir
    e. Suspension
    f. Intraocular disk
    g. Lotion
21. Commonly abused over-the-counter medications include aspirin and cough and cold medicines.

22. Noncompliance or nonadherence may be related to a dislike of the side effects, the cost of the medication, or a busy lifestyle.
23. Faster absorption or action is found with:
    a. IV
    b. IM
    c. Acidic oral medication
    d. Solutions
    e. Large surface area
    f. Highly lipid soluble medication
    g. Non–albumin binding medication
24. This is the peak action of the drug.
25. Oral medications are contraindicated for the patient who has an NPO order, GI alterations, dysphagia, nausea, vomiting, gastric suction, NG tube, or received anesthesia.
26. The problem with this order is that the decimal point may be missed and the patient would receive 10 times the actual dose.
27. The equivalents are:
    a. 15 gtt
    b. 2 ounces
    c. 1 L
    d. 3000 mg
    e. 250 ml
    f. 5 ml
28. The Braslow tape uses color and the child's height to determine the safe dosage range.
29. Verbal orders are to be signed within 24 hours.
30. This number of tablets is not common, so the nurse should recheck the calculation to determine accuracy. Another nurse may be asked to verify the final calculation.
31. If the patient identifies that the medication looks different, it is important for the nurse to check and make sure that the medication and the order are correct.
32. False
33. True
34. False
35. True
36. A patient with dysphagia will benefit from a liquid form of the medication or one that can be crushed.
37. Techniques for administering medications to children include:
    a. Oral medications—give frozen juice bars, juice, or soft drinks after the medication is swallowed (as allowed)
    b. Injections—wake the child up before an injection, ask for assistance in holding the child, distract the child during the injection, give the medication quickly, avoid calling the injection a "shot," and inform the child that it may "pinch"
38. The discomfort of an injection may be minimized by:
    - Using a sharp-beveled needle of the smallest possible size
    - Positioning the patient comfortably
    - Selecting the proper site
    - Diverting the patient's attention away from the procedure
    - Inserting the needle quickly and smoothly
    - Holding the syringe steady while injecting the solution
    - Injecting the medication slowly and steadily
    - Using the Z-track technique
    - Massaging the site, unless contraindicated
39. The Z-track technique should be used for medications that are irritating to the tissues.
40. a. Intramuscular—90-degree angle
    b. Subcutaneous—45-degree angle
    c. Intradermal—5-degree to 15-degree angle
41. Medication may be administered intravenously via mixtures with large volumes of IV fluids, by injection (bolus) or intermittent access devices, or by piggyback through an existing IV line.
42. a. $\frac{\text{Dose ordered}}{\text{Dose on hand}} \times \text{Amount on hand}$
    $= \text{Dose to be administered}$

    b. $\frac{\text{Child's surface area}}{1.7\ \text{m}^2} \times \text{Adult dose}$
    $= \text{Dose to be administered}$
43. a. ac = before meals
    b. bid = twice a day
    c. prn = as necessary
    d. q4h = every 4 hours
    e. stat = immediately

44. a. $\frac{150\ \text{mcg}}{75\ \text{mcg}} \times 1\ \text{tablet}$
    = 2 tablets should be given

    Conversion of 0.150 mg to mcg: multiply 0.150 by 1000
    b. $\frac{150\ \text{mg}}{50\ \text{mg}} \times 1\ \text{ml} = 3\ \text{ml}$ should be given

c. $\frac{20\text{ mg}}{10\text{ mg}} \times 1\text{ ml} = 2\text{ ml}$ should be given

d. $\frac{250\text{ mg}}{125\text{ mg}} \times 1$ tablet
= 2 tablets should be given

e. $\frac{75\text{ mg}}{25\text{ mg}} \times 0.5\text{ ml}$
= 1.5 ml should be given

f. 100 units = 1 ml
24 units/100 units = 0.24 ml

g. $\frac{1.25\text{ m}^2}{1.7\text{ m}^2} \times 25\text{ mg}$
= 18.4 mg should be given

45. Patient assessments that should be completed before medication administration include:
    a. Parenteral injections—the size of the patient, condition of the injection site (integument and muscle condition), circulatory status

    For all patients, the type of medication and its effect on the patient are to be evaluated by the nurse.

46.

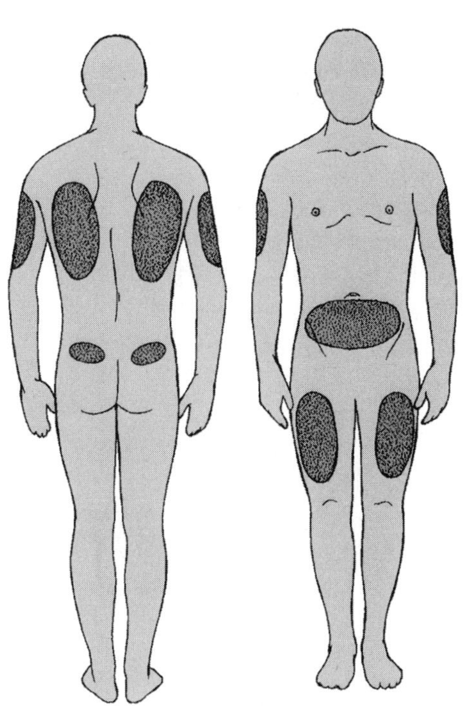

47. The correct techniques for administration of medications to patients with dysphagia are listed in answers b, c, and f.
48. Proper placement of the nasogastric tube is a priority assessment.
49. The nurse should apply clean gloves before administering topical medications. Sterile gloves may be indicated for medications applied to open wounds.
50. For administration of ear drops:
    a. Position the patient side-lying or sitting in a chair with the head tilted to the side.
    b. Pull the outer ear of an adult up and back.
    c. Irrigate with 50 ml of solution at room temperature.
51. For a metered-dose inhaler:
    a. A spacer should be used.
    b. This canister should last for 20 days (8 puffs/day, 160 total puffs in the canister).
52. The patient should be placed in left Sims' position, if tolerated.

53.	2	59.	1	65.	2
54.	3	60.	2	66.	1
55.	2	61.	3	67.	3
56.	4	62.	4	68.	2
57.	4	63.	2	69.	3
58.	4	64.	3	70.	1

CHAPTER 15: Fluid, Electrolyte, and Acid-Base Balances

Case Studies

1. A patient taking both digoxin and Lasix is more susceptible to fluid volume deficit (FVD) and hypokalemia. Digoxin strengthens the contraction of the heart muscle, improving the cardiac output and circulatory volume. Lasix is a potent diuretic that does not have a potassium-sparing effect. The patient should be instructed to be alert to the signs of both decreased fluid and decreased potassium levels as follows:
- Hypokalemia—weakness, fatigue, decreased muscle tone, intestinal distention, change in pulse rate or rhythm
- FVD—poor skin turgor, thirst, sunken eyeballs, dryness, weakness, change in pulse rate or rhythm

The patient also should be instructed in the technique for taking her own pulse rate and on the importance of dietary replacement of potassium (e.g., bananas, oranges, potatoes) or administration of prescribed supplements.

2. The patient on prolonged immobility is prone to hypercalcemia as a result of calcium being released from the bones into the bloodstream. The nurse is alert to changes in the cardiac rate and rhythm (e.g., tachycardia) and increases in the BUN and serum calcium levels. If the patient is conscious, there may be anorexia, nausea, vomiting, low back pain, and a reduction in the level of consciousness.

   Alcoholic patients are more susceptible to malnutrition and hypomagnesemia. The nurse is alert to muscle tremors, hyperactive reflexes, confusion, disorientation, dysrhythmias, positive Trousseau's/Chvostek's signs, and a serum magnesium level below 1.5 mEq/L.

3. a. The nurse may anticipate that this patient will have signs and symptoms of diminished oxygenation, including dyspnea, wheezing, coughing, activity intolerance, restlessness, pallor/cyanosis, and possible lack of concentration.
   b. This patient most likely will experience respiratory acidosis.

Chapter Review

1. e	5. b	9. h
2. f	6. a	10. d
3. i	7. c	
4. g	8. j	

11. a. Extracellular fluid
    b. Interstitial fluid
    c. Intracellular fluid
12. a. Sodium: cation, extracellular—maintenance of water balance, nerve impulse transmission, regulation of acid-base balance, and participation in cellular chemical reactions
    b. Potassium: cation, intracellular—necessary for glycogen deposits in the liver and skeletal muscle, transmission and conduction of nerve impulses, cardiac rhythm, and skeletal and smooth muscle contraction
    c. Calcium: cation, intracellular—bone and teeth formation, blood clotting, hormone secretion, cell membrane integrity, cardiac conduction, transmission of nerve impulses, and muscle contraction
    d. Magnesium: cation, intracellular—enzyme activities, neurochemical activities, and cardiac and skeletal muscle excitability
    e. Chloride: anion, extracellular—follows sodium
    f. Bicarbonate: anion, both intracellular and extracellular—major chemical base buffer
13. The three types of acid-base regulators within the body are chemical, biological, and physiological.
14. Infants, young children, and older adults are most susceptible to fluid and acid-base disturbances.
15. a. Isotonic
    b. Hypotonic
    c. Isotonic
    d. Isotonic
    e. Hypertonic
16. The types of medications that may cause fluid, electrolyte, or acid-base disturbances include diuretics, steroids, potassium supplements, depressants, antibiotics, and antacids.
17. Nursing diagnoses for imbalances include:
    Ineffective breathing pattern
    Decreased cardiac output
    Deficient fluid volume
    Excess fluid volume
    Impaired gas exchange
    Impaired skin integrity
    Impaired tissue integrity
    Ineffective tissue perfusion
18.

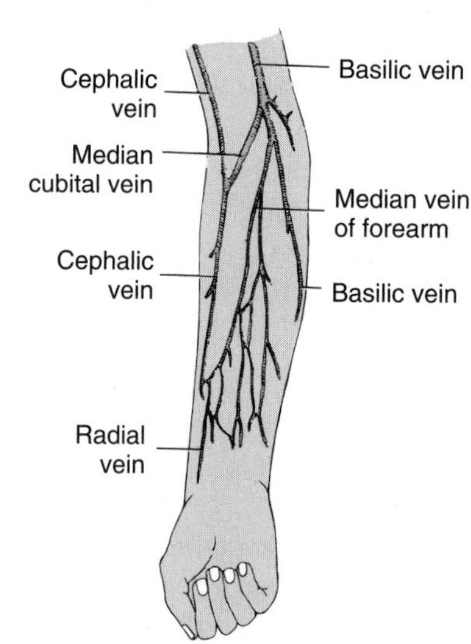

19. A patient who is NPO nd receiving IV fluids needs to have potassium added to the solution.
20. A patient with a PICC line who develops a fever and increased WBCs will have the PICC line discontinued and receive an order for antibiotic therapy.
21. Before a blood transfusion, the nurse checks the blood/blood product with another nurse to determine that the identification and blood type are correct.
22. Transfusion of a patient's own blood is an autologous transfusion.
23. a. Hyponatremia
    b. Hyperkalemia
    c. Hypocalcemia
    d. Hypomagnesemia
24. a. $\frac{500 \text{ ml}}{5 \text{ hours}} = \frac{500 \text{ ml} \times 15 \text{ gtt/ml}}{5 \text{ hours} \times 60 \text{ min/hour}}$
    $= 25$ gtt/min
    b. $\frac{1000 \text{ ml}}{8 \text{ hours}} = \frac{1000 \text{ ml} \times 10 \text{ gtt/ml}}{8 \text{ hours} \times 60 \text{ min/hour}}$
    $= 21$ gtt/min
    c. $\frac{200 \text{ ml}}{4 \text{ hours}} = \frac{200 \text{ ml} \times 60 \text{ gtt/ml}}{4 \text{ hours} \times 60 \text{ min/hour}}$
    $= 50$ gtt/ml
    d. $\frac{2000 \text{ ml}}{18 \text{ hour}} = 111$ ml/hour
25. a. Pituitary hormone—ADH (antidiuretic hormone)
    b. Adrenal hormone—aldosterone
26. True
27. Arterial pH is an indirect measurement of the hydrogen ion concentration.
28. Oxygen moves into the lungs by diffusion.
29. An average adult's daily intake of fluid is approximately 2200 to 2700 ml.

30.	1	40.	4	50.	1
31.	2	41.	3	51.	2
32.	3	42.	2	52.	2
33.	3	43.	4	53.	3
34.	3	44.	4	54.	4
35.	1	45.	3	55.	3
36.	2	46.	4	56.	3
37.	3	47.	3	57.	3
38.	4	48.	1		
39.	3	49.	4		

CHAPTER 16: Caring in Nursing Practice

Case Study

One of the most important things that the nurse can do for the patient's daughter and her family is to sit with them and allow them to verbalize their feelings about the situation. Listening to the family and acknowledging their emotions lets them know that their feelings and concerns are important. It also demonstrates that the nurse is responsive to their needs and is involved in the holistic care of the patient. The nurse should explain how the patient's condition has progressed and the treatments that currently are being provided for comfort and support. The nurse may provide the daughter with the opportunity to assist with or observe the physical care that is being given to the patient. Providing information on available resources, such as hospice, is also important in demonstrating caring and concern for the well-being of the patient and her family.

Chapter Review

1. The theories of caring are:
   a. Swanson
   b. Watson
   c. Benner and Wrubel
   d. Leininger
2. Examples of clinical interventions for the following are:
   a. Providing presence—staying with the patient while waiting for a procedure or test results
   b. Comforting—holding the patient's hand, giving a massage, skillfully and gently performing a procedure
   c. Listening—opening the lines of communication, attentively listening to what the patient is saying, and responding appropriately
   d. Knowing the patient—centering on the patient and providing information that is relevant to the patient's circumstances
3. The nurse demonstrates caring behaviors during an IV insertion by explaining the procedure to the patient in advance and during the intervention, using skillful and

gentle technique, and maintaining eye contact.

4. 1
5. 3
6. 3
7. 4
8. 4
9. 3
10. 2
11. 2

CHAPTER 17: Cultural Diversity

Case Study

a. For a patient from a culture that has a matriarchal organization, the nurse may involve the wife, mother, or sister in the plan of care and decision-making process.
b. Involvement of the family is important in assisting the patient to achieve an optimal level of well-being, but there may need to be limits placed on the number of family members who may stay in the room, a reasonable time frame for visiting to allow the patient to rest and receive treatment, and the determination of where the family may gather to conduct discussions.
c. The therapeutic diet may need to be adapted to avoid meat and meat products but still provide necessary nutrients (protein) or avoid unwanted ingredients (sodium). In an acute or restorative care setting, the dietitian should be involved in providing a menu that meets the patient's cultural preferences but is also tasteful, satisfying, and within therapeutic guidelines.
d. A healer may provide emotional as well as health care support for the patient. The nurse should work with the health care team to integrate, as much as possible, the actions of the healer. Traditional remedies or treatments should be investigated, however, to determine if there may be any interaction with the prescribed medications or therapies.
e. To promote communication with individuals and families who speak another language, the nurse should obtain an interpreter who is proficient in that language, use word signs or charts, refrain from speaking loudly, use appropriate titles and greetings, be attentive to nonverbal communication, and clarify uncertain areas.

Chapter Review

1. e
2. c
3. j
4. g
5. a
6. b
7. h
8. f
9. d
10. i
11. The largest minority group currently in the United States is Hispanic, and the largest growth rate is seen in the Asian population.
12. False
13. Ways that a variant culutre may approach illness causation and treatment include answers a and d.
14. Nursing diagnoses related to cultural needs may include:
    Impaired verbal communication
    Compromised family coping
    Ineffective health maintenance
    Impaired social interaction
    Noncompliance
15. False
16. A patient with a present time orientation may be late for scheduled appointments.
17. The correct cultural beliefs of pregnancy and childbirth are answers c and d.
18. True
19. 1
20. 2
21. 1
22. 4
23. 3
24. 1
25. 1
26. 4
27. 1

CHAPTER 18: Spiritual Health

Case Study

a. The nurse should obtain information about the extent to which the patient practices Buddhism, including whether he or she is a vegetarian, fasts and refuses treatment on holy days, avoids alcohol, and hesitates to use medications. In addition, the patient's advance directives should be obtained because life support may be removed, if indicated.
b. Dependent on the degree to which the patient practices his or her faith, adaptations may need to be made as follows:
    - Special dietary request for a vegetarian diet
    - Scheduling of treatments or tests, for example, on days that are not considered holy

- Determination of medications that may be acceptable
- Use of medications, use of a mouthwash that contains alcohol
- Provide contact with a Buddhist priest

Chapter Review

1. d
2. a
3. e
4. b
5. f
6. g
7. c
8. The four themes of spirituality are:
   - Existential reality
   - Transcendence
   - Connectedness
   - Power/force/energy
9. Nursing interventions for patients who have had near death experiences include the following: promoting open communication, providing a chance for the patient to explore the experience, supporting the patient's discussion with family/significant others.
10. Possible nursing diagnoses include:
    Readiness for enhanced spiritual well-being
    Spiritual distress
    Ineffective coping
    Readiness for enhanced family coping
    Interrupted family processes
    Dysfunctional grieving
    Anxiety
    Hopelessness
    Situational low self-esteem
11. The acronym stands for:
    B—Belief systems
    E—Ethics or values
    L—Lifestyle
    I—Involvement in a spiritual community
    E—Education
    F—Future events
12. Questions to determine a patient's spiritual belief system include:
    "What is most important in your life?"
    "What gives your life meaning or purpose?"
13. 4
14. 1
15. 4
16. 1
17. 3
18. 1
19. 4
20. 3

CHAPTER 19: Growth and Development

Case Studies

1. Promotion of growth and development for the hospitalized infant may include the following:
   - Having the parents/guardians provide most of the care to avoid interfering with the attachment process
   - Limiting the number of caregivers and following the parents' directions for care to promote trust
   - Limiting negative experiences and providing pleasurable sensations

   Promotion of growth and development for the hospitalized 5-year-old child may include the following:
   - Creating a comfortable environment for the child and parents
   - Providing consistent and appropriate care, if the parents are not available
   - Limiting the number of caregivers
   - Providing an environment of acceptance for regressive behavior and reassuring parents that the behavior is normal for children in this situation
   - Allowing children to examine equipment that may be used and participate in procedures, as appropriate
   - Providing comfort items, such as a tape with the parents' voice, pictures of family members, and favorite toys
   - Providing opportunities for play and social interaction with other children
   - Explaining routines in understandable language
   - Incorporating activities of daily living into the hospital routine

2. This patient may benefit from reality orientation, which includes the following:
   - Using time, date, place, and name in conversation
   - Reinforcing reality and providing meaningful things to do
   - Encouraging participation in activities

- Ensuring that hearing aids or glasses, for example, are working or fitted correctly
- Providing bowel and bladder training
- Reinforcing positive behaviors
- Being patient and allowing sufficient time for completion of activities
- Speaking slowly and clearly, repeating as necessary
- Providing clear, simple directions
- Maintaining a caring and stimulating environment

3. Children in this age-group usually are interested in games and sports. For indoor recreation, board games, electronic games, or word games may be suggested. Hobbies and crafts are also appropriate if they stimulate and maintain the children's interest. If the children will be outdoors, supervised games such as volleyball, softball/baseball, kickball, tennis, or relay races may be organized. Some sports may need to be modified to meet the physical abilities of the age-group. Swimming, bicycling, rowing/canoeing, walking, and hiking are activities that do not have to involve competition but promote exercise.

4. Suicide is one of the main causes of death in adolescents and young adults. Parents should be aware of the following warning signs:

- Diminished performance in school
- Withdrawal from social activities with family and friends
- Substance abuse
- Changes in personality
- Disturbances in sleep, appetite, and usual activity levels
- Talking about death or suicide
- Giving away personal items

Chapter Review

1. d 3. c 5. e
2. a 4. f 6. b
7. Teratogens include communicable diseases, alcohol and drugs, smoking, and pollutants.
8. The leading cause of death in the toddler and preschool age-group is accidents.
9. The behaviors are associated with the following age-groups:
   a. Toddler
   b. Infant
   c. School Age
   d. Infant
   e. Young Adult
   f. Toddler
   g. Adolescent
   h. Middle Adult
   i. Toddler
   j. School Age
   k. Preschool Age
   l. Older Adult
   m. School Age
   n. Adolescent
   o. Young Adult
   p. Older Adult
   q. Middle Adult
10. To promote awareness of time, place, and person, the nurse should implement reality orientation.
11. Prescription or use of more medications than indicated is called polypharmacy.
12. Safety concerns in the home environment include:
    a. Toddler—access to poisons, such as cleaning supplies; electrical outlets; ability to exit the home; swimming pools; kitchen appliances; auto accidents; choking on small objects
    b. Older adult—poor lighting, slippery floors and unsecured rugs, excessive water temperature, stairs

13. 4 18. 4 23. 4
14. 2 19. 3 24. 4
15. 2 20. 3 25. 1
16. 4 21. 1
17. 4 22. 4

CHAPTER 20: Self-Concept and Sexuality

Case Studies

1. a. This adolescent patient most likely will experience alterations in his self-concept, especially the perception of his body image and identity. Adolescents may be very sensitive about their physical appearance and social status, and now the patient will have to cope with an alteration in his social and athletic activity in school. In addition, the paraplegia will significantly influence his sexual functioning, an area where he may have been exploring and now will have to adapt.

b. Sample care plan:

Nursing Diagnosis	*Expected Outcome*	*Nursing Interventions*
Potential body image disturbance related to accidental injury and resultant lack of mobility and sensation to lower extremities (as manifested by his frequent verbalization of prior involvement in athletics and other school activities).	Patient will adapt to change in body image by: • Discussing feelings about his injury and change in activity status • Participating in care as much as possible • Reflecting on personal strengths	Provide time for talking with the patient and discussing feelings; explore coping skills that the client has used before, and encourage and support those skills; involve the client in health care activities.
Altered sexuality patterns related to accidental injury and resultant lack of mobility and sensation to lower extremities.	Patient will learn/utilize measures to attain sexual satisfaction within limitations by: • Discussing feelings about sexual function and adaption • Participating in educational program on alternative measures to promote sexual response. • Sharing response to measures utilized and suggesting possible alternatives.	Provide time to talk with the patient and discuss feelings and concerns; provide information on sexual response and stimulation for patients with paraplegia; obtain a referral/consultation, if indicated, for addtional support and information; have another young male paraplegic individual speak with the patient; provide for patient privacy.

2. a. The patient who you suspect may be a victim of sexual abuse may be found to have:
- Physical signs—bruises, laceration, abrasions, burns, headaches, GI problems, eating disorders, abdominal or vaginal pain
- Behavioral signs—sleep-pattern disturbances, nightmares, insomnia, depression, anxiety, fear, decreased self-esteem, substance abuse, frequent visits to health care providers

b. Examples of questions that should be asked include:
- “Are you in a relationship where someone is hurting you?”
- “Have you ever been forced to have sex when you didn’t want to?”
- “Are you afraid of the situation that you are in?”

Chapter Review

1. b
2. f
3. e
4. d
5. h
6. a
7. c
8. g
9. General positive influences on self-concept include words and actions of approval, interest, and acceptance; recognition and inclusion in decision-making; trust; and support. Stressors that may influence self-concept include those that threaten body image, self-esteem, role, or identity such as the effects of traumatic accidents, surgery, and acute or chronic diseases.
10. Behaviors that may indicate an altered self-concept include: (c) hesitant speech,

(d) overly angry response, (f) passive attitude, and (h) unkempt appearance.

11. Potential concerns related to self-concept include:
    a. Alteration in body image—removal of breast can lead to question of feminine image and sexual desirability
    b. Alteration in body image and role—loss of hair from chemotherapy, possible hospitalizations and diminished strength may interfere with role as mother
    c. Alteration in body image and identity—physical changes in appearance and function (ability to play with others)
    d. Alteration in role and self-esteem—possible inability to maintain current occupation, dependence on others
12. Ways in which the nurse may promote self-concept in an acute care setting include the following:
    - Arranging visits with someone who has experienced similar/problems changes
    - Being sensitive to and supporting the patient's needs
13. Alterations in sexual health include infertility, sexual abuse, sexual dysfunction, and personal and emotional conflicts.
14. Client teaching for the promotion of sexual health may include instruction about:
    - Refraining from drinking alcohol 1 to 2 hours before sexual activity
    - Discussing behavior that provides the most sexual stimulation and satisfaction
    - Options available for contraception
    - Side effects of medications that alter sexual function and response
    - Use of usual positions and selection of times when client feels rested (for individuals with cardiac dysfunction)
    - Safe sex practices
15. For the nursing diagnosis, *Situational Low self-esteem related to being unable to pass a required college course*, examples are as follows:
    - Patient goal; Increased self-esteem
    - Outcome: Discusses positive aspects of self and future plans
    - Nursing interventions: Spend time with the patient to allow for discussion of feelings and concerns, establish sense of trust
16. False
17. False
18. Promotion of self-concept for an older adult may include:
    - Clarifying what life changes mean
    - Being alert to preoccupation with physical complaints and encouraging verbaalization of needs
    - Identifying positive and negative coping mechanisms and supporting effective strategies
    - Encouraging the use of storytelling
    - Communicating that the individual is worthwhile by actively listening to and accepting the person's feelings and concerns
    - Allowing additional time to complete tasks and reinforcing the person's efforts at independence

19.	3	24.	1	29.	2
20.	4	25.	2	30.	3
21.	4	26.	4	31.	4
22.	4	27.	4	32.	3
23.	1	28.	4	33.	2

CHAPTER 21: Family Context in Nursing

Case Study

a. The patient, who provides the major financial support to the family, has been hospitalized with a serious health problem. His wife has maintained a traditional role as "homemaker" while her husband has worked. The younger daughter has assumed a family life that appears to be more acceptable to her parents, whereas the older son is involved in an alternative family form. The younger daughter may be more involved in her parents' life because of her family pattern.

b. The family is apparently progressing from "Launching children and moving on" to the "Family in later life" stage. There are elements of both stages within this situation.
c. The nurse may begin discussions with the father and mother initially, moving toward a total family meeting at a later date. Providing opportunities for family members to express their feelings about both the health care and the family situation may facilitate open communication about family structure and relationships. The family may need to be referred for ongoing counseling if there is a negative impact on the health/recovery of the patient.
d. The patient may have feelings about his business and family roles and his ability to resume them when he is discharged. His wife will need to be involved in the educational process to follow through with the plan of care. The patient's wife may need to assume a greater decision-making role with the patient to maintain the economic and emotional status of the family.
e. Possible family-oriented nursing diagnoses include:
   - *Family processes*
   - *Ineffective role performance*
   - *Compromised family coping*

Chapter Review

1. b
2. d
3. a
4. e
5. c
6. A possible nursing diagnosis is: *Caregiver role strain.*
7. The correct statements are b, d, f, and g.
8. Inadequate functioning can have many effects on the family, including stress, impaired cardiovascular and neuroendocrine functioning, and interference with decision making and problem solving.
9. 3
10. 4
11. 3
12. 1
13. 3
14. 4
15. 4
16. 3
17. 4
18. 1

CHAPTER 22: Stress and Coping

Case Study

a. This patient may demonstrate the following:
   - Physical signs—increased heart rate, respirations, and blood pressure; headaches; fatigue; sleep disturbances; restlessness; gastrointestinal distress; weight gain or loss; backaches; amenorrhea; frequent or prolonged colds or flu
   - Psychological signs—forgetfulness, preoccupation, increased fantasizing, decreased creativity, slower reactions and thinking, confusion, decreased attention span
   - Emotional signs—crying tendencies, lack of interest, irritability, negative thinking, worrying
   - Behavioral signs—diminished activity or hyperactivity, withdrawal, suspiciousness, substance abuse, change in communication or interaction with others
b. Possible nursing diagnoses for this patient include:
   - *Anxiety*
   - *Ineffective coping*
c. A number of alternatives may be presented to this patient so that she may select those that are most beneficial to her. The nurse may use guided imagery, biofeedback, progressive muscle relaxation, hypnosis, music/art therapy, humor, assertiveness training, or journal/diary entry.

Chapter Review

1. Evaluating an event for its personal meaning is called primary appraisal.
2. The correct statements about stress are a, d, and e.
3. A priority nursing intervention for patient safety is to determine if the patient is suicidal or homicidal.
4. True
5. Positive benefits from exercise include increased muscle tone, decreased tension, increased relaxation, weight control,

increased circulation, improved posture, and endorphin release.

6. a. Maturational
   b. Sociocultural
   c. Posttraumatic stress disorder
   d. Sociocultural
   e. Situational
   f. Maturational
   g. Situational
   h. Maturational
   i. Posttraumatic stress disorder
   j. Sociocultural
7. a. Cognitive—forgetfulness, denial, increased fantasy life, poor concentration, inattention to detail, orientation to the past, decreased creativity, slower thinking and reactions, learning difficulties, apathy, confusion, decreased attention span, calculation difficulties
   b. Cardiovascular—increased heart rate, increased blood pressure, tightness in chest
   c. Gastrointestinal—nausea, diarrhea, vomiting, weight gain or loss, change in appetite, bleeding
   d. Behavioral—change in activity level, withdrawal, suspiciousness, change in communication and interaction with others, substance abuse, excessive humor or silence, no exercise, hyperactivity
   e. Neuroendocrine—headaches/migraines, fatigue, insomnia/sleep disturbances, feeling of being uncoordinated, restlessness, tremors, profuse sweating, dry mouth

8.	1	11.	3	14.	4
9.	2	12.	4	15.	1
10.	1	13.	3	16.	2

CHAPTER 23: Loss and Grief

Case Study

a. Mrs. R. may demonstrate the following behaviors indicative of complicated bereavement:
   - Overactivity without a sense of loss
   - Alteration in relationships with friends and family
   - Anger against particular people
   - Agitated depression—tension, guilt, feelings of worthlessness
   - Decreased participation in religious or cultural activities
   - Inability to discuss the loss without crying (a year or more after the loss)
   - False euphoria
   - Eliminating all signs of the deceased (e.g., pictures) or creating a "shrine"
   - Alterations in eating and sleeping patterns
   - Regressive behavior
b. Possible nursing diagnoses for Mrs. R. may be:
   - *Dysfunctional grieving related to sudden loss/suicide of husband*
   - *Ineffective individual coping related to inability to deal with husband's loss/suicide*

   Possible goals may be:
   - Mrs. R. will accept the reality of her husband's death
   - Mrs. R. will renew activities of daily living and complete a normal grieving process

   Nursing interventions may include:
   - Using therapeutic communication to promote Mrs. R.'s verbalization of feelings concerning her husband's suicide
   - Demonstrating support of the patient by staying with her and using comfort measures, such as touch
   - Referring the patient to support groups, clergy, and/or counseling as appropriate for her needs

Chapter Review

1.	f	3.	a	5.	e
2.	c	4.	b	6.	d

7. Special circumstances that may influence grief resolution include suicide, sudden death, miscarriage/child's death, and AIDS.
8. True
9. Interventions that should be implemented for a family dealing with a patient's terminal illness include involving everyone in

discussions, promoting open communication, answering questions, and providing caregiver support.

10. The correct interventions are c and d.

11.	2	16.	3	21.	1
12.	2	17.	2	22.	4
13.	3	18.	1	23.	3
14.	4	19.	3	24.	1
15.	4	20.	1		

CHAPTER 24: Managing Patient Care

Case Studies

1. a. After determining what needs to be done and prioritizing your interventions, you can delegate to the nursing assistant activities such as vital sign measurements, evening hygienic care, basic procedures (catheter care), and assistance with meals. The nursing assistant may also be asked to obtain necessary supplies and equipment for patient care. You also may have the assistant check on the general status of the patients and report back any immediate problems.
   b. To safely delegate activities, you need to determine the level of acuity of the patients and the knowledge and ability of the aide. If some of the patients are having abnormal vital signs, such as dysrhythmias, then it would not be appropriate to delegate pulse rate measurement to the nursing assistant.
2. Possible areas for QI projects on the surgical unit may include patient satisfaction, postoperative infection rates, success of preoperative teaching and postoperative exercises, and frequency of respiratory or circulatory complications.
3. To become a nurse practitioner, this individual will need to complete the bachelor's degree in nursing and progress on to a graduate program in nursing to obtain a master's degree. Advanced practice nurses, such as nurse practitioners, require additional education in advanced physical assessment, pharmacology, and clinical care, as well as expertise in their field. The individual also will need to be licensed in the state where she will practice.

Chapter Review

1. Upon completion of a nursing program, graduates will take the NCLEX-RN® or NCLEX-PN® licensure examination.
2. A person who is reasonably independent in decision making is demonstrating autonomy.
3. The most important aspect of delegation is consideration of the qualifications of the person to whom the responsibility is being delegated.
4. The correct terms are:
   a. Responsibility
   b. Authority
   c. Accountability

5.	4	10.	4	15.	1
6.	2	11.	2	16.	1
7.	1	12.	4	17.	2
8.	1	13.	3	18.	3
9.	4	14.	4		

CHAPTER 25: Exercise and Activity

Case Study

a. Mrs. T. should be assessed for her ability to move independently, including her posture, muscle strength, range of motion, gait (if able), balance, activity tolerance, and cognitive status. If Mrs. T. is able to bear weight on both legs and maintain an erect position, the nurse must determine if she is capable of ambulating safely. Initial assessment of Mrs. T.'s transfer out of bed should be accomplished with assistance in the event that the patient is unable to maintain a standing position.

b. If Mrs. T. is not able to ambulate independently, she may be able to use an assistive device, such as a cane or walker. If possible, one or more nurses may use a gait belt to assist Mrs. T. in ambulating. Should Mrs. T. not be able to ambulate safely, even with assistance, a wheelchair may be necessary. To assist Mrs. T.

in gaining muscle strength, a program of exercise may be implemented.

Chapter Review

1. j
2. h
3. i
4. g
5. e
6. b
7. f
8. d
9. a
10. c
11. Assessment of a patient's mobility includes range of joint motion, gait, and exercise.
12. The correct principles of body mechanics are options b, d, and f.
13. False
14. Before ambulation, the patient should be placed in a sitting position with the legs dangled over the side of the bed.
15. True
16. Examples of physiological factors that may influence activity tolerance are musculoskeletal abnormalities, diminished cardiovascular function, and diminished respiratory function.
17. Possible nursing diagnoses associated with a change in a patient's ability to maintain physical activity include:
    - *Activity intolerance*
    - *Disturbed body image*
    - *Risk for injury*
    - *Impaired physical mobility*
    - *Impaired skin integrity*
    - *Acute or chronic pain*
18. The priority for this patient is pain relief.
19. The patient should be in Fowler's position—the head of the bed elevated 45 to 60 degrees above level.
20. Safety during transfers is the priority.
21. a. Supine
    b. Prone
    c. Lateral
22. Expected findings are answers a and g.
23. The correct techniques are answers d and e.
24. 3
25. 2
26. 4
27. 1
28. 1
29. 2
30. 4
31. 4
32. 2
33. 1
34. 4
35. 2
36. 4
37. 4

CHAPTER 26: Safety

Case Studies

1. a. You should assess some of the following areas regarding home safety:
- Location of the home in the community
- Security measures within the home
- Environmental conditions—lighting, temperature, sanitation, stairways, floors/carpeting
- Fire and electrical safety measures/hazards
- Exposure to pollutants/pathogens

b. With a toddler and a preschool child in the home, safety measures are extremely important. Accidents are one of the major problems for children, including falls and poisoning. If there are stairs in the home, gates should be in use or doors to the outside should be locked. For upper level apartments or rooms, child-safety devices should be in place on the windows. Any household chemicals or medications should be out of reach and/or in a locked compartment. There also may be locks on other kitchen cabinets, drawers, and the refrigerator to prevent access. Electrical outlets should have covers, and plugs should be out of sight of the children. The family should have a fire safety plan, fire extinguishers, and smoke/fire alarms. Items that may be swallowed or broken should be out of reach. Additional safety measures may be in place in the kitchen and bathroom, such as faucet covers.

2. a. For the patient in the home who has diabetes mellitus and requires insulin injections, the following precautions should be taken:
- Perform hand hygiene and maintain sterile asepsis for the injections
- Store the insulin properly
- Maintain an adequate supply of insulin and injection supplies

- Dispose of used needles and syringes appropriately—do not reuse the injection supplies
- Have adequate light for preparation and administration of the injection
- Wear eyeglasses, if needed

Chapter Review

1. Basic human needs in a safe environment and examples of what may affect them are:
   - Oxygen—carbon monoxide, improper ventilation, pollutants
   - Degree of humidity—excessive dryness
   - Nutrition—improper storage/refrigeration, inadequate cleaning of cooking surfaces
   - Optimal temperature—excessive heat or cold
2. Inadequate lighting, clutter, lack of security, fire/electrical hazards, and temperature extremes are examples of physical hazards in the home.
3. Diminished vision, hearing, mobility, reflexes, and circulation are some of the reasons that older adults are predisposed to accidents.
4. The following are examples of how the nurse may prevent health care agency risks:
   a. Falls—complete a risk assessment, provide supervision, place the patient close to the nurse's station, orient the patient to the surroundings, use physical restraints if absolutely necessary
   b. Patient-inherent accidents—institute seizure precautions, remove foreign substances or hazardous items (sharps), provide supervision of the patient's activities
   c. Procedure-related risks—follow policies and procedures carefully, use appropriate technique for performing procedures
   d. Equipment-related risks—learn how to operate the equipment, have it checked regularly for proper functioning
5. Motor vehicle accidents are the leading cause of unintentional death.
6. Active immunity is obtained through the injection of weakened or dead organisms and modified toxins.
7. Potential hazards include:
   a. Infant, toddler, preschool: injuries, accidents, poisoning
   b. School-age child: sports, after-school activities, bicycle accidents, school bus injuries
   c. Adolescent: smoking, substance abuse, motor vehicle accidents, stress, sexual activity
   d. Adult: alcohol/substance abuse, motor vehicle accidents, stress-related activities
   e. Older adult: falls, medication misuse
8. Patients experiencing impaired mobility, diminished sensation and/or cognition, and decreased safety awareness are a high risk for injury.
9. Potential agents that may be used are:
   a. Biological—anthrax, smallpox, typhoid, plague, botulism
   b. Chemical—cyanide, mustard gas, chlorine, nerve agents
   c. Radiological—nuclear device, "dirty bomb"
10. A risk for poisoning exists in the home of an older adult with multiple medications, especially from a variety of prescribers.
11. Teaching areas for a school-age child include crossing the street, stranger safety, bicycle safety, sport/activity safety, and personal hygiene.
12. The primary goal of restraints (safety reminder devices) is to prevent falls.
13. A nursing home is required to obtain informed consent from the patient and/or family, along with a health care provider's order.
14. False
15. An older adult having difficulty with medication administration in the home may benefit from the use of a medication organizer device or system.
16. In a health care agency, medication safety is promoted by using the "seven rights,"

including properly identifying the patient, maintaining accurate labeling and storage, and documenting promptly.

17. Environmental adjustments include:
    a. Tactile deficit—check/adjust the water heater temperature, clearly label the settings on the stove/oven, obtain easy-open medication containers
    b. Visual deficit—maintain adequate lighting, use stair treads and handrails, decrease clutter, use distinct colors, have large print on labels
18. The following alternative measures may be implemented:
    - Orienting patients/families to the surroundings
    - Explaining routines and procedures
    - Encouraging family and friends to stay with the patient
    - Providing adequate stimulation, diversional activity
    - Using relaxation techniques
    - Instituting exercise and activity plans
    - Eliminating bothersome therapies as soon as possible
    - Maintaining toileting routines
    - Evaluating the effect of medications
    - Performing regular assessments of the patient's status
    - Using electronic bed and chair alarm devices
    - Placing the patient in a room near the nurses' station
19. Possible nursing diagnoses include:
    - *Risk for imbalanced body temperature*
    - *Impaired home maintenance*
    - *Risk for injury*
    - *Deficient knowledge*
    - *Risk for poisoning*
    - *Disturbed sensory perception*
    - *Risk for suffocation*
    - *Disturbed thought processes*
    - *Risk for trauma*

20. 4
21. 3
22. 2
23. 1
24. 3
25. 2
26. 4
27. 3
28. 3
29. 4
30. 4

CHAPTER 27: Hygiene

Case Studies

1. For the patient with diabetes mellitus, you should include the following instructions:
    - Carefully inspect the skin surfaces, particularly the extremities
    - Perform daily foot care using lukewarm water, with no soaking—
      dry the feet well, especially between the toes
    - Do not cut corns or calluses
    - Apply bland powder if the feet perspire
    - File the toenails straight across, no cutting
    - Wear clean, dry socks daily
    - Do not walk barefoot
    - Wear properly fitting, flexible shoes
    - Exercise regularly
    - Avoid application of hot water bottles or heating pads to the extremities
    - Clean minor cuts immediately and apply only mild antiseptics, if necessary
    - Avoid wearing elastic stockings, tight hose, or noncotton socks
    - Avoid crossing the legs
    - Avoid the use of commercial preparations for corn/callus removal, athlete's foot, or ingrown toenails
    - Consult a podiatrist as needed for foot problems
2. The older adult patient may be experiencing changes in their skin integrity. The skin is more fragile, so hot water and strong cleansing agents should be avoided. Older adults usually perspire less, so bathing need not be as frequent (unless personally desired). There may be an increased sensitivity or itching that may be relieved with the use of hydrocortisone cream, moisturizing soaps, or petrolatum jelly. Humidity should be higher in the environment to alleviate skin dryness. Care should be taken to avoid injury to the skin as wound healing is slower in this population.

Chapter Review

1. e
2. b
3. d
4. a
5. f
6. c
7. g
8. Appropriate techniques are answers d, e, f, h, and i.
9. A nurse-initiated treatment for a rash is a warm soak.
10. Plain water is used on the patient's eyes.
11. Eyeglasses should be kept in a case on top of the bedside table or in a drawer of the bedside table when not in use.
12. Ear irrigation is contraindicated in the presence of a perforated tympanic membrane (eardrum).
13. Asepsis is maintained during linen changes by:
    - Keeping soiled linen away from the uniform and off the floor
    - Placing soiled linen in the proper container
    - Avoiding fanning or shaking of linens
    - Discarding clean items that fall on the floor
14. The nurse prepares a comfortable environment for the patient by controlling the room temperature, providing for adequate ventilation and lighting, limiting noise, reducing odors, and keeping the room neat.
15. The best type of light to use for skin assessment is natural or halogen light.
16. 3
17. 1
18. 4
19. 4
20. 3
21. 2
22. 1
23. 3
24. 3

CHAPTER 28: Oxygenation

Case Study

a. To gather further information from the patient about her current respiratory status, the nurse should ask the following questions:
    - "When do you experience shortness of breath/difficulty breathing?"
    - "What activities bring on the shortness of breath?"
    - "Does the shortness of breath interfere with your activities of daily living?"
    - "Do you find that it is hard to inhale or exhale?"
    - "Do you sleep with extra pillows at night?"
    - "Are you more tired than usual?"
    - "Do you smoke?"
    - "Are you exposed to smokers or other environmental hazards at home or at work?"
    - "When does the cough start?"
    - "Are there times when your breathing/coughing is better or worse?"
    - "What are you bringing up when you cough?"
    - "Have you been exposed to anyone with a respiratory infection?"
    - "Have you recently had an upper respiratory infection?"
    - "Have you had pain in your chest when you breathe?"
    - "Are you currently taking any medications?"

b. Based on additional information from the patient, possible nursing diagnoses for this patient may be:
    - *Activity intolerance*
    - *Ineffective airway clearance*
    - *Impaired gas exchange*
    - *Risk for infection*

c. Nurse-initiated actions may include measurement of vital signs, auscultation of lung sounds, inspection of sputum, positioning for optimum respiratory function and comfort, and preparation of oxygen and suctioning equipment in case severe respiratory distress develops.

d. General teaching for health promotion should include the importance of:
    - Receiving the pneumococcal and influenza vaccines (if she has not had them)
    - Limiting exposure to crowds and environmental pollutants
    - Avoiding smoking or secondhand smoke
    - Covering the mouth and nose if exposed to cold air
    - Determining and improving activity and exercise tolerance

- Taking medications regularly
- Performing breathing/coughing exercises

Chapter Review

1. c
2. e
3. f
4. d
5. b
6. k
7. a
8. h
9. g
10. i
11. The average resting heart rate for an adult is 60 to 80 beats per minute.
12. Conditions that may affect chest wall movement include pregnancy, obesity, musculoskeletal abnormalities, abnormal structural configuration, trauma, muscle diseases, and nervous system diseases.
13. a, b—Right ventricular heart failure
    c, d—Left ventricular heart failure
14. Hyperventilation may be caused by answers a, b, and d.
15. a. Decreased oxygen carrying capacity: anemia, inhalation of toxic substances (carbon monoxide)
    b. Decreased inspired oxygen concentration: airway obstruction, higher altitudes
    c. Hypovolemia: fluid loss, dehydration, shock
    d. Increased metabolic rate: fever, pregnancy, hyperthyroidism
16. A premature infant may have a deficiency of surfactant.
17. Modifiable risk factors include smoking, substance abuse, poor nutrition, lack of exercise, and stress.
18. Changes that occur in the cardio-pulmonary system as a result of aging include answers b, e, and g.
19. This condition is noted by the nurse as paroxysmal nocturnal dyspnea (PND).
20. Wheezing is a high-pitched, musical lung sound that is heard on inspiration and/or expiration.
21. a. Premature ventricular contractions (PVCs)
    b. Ventricular tachycardia
22. a. Retraction is the visible sinking in of the soft tissues of the chest between and around firmer tissue and ribs; seen often in the intercostal spaces.
    b. Paradoxical breathing is asymmetrical or asynchronous breathing where the chest contracts during inspiration and expands during expiration.
23. Surgical asepsis or sterile technique is used to suction the trachea.
24. Continuous bubbling in the chest tube water-seal chamber indicates an air leak.
25. Nursing interventions to achieve the following include:
    a. Dyspnea management—administration of medications (e.g., bronchodilators), supervision of oxygen therapy, and instruction in breathing and coughing techniques and relaxation measures
    b. Patent airway—instruction in coughing techniques, suctioning, and airway placement
    c. Lung expansion—positioning, administering chest physiotherapy, instruction in the use of incentive spirometry, and management of chest tubes
    d. Mobilization of secretions—hydration of the patient, humidification/nebulization of oxygen therapy, and administration of chest physiotherapy
26. a. Simple face mask: 30% to 60% (6 to 8 L/min)
    b. Venturi mask: 24% to 55% (2 to 14 L/min)
27. For tuberculin (Mantoux) testing:
    a. Forearm
    b. 72 hours
    c. Negative reaction
28. For chest percussion, vibration, and postural drainage:
    a. Bleeding disorders, osteoporosis, fractured ribs
    b. Exhalation
    c. Positioned on the nurse's/parent's lap
29. For CPAP:
    a. Sleep apnea, postpolio syndrome, congestive heart failure, neuromuscular and pulmonary diseases
    b. 5 to 20 cm H_2O
    c. Hypercapnea, gastric distention, discomfort, risk for skin irritation, noise

30. An indication for home oxygen therapy is an SaO_2 of 88% or less.
31. The ABCs of CPR:
    A—airway
    B—breathing
    C—circulation
32. Defibrillation is recommended within 5 minutes inside and 3 minutes outside of a hospital/medical center.
33. True
34. The nurse instructs the patient/family and/or implements the following safety measures for home oxygen therapy:
    - Place "no smoking" signs around the patient area, with visitors informed that smoking is prohibited where the oxygen is being used
    - Check the electrical equipment to determine that it is functioning properly and will not create sparks
    - Review fire procedures and location of extinguishers
    - Check the oxygen level to ensure a sufficient amount is present (an additional source may be obtained as a backup)
    - Have an alternative source of oxygen in case of a power failure
35. For the nursing diagnosis *Ineffective airway clearance related to the presence of tracheobronchial secretions*, possible patient outcomes and nursing interventions are:
    Patient outcomes:
    - Sputum will be clear within 24 to 36 hours
    - No adventitious lung sounds auscultated
    - Respiratory rate of 16 to 24 breaths/min
    - Coughing and clearing airway within 24 hours

    Nursing interventions:
    - Instruct patient on coughing and deep breathing
    - Assist with position changes and ambulation
    - Provide 2000 to 2500 ml of fluid, if not contraindicated
    - Monitor vital signs
    - Suction prn
    - Provide chest physiotherapy, if indicated

36.	4	42.	4	48.	1
37.	3	43.	2	49.	3
38.	3	44.	3	50.	1
39.	4	45.	3	51.	4
40.	1	46.	4	52.	4
41.	2	47.	1	53.	2

CHAPTER 29: Sleep

Case Study

a. A possible nursing diagnosis for this patient is *Disturbed sleep pattern related to current life situation: stress at home and work.* Goals include:
    - Patient will achieve an adequate amount of nightly sleep within 1 month
    - Patient will identify and verbalize about current life stressors
    - Patient will practice stress reduction/relaxation techniques as needed

b. The nurse may implement the following:
    - Sit with the patient and offer an opportunity for her to vent about her feelings and concerns
    - Instruct the patient on stress reduction/relaxation techniques
    - Advise about the value of exercise and activity before sleep
    - Discuss manipulation of the environment to provide maximum comfort and minimum distraction
    - Instruct the patient on the avoidance of heavy meals before bedtime and excessive caffeine or alcohol intake
    - Have the patient maintain a log of sleep/rest patterns

Chapter Review

1.	f	4.	a	7.	d
2.	b	5.	h	8.	e
3.	g	6.	c		

9. Sleep may be affected by physical illness, medications/substances, lifestyle changes, sleep pattern alterations, emotional stress, environmental variations, exercise, fatigue, and food and caloric intake.
10. The correct responses are c and f.

11. The nurse may promote a restful environment by checking that the:
    - Patient's bed is clean and dry
    - Lights are lowered and not directed at patient's eyes
    - Temperature and ventilation in the room are at comfortable levels
    - Amount of noise is decreased
    - Number of distractions is decreased
12. True
13. False
14. A sleep log usually includes information on waking and sleeping activities such as: exercise, work, mealtimes, alcohol and caffeine intake, the time and length of naps, evening and bedtime routines, the time the patient tries to fall asleep, time and number of awakenings, and the time of morning awakening.

15. 3	22. 2	29. 4
16. 4	23. 3	30. 1
17. 1	24. 3	31. 4
18. 2	25. 1	32. 1
19. 2	26. 4	33. 3
20. 3	27. 1	34. 3
21. 3	28. 1	

CHAPTER 30: Promoting Comfort

Case Study

a. To successfully use a PCA pump, the patient must understand the purpose and use of the medication and pump, as well as be able to locate and push the button on the pump that controls the administration of the medication.
b. Teaching for this patient should include:
    - Use of the equipment
    - Purpose of PCA, action(s) of the medication, expected pain relief, precautions, and potential side effects of the medication (CNS depression)
    - General precautions for an IV infusion
    - Caution against family members/visitors operating the device for the patient

Chapter Review

1. k	5. e	9. f
2. a	6. g	10. h
3. d	7. c	
4. j	8. b	

11. The first structure in the brain to process pain is the thalamus.
12. The gate control theory suggests that heat, cold, transcutaneous electrical nerve stimulation (TENS), and pharmacological interventions will reduce pain.
13. The physiological responses to pain as a result of sympathetic stimulation include an increased heart rate (b), increased blood glucose level (d), and diaphoresis (e).
14. The influence of chronic pain on an individual's lifestyle can include the following: change of sleep patterns, inability to perform hygienic care, sexual dysfunction, alteration in home or work management, and interruption of social activities.
15. An infant may respond to pain by crying and by exhibiting changes in vital signs, facial expressions, or extremity movement. A child may respond to pain with crying, irritability, loss of appetite, quietness or restlessness, disturbed sleep patterns, or rigid body posture.
16. The single most reliable indicator of pain is the patient's self-report.
17. For the PQRSTU assessment:
    a. **Quality**—suggest a change in medications if the quality of pain changes
    b. **Region**—position the patient so body weight is shifted away from area of pain; apply heat/cold directly to the site
    c. **Timing**—administer medication so the peak effect occurs when pain is most acute
18. a. Toddler—use of words that the child can understand ("boo-boo"), pictures ("Oucher" scale), dolls to act out with, pointing at areas of discomfort
    b. Person who speaks English as second language—use of an interpreter, pictures (pain scale), gestures, and pointing to areas of discomfort
19. In determining the location of the pain, the nurse should ask the patient to point to the area, or draw or trace the extent of the pain.

20. A pain rating of 7 on a scale of 1 to 10 is an emergency.
21. The nurse should administer the pain medication about 30 minutes before painful activities.
22. Individualizing a patient's pain management may include:
    - Using different types of pain relief measures
    - Providing pain relief measures before the pain becomes severe
    - Using measures that the patient believes are effective
    - Using the patient's ideas for pain relief and scheduling
    - Suggesting measures that are within the patient's capability
    - Choosing pain relief measures on the basis of the patient's responses
    - Encouraging the patient to try measures more than once to see if they may work
    - Keeping an open mind about nontraditional measures
    - Protecting the patient from more pain
    - Educating the patient about the pain
23. The following statements are correct regarding TENS: it requires a health care provider's order (b), skin preparation is required before electrode placement (c), and controls should be adjusted until the patient feels a buzzing sensation (e).
24. Medications used for mild to moderate pain include Motrin (a), Ultram (d), and Tylenol (f).
25. Nonpharmacological interventions for pain relief include reduction/removal of painful stimuli, cutaneous stimulation, distraction, relaxation, guided imagery, anticipatory guidance, biofeedback, and hypnosis.
26. Adjuvant medications that may be used in conjunction with analgesics to manage pain are sedatives, anticonvulsants, steroids, antidepressants, antianxiety agents, and muscle relaxants.
27. The usual dosage of on-demand morphine for PCA is 1 mg every 6 minutes to a maximum dosage of 10 mg per hour.
28. Priority nursing interventions for the patient with an epidural infusion include assessment of the site and patency of the tube along with maintenance of aseptic technique in site care.

    A priority assessment before and during administration of all analgesics is the patient's respiratory status.
29. The nurse may adapt/alter the patient's environment to increase comfort by:
    - Straightening wrinkled bed linen
    - Repositioning the patient
    - Loosening tight clothing or bandages (unless contraindicated)
    - Changing wet dressings or bed linens
    - Checking the temperature of hot/cold applications and bath water
    - Lifting the patient up in bed, not pulling
    - Positioning the patient correctly on the bedpan
    - Avoiding exposure of the skin or mucous membranes to irritants (e.g., urine)
    - Preventing urinary retention by keeping the catheter patent
    - Preventing constipation by use of fluids, diet, and exercise
    - Reducing lighting that glares/shines directly on the patient
    - Checking the temperature of the room and the sensation of the patient
    - Reducing the level of noise and traffic
30. a. True d. False g. False
    b. True e. True h. True
    c. False f. False

31. 3
32. 2
33. 4
34. 3
35. 2
36. 4
37. 3
38. 1
39. 1
40. 1
41. 4
42. 4
43. 2
44. 3
45. 1

CHAPTER 31: Nutrition

Case Study

a. To assist this patient and the family with dietary planning, it is important to find out the following information:
    - Who prepares the food in the home?
    - Who buys the food, and where is the food purchased?

- What foods are regularly eaten? Are there special foods for holidays or family occasions?
- What are the patient's food preferences?

In addition, the patient should keep a record of dietary intake (usually recorded over 3 to 7 days).

b. Teaching about foods that are high in sodium and saturated fat is an important part of the plan for this patient. Reading labels and menus (if the patient eats out) will help in the selection of appropriate foods. The patient and family also may be informed about possible substitutions for foods, spices, and oils that are high in sodium and fat. Alternatives, such as polyunsaturated oils, lean meats, and egg substitutes, may be incorporated into meal preparation. A separate meal plan for the patient is usually not necessary because flavorings, such as lemon, can make foods attractive (as well as healthy) for the entire family. The most difficult times are often during holidays and special occasions, when food plays a central role in the family's activities. Low-salt and low-fat substitutions, wherever appropriate, should be used. Fresh or frozen fruits and vegetables, without sodium or fat-based sauces or additives, may be more flavorful than low-sodium canned foods. The patient also may be able to eat traditional foods, in moderation, on these occasions. Realistic expectations may work best for the patient rather than offering harsh, uncompromising restrictions.

Chapter Review

1.	i	5.	j	9.	b
2.	c	6.	g	10.	d
3.	a	7.	f		
4.	h	8.	e		

11. The goals are for individuals to increase their daily intake of fruits, vegetables, and grain products and decrease their intake of sodium and fat.
12. Vitamin K is synthesized by the body.
13. a. Carbohydrates
    b. Proteins
    c. Fats
    d. Carbohydrates
    e. Fats
    f. Proteins
    g. Carbohydrates
14. Some general nutritional guidelines to share are:
    - Eat a variety of foods—consume plenty of grains, fruits, and vegetables
    - Balance the intake of food with the amount of physical activity
    - Reduce the intake of sugar, sodium, fat/saturated fat, and cholesterol
    - Moderate the intake of alcoholic beverages
    - A copy of MyPyramid may be provided and discussed with the patient
15. Examples of alternative dietary patterns include vegetarians, ovolactovegetarians, and lactovegetarians. In addition, patients from diverse sociocultural backgrounds may have dietary patterns that are unique.
16. For the nutritional assessment:
    a. Food and nutrient intake: 24-hour recall, percentage of meals consumed, food preferences, allergies, dislikes, and physical barriers to eating (oral discomfort, dysphagia)
    b. Physical examination: signs and symptoms of nutrient deficiencies, fat deposits, and poor muscle tone and skin turgor
    c. Anthropometric measurements: height, weight, and any changes in height or weight
17. Indicators of malnutrition include listlessness (a), paresthesias (d), loss of ankle reflexes (e), rapid heart rate (f), apathy (h), dry, scaly skin (i), spongy gums (k), pale conjunctivae (m), corneal xerosis (n), and calf tenderness (p).
18. The nurse calculates this individual's BMI as 24.5, within the expected range of 18.5 to 24.9. The weight in pounds is rounded to 82 kg and the 6-foot height is 3.34 m^2.
19. Neurogenic causes of dysphagia include stroke, cerebral palsy, Guillain-Barré syndrome, multiple sclerosis, ALS, diabetic neuropathy, and Parkinson's disease.

Myogenic causes include myasthenia gravis, aging, muscular dystrophy, polymyositis, and dermatomyositis.

20. A common sign of food-borne illnesses is diarrhea, often accompanied by cramping, nausea, and vomiting.
21. To promote a patient's appetite in the acute care setting, the nurse should:
    - Enhance food presentation
    - Remove food covers from the patient's food tray
    - Clean the area and remove odors
    - Provide oral care
    - Provide for the best temperature and seasoning of the food
    - Include food preferences, as appropriate, within the diet
22. The patient with dysphagia should be positioned upright, with support as necessary.
23. Advantages of enteral nutrition include the following: decreased prevalence of hypoglycemia and electrolyte imbalances, increased utilization of nutrients, maintenance of structure and function of the GI tract, safer and less costly than parenteral nutrition.
24. The most serious complication associated with tube feedings is aspiration, and this can be avoided by positioning the patient upright (head of bed elevated at least 30 degrees).
25. The method of choice for long-term enteral feeding is a gastrostomy.
26. The pH of gastric aspirate for a fasting patient is usually between 1 and 4.
27. A central venous line is used for a hyperosmolar solution.
28. a. PN is used because the patient is unable to ingest or digest enteral feedings.
    b. Nursing goals for PN are to prevent infection, maintain the PN system, prevent complications, and promote the patient's well-being.
    c. Nursing interventions to prevent complications of PN therapy include weighing the patient daily, monitoring I&O and caloric intake, testing urine or blood for glucose, obtaining blood samples for nutritional assessment, observing for fluid and electrolyte balance, and maintaining the correct infusion rate.
    d. The recommended infusion rate for lipids is 1 ml/min. Solutions should not be used if there is a separation of contents (oil/creamy layer on top) or if the solution is more than 12 hours old.
29. For patients without teeth or with ill-fitting dentures, a soft diet may be ordered. Patient preferences for foods should be taken into account, as well as consistencies, flavors, and colors.
30. For the patient who is underweight, a nursing diagnosis of *Imbalanced nutrition: less than body requirements* is indicated. An expected outcome for this patient is that he or she will achieve optimum weight for age and size, gaining ½ to 1 pound per week.

31.	1	39.	2	47.	4
32.	1	40.	4	48.	1
33.	2	41.	1	49.	2
34.	2	42.	4	50.	1
35.	4	43.	2	51.	3
36.	1	44.	3	52.	2
37.	2	45.	1	53.	3
38.	2	46.	4		

CHAPTER 32: Urinary Elimination

Case Studies

1. a. Before the IVP, the patient should be assessed for:
   - Allergies to shellfish, iodine, or contrast dyes
   - Fluid status (avoid dehydration from bowel preparation because this may increase the potential toxicity of the contrast dye)
   - Medical conditions that increase risk (e.g., renal insufficiency)
   - Recent barium studies (tests within 2 to 3 days of the IVP will obscure findings)

   The patient should be instructed to:
   - Take the cathartic the evening before the IVP

- Remain NPO after midnight
- Expect an IV infusion to be started for the injection of the dye
- Expect a flushing sensation and a feeling of warmth, dizziness, or nausea when the dye is injected
- Expect that a number of x-rays will be taken during the test and that voiding will be done near the end of the test

b. Following the IVP, the nurse will monitor I&O and report decreased or absent urination. The patient is informed that a normal diet may be resumed, fluid intake is encouraged, and any signs of an allergic reaction (e.g., itching or hives) should be reported.

2. The nurse may safely delegate the following urinary care measures: assisting the patient with the use of the bedpan/urinal, monitoring I&O, maintaining aseptic technique, and promoting patient privacy and dignity. In some institutions, the established policy may allow for additional measures to be delegated, such as routine catheter care and specimen collection. Delegation to unlicensed assistive personnel requires that the nurse evaluate their ability to safely and accurately perform the specified measures.

3. The action proposed by the primary nurse is unsafe because it could result in serious damage to the patient's urethra. The correct procedure requires that you prepare a clean disposable towel, gloves, and a sterile syringe (same volume as the fluid in the catheter balloon). The patient is positioned in the same way as for catheter insertion, the syringe is attached to the balloon port, and the entire amount of fluid is aspirated. The catheter then is pulled out slowly and smoothly. If resistance is encountered, an additional attempt is made to remove fluid from the balloon. The catheter then is wrapped in a waterproof pad and disposed of in an appropriate container, along with the drainage tubing and bag (after emptying and measuring the remaining amount of urine). Perineal care then is provided to the patient, and the nurse will monitor the urinary output carefully.

4. The patient is provided with a sterile specimen cup, sterile disinfectant wipes, and clean gloves. He is instructed to apply the gloves and wipe the urinary meatus in a circular motion, moving up from the meatus to the glans penis. He also is cautioned against using the contaminated wipe repeatedly. After cleansing, the patient should discard the initial urination and begin collection in the sterile cup at the midstream portion of voiding. The cover of the specimen cup then is replaced, and the specimen is sent to the lab within 1 hour of the collection. If necessary to promote patient understanding, the use of more understandable terms, other than meatus and voiding, may be more effective.

Chapter Review

1. d
2. g
3. i
4. h
5. a
6. j
7. e
8. b
9. f
10. c
11. Noninvasive procedures for examination of urinary function include abdominal roentgenogram (radiograph of kidneys, ureters, and bladder [KUB]), intravenous pyelogram (IVP), renal scan, and computerized axial tomography (CAT).
12. Intermittent catheterization is used for immediate relief of bladder distention, long-term management of patients with incompetent bladders, sterile urine specimen collection, assessment of residual urine, and instillation of medication. Indwelling catheters are used for urinary outflow obstructions, patients having surgery of the urinary tract or surrounding structures, prevention of obstruction from blood clots, accurate monitoring of I&O and prevention of skin breakdown in critically ill or comatose patients, and provision of bladder irrigations.
13. A female patient may be placed in the lithotomy or Sims' position for catheterization.

14. The recommended daily fluid intake is 2000 to 2500 ml. The minimum urinary output for an adult is 30 ml/hr.
15. a. Sociocultural—privacy needs for urination and expectations (e.g., intermissions/recesses)
    b. Fluid intake—increased intake will increase output (if fluid/electrolyte balance exists); alcohol, caffeine, and foods with high fluid content promote urination
    c. Pathological conditions—diabetes mellitus and multiple sclerosis cause neuropathies that alter bladder function, arthritis and joint diseases interfere with activity, renal disease influences amount and characteristics of urine, fevers reduce urinary output, and spinal cord injuries disrupt voluntary bladder emptying
    d. Medications—diuretics promote excretion of fluid and selected electrolytes, some drugs change the color of the urine, and some medications influence the ability of the bladder to relax and empty
16. Stress incontinence
17. a. pH 10 = unexpected
    b. Protein 4 mg = expected
    c. Presence of glucose = unexpected
    d. Specific gravity 1.2 = unexpected
    e. Amber color = expected
18. The condom catheter should be changed every day, with the skin checked for signs of irritation and breakdown. Perineal care is provided with each catheter change. The tubing must be checked frequently to ensure that there are no kinks or other obstructions.
19. To maintain the patient's dignity when assisting with urinary elimination, the nurse should:
    - Provide comfort, privacy, time, access, and appropriate positioning
    - Provide gender-congruent care
    - Recognize cultural practices
    - Explain procedures
20. Manual compression of the bladder is called Credé's method.
21. Correct statements about urinary diversions are answers b and c.
22. For strict intake and output measurement, the nurse should provide the patient with a urinal, bedpan, or urinary hat for the toilet.
23. To stimulate the patient to void, the nurse should run water near the patient, place the patient's hand in warm water, or stroke the inner thigh of a female patient.
24. To assist the patient to strengthen the pelvic floor muscles, the nurse teaches the patient Kegel exercises.
25. The length of catheter insertion is:
    a. Female patient: 2 to 3 inches (5 to 7.5 cm)
    b. Male patient: 7 to 9 inches (17.5 to 22.5 cm)
26. Correct indwelling catheter care techniques are listed in options a, f, and g.
27. With regard to a cystoscopy, answers a, c, e, g, h, and i are correct.

28.	1	35.	4	42.	3
29.	3	36.	2	43.	2
30.	4	37.	3	44.	3
31.	3	38.	4	45.	2
32.	3	39.	2	46.	3
33.	1	40.	4	47.	2
34.	4	41.	4		

CHAPTER 33: Bowel Elimination

Case Studies

1. Nursing diagnosis: *Constipation related to overuse of laxatives/enemas and inadequate dietary fiber* (as manifested by patient's statement that she is having difficulty with bowel elimination)

Goal: Patient will establish a regular defecation pattern within 1 to 2 months

Outcomes:

- Patient will have a regular bowel movement within 3 days
- Patient's abdomen will be nondistended and nontender
- Patient will pass soft, formed stools at least every 2 to 3 days

Goal: Patient will maintain a diet that incorporates an adequate amount of fiber and fluids

Outcome:
- Patient will identify and eat foods that are high in fiber and drink an adequate amount of fluid on a daily basis

Nursing interventions:
- Provide instruction about foods high in fiber
- Provide instruction on the importance of an adequate fluid intake
- Encourage allowing ample/regular time for defecation
- Provide instruction on the adverse effects of reliance on laxatives/enemas
- Investigate family and social contacts for stimulation of appetite
- Identify that daily bowel movements are not absolutely necessary

2. Before the colonoscopy, the patient should be instructed to:
   - Drink clear liquids the day before
   - Take some form of bowel cleanser (GoLYTELY)
   - Take enemas until clear, if ordered

Chapter Review

1. d
2. e
3. a
4. b
5. c
6. Constipation in the older adult is usually the result of decreased fiber and fluid in the diet.
7. Patients should be cautioned against straining (Valsalva's maneuver) on defecation if they have cardiovascular disease, glaucoma, increased intracranial pressure, or a new surgical wound.
8. As a result of diarrhea, the patient is at risk for fluid and electrolyte disturbances and anal irritation.
9. Fecal incontinence can create skin breakdown, embarrassment, a change in body image, social isolation, depression, and diminished sexuality.
10. The following factors will decrease peristalsis: slower esophageal emptying (a), immobilization (c), consumption of lean meats (d), emotional depression (f), abdominal surgery (g), Parkinson's disease (j), and use of narcotic analgesics (k).
11. Individuals from the following backgrounds will usually try to avoid exposure of the lower torso: Asians, Africans, Hispanics, Hindus, Muslims, Arabs, Orthodox Jews, and Amish.
12. Risk factors for colon cancer include:
    - Age older than 50 years
    - Family history of colorectal cancer
    - Ethnocultural background
    - Personal history of inflammatory bowel disease
    - Urban residence
    - High dietary intake of fats, with low fiber intake
13. Examples of nursing interventions include:
    a. Constipation—increase intake of fiber (vegetables, fruits, whole grain cereals) and fluids, reduce caffeine intake, elevate the toilet seat, establish a routine, promote exercise, allow for privacy and time, provide chopped foods, rather than pureed (for poor dentition), provide mashed foods with fruit juices and hot tea (for difficulty swallowing)
    b. Diarrhea—increase intake of low fiber foods, replace fluids and electrolytes, reduce intake of milk/milk products and spicy foods, and provide perineal/perianal care
14. a. Positioning—squatting or sitting allows for intraabdominal pressure to be exerted and thigh muscles to be contracted to aid in defecation
    b. Pregnancy—constipation commonly occurs because of pressure of the fetus on the rectum
    c. Diagnostic tests—some tests require NPO or enemas in advance, and barium can harden and cause constipation if not eliminated after the test
15. The nurse may provide local application of heat, sitz baths, or topical medications (as prescribed) to promote comfort for the patient with hemorrhoids.
16. Increased total bilirubin and increased alkaline phosphatase levels can be indicative of obstructive biliary disease.
17. The correct position for an adult patient is left Sims' position.

18. Kayexalate enema
19. a. A hypertonic enema works by exerting osmotic pressure, pulling fluid from the interstitial spaces, and filling the colon with fluid. The distention in the colon promotes defecation.
    b. Fleet enema
20. The hyperosmolarity of enteral solutions draws fluid into the intestine and promotes defecation
21. A focused assessment of a patient's bowel function should include:
    - Chewing—check the condition of teeth, gums, and mouth and ability to eat
    - Mobility—observe the gait, ability to assist with transfer, positioning, activity, and use of toilet facilities
    - Anal sphincter function—check for abdominal distention, impaction
    - Abdominal muscle contractility—observe muscle contraction (bearing down) while palpating lower abdomen
22. a. Colorectal cancer—end colostomy
    b. Diverticulitis—temporary end colostomy with pouch
23. The teaching plan for a patient with an ostomy should include the following: emptying the pouch when it is less than half full (b), applying Kenalog spray (d), using the same manufacturer's supplies (g), cutting the pouch opening slightly larger than the stoma (h), and applying a skin barrier (i).
24. a. Expected d. Unexpected
    b. Unexpected e. Expected
    c. Unexpected f. Expected
25. Before giving a patient a bedpan, the nurse should position the patient with the head of the bed elevated at least 30 degrees, warm a metal bedpan, and provide privacy.
26. Enema administration may be delegated to assistive personnel, if indicated in agency policy.
27. For an adult patient, the enema tube is inserted 3 to 4 inches and the height of the bag is 12 inches above the anus.

28.	3	33.	3	38.	1
29.	4	34.	3	39.	1
30.	4	35.	1	40.	2
31.	3	36.	2	41.	2
32.	4	37.	4	42.	1

CHAPTER 34: Immobility

Case Study

Mrs. B. may benefit the most from discussing her feelings, needs, and concerns with the nurse, and being involved, as much as possible, in the decision-making process for her plan of care. In addition, Mrs. B. may benefit from the following interventions:

- Orienting her to the environment, routine/schedule, and staff members
- Placing her with mobile patients who can interact with her
- Encouraging frequent visits from family members and friends
- Providing her with materials she enjoys, such as books and magazines
- Providing stimulating diversional activity for her, such as music and games
- Engaging in conversation with her during meals and implementation of nursing actions
- Encouraging her to use any necessary assistive aids, such as glasses
- Encouraging and assisting her (as necessary) to attend to daily grooming
- Providing a stimulating physical environment, such as changing her view or decorating with personal objects

Chapter Review

1.	i	5.	c	9.	a
2.	e	6.	b	10.	g
3.	d	7.	f		
4.	j	8.	h		

11. The objectives of bed rest are to decrease physical activity and oxygen needs, allow the ill/debilitated patient to rest, and prevent further injury.
12. The pathophysiological changes that occur with immobility include answers b, c, f, h, i, k, and m.

13. Fluid and electrolyte imbalances that occur with immobility include hypercalcemia and hypovolemia (initial phases).
14. An immobilized patient may react to the experience by exhibiting hostility, belligerence, inappropriate moods, altered sleeping patterns, withdrawal, confusion, anxiety, sadness, hopelessness, and depression.
15. The heart rate of an immobilized patient is generally 4 to 15 beats per minute faster.
16. Virchow's triad refers to thrombus formation, and the three associated problems are (1) loss of integrity of the vessel wall, (2) abnormal blood flow, and (3) altered blood cells and clotting factors.
17. The nurse's focus for an immobilized child is on providing physical and psychosocial stimulation in order to keep pace with motor and intellectual development.
18. To maintain the patient's autonomy, the nurse encourages the patient to do as much as possible, demonstrate activities, and participate in goal setting and decision making.
19. Cardiovascular system changes include:
    - Orthostatic hypotension—move the patient slowly from one position to another
    - Increased cardiac workload—place the patient in an upright position (if possible), provide regular exercise and adequate fluid intake
    - Thrombus formation—provide regular exercise, adequate fluid intake, and antiembolitic stockings
20. Respiratory system changes include hypostatic pneumonia and atelectasis. Nursing interventions include encouraging coughing and deep breathing, adequate fluid intake, and exercise; turning; upright positioning; and chest physiotherapy.
21. Focused assessment of the patient's mobility includes joint range of motion (JROM), pain, endurance, and activity.
22. a. Rotation of the neck
    b. Abduction of the arm
    c. Supination of the forearm
    d. Circumduction of the arm
    e. Hyperextension of the hip
23. To evaluate muscle atrophy, the nurse should perform anthropometric measurements—height, weight, and triceps skin folds.
24. The nurse checks for edema in the immobilized patient at the sacrum, hips, legs, and feet.
25. Assessment frequency (unless indicated by agency policy or changes in patient status):
    a. Respiratory status—every 2 hours
    b. Anorexia—at meals
    c. Urinary elimination—at the beginning or end of every shift
    d. Intake and output—every shift for daily measurement
26. Specific exercises to prevent thrombus formation include ankle pumps, foot circles, knee flexion, and hip rotation.
27. For antiembolitic stockings:
    a. Contraindications for use include dermatitis, open skin lesions, new skin grafts, and decreased circulation.
    b. The stockings are removed every shift.
    c. The stockings should not be partially rolled down or wrinkled, and the toes should not be uncovered.
28. For a sequential compression device, options a and d are correct.
29. Heparin (anticoagulant) is usually given every 8 to 12 hours by the subcutaneous route.
30. For the immobilized patient with a suspected pulmonary emboli, the nurse should (b) place the patient in high-Fowler's position and (e) check the patient's oxygen saturation level.
31. a. Integumentary—Pressure is exerted, with decreased circulation to the tissues leading to pressure ulcers. Nursing interventions include assessment of the skin, use of supportive devices, provision of adequate nutrition and hydration, change of position every 1 to 2 hours, and provision of meticulous skin care.
    b. Gastrointestinal—Reduced appetite (anorexia), nutritional imbalance, decreased peristalsis leading to constipation and possible impaction. Nursing interventions include provision of adequate nutrition (fruits,

vegetables, fiber) and hydration, measurement of I&O, administration of prescribed cathartics, promotion of activity or movement, and institution of bowel program.

c. Urinary—Urinary stasis resulting in greater risk for infection and calculi. Nursing interventions include provision of adequate hydration and promotion of activity or movement.

d. Musculoskeletal—Loss of strength and endurance, reduced muscle mass, decreased stability and balance, with possible contractures and disuse osteoporosis. Nursing interventions include provision or encouragement of range-of-motion exercises, turning every 1 to 2 hours, position changes, and referral to physical therapy.

32. 2
33. 3
34. 2
35. 3
36. 2
37. 4
38. 3
39. 4
40. 2
41. 3
42. 1
43. 4
44. 2
45. 2

CHAPTER 35: Skin Integrity and Wound Care

Case Study

Nursing diagnosis: *Risk for impaired skin integrity related to prolonged pressure on bony prominences* (as manifested by reddened areas [reactive hyperemia] on sacrum, elbows, and heels)

Goal: Integrity of skin and underlying tissues will be maintained

Outcomes:

- Reactive hyperemia will subside and patient's normal skin coloration will return within 2 days
- Patient will assist, as possible, with turning and positioning every 1 to 2 hours

Nursing interventions:

- Reposition or assist with repositioning every 1 to 2 hours
- Encourage the patient to shift weight when out of bed and in a chair
- Assess skin and underlying tissues with each position change
- Use supportive devices— padding for mattress and bony prominences
- Keep sacral area clean and dry
- Measure, document, and report reddened areas

Chapter Review

1. h
2. i
3. b
4. c
5. k
6. a
7. j
8. d
9. e
10. f
11. Sites marked should include occipital bone, scapula, spine, elbow, iliac crest, sacrum, ischium, Achilles' tendon, and heel.
12. a. Stage I b. Stage III
13. The following increase a patient's risk for pressure ulcer development: shearing force, friction, moisture on the skin, poor nutrition, cachexia, infection, impaired peripheral circulation, obesity, and advanced age.
14. Infants, young children, and older adults are most susceptible to pressure ulcer development and sensitivity to heat and cold therapy.
15. Dryness of the older adult's skin makes it less tolerant to pressure, friction, and shearing forces.
16. a. Primary intention
    b. Secondary intention
17. a. True b. False c. False
18. a. Dehiscence
    b. Hematoma/bleeding
    c. Infection
    d. Infection
    e. Bleeding/shock
    f. Evisceration
    g. Infection
19. a. Lighting source: natural or halogen light, avoid fluorescent light
    b. Unexpected consistency: firm, taut (edema, induration), diminished turgor
    c. Unexpected color: different from other skin tones, darker, purple or bluish
20. a. Age—Infants and older adults may have decreased circulation, oxygen delivery, clotting, and inflammatory responses, with an increased risk of infection. Older adults have slower cell

growth and differentiation, and scar tissue is less pliable.
   b. Obesity—Obese individuals have a decreased supply of blood vessels in fatty tissue (impaired delivery of nutrients to the site), and suturing of adipose tissue is more difficult.
   c. Diabetes—These individuals have small blood vessel disease (reduced oxygen delivery), and elevated glucose levels impair macrophage function.
   d. Immunosuppression—A reduced immune response leads to poor healing. Steroids also mask signs of inflammation/infection, and chemotherapeutic agents interfere with leukocyte production.

21. a. 3, serous
    b. 4, sanguineous
    c. 1, serosanguineous
    d. 2, purulent
22. a. Pressure reduction: Use of a supportive surface, regular and frequent turning and repositioning in the bed (q2h) and chair (q1h)
    b. Skin care: Keep skin clean and dry after incontinence, use skin barriers/protectants, turn or lift sheets to reduce friction and shear, maintain head of the bed at 30 degrees or lower, avoid vigorous massage of bony prominences or areas of redness
23. To obtain an aerobic wound culture, the nurse should:
    1. e   3. d   5. a
    2. c   4. b
24. The patient who has a dirty, penetrating wound may require a tetanus toxoid injection.
25. The nurse determines wound healing by measuring the wound diameter and depth, assessing the wound tissue, checking the periwound skin condition, and observing for exudate.
26. A patient who is out of bed in a chair should be limited to 2-hours sitting and repositioned every 1 hour.
27. The nurse reduces friction or shear by using a draw sheet, trapeze bar, and/or support when moving the patient and by providing skin care to maintain integrity.
28. Care of an abrasion or laceration includes control of any bleeding, rinsing of the wound under running water, gentle cleansing with mild soap, application of a prescribed or over-the-counter antiseptic, and protection with a bandage.
29. For a wound VAC system:
    a. The purpose is to remove excess fluid, stimulate granulation tissue growth, and reduce wound bacteria.
    b. The VAC tube is attached to suction to provide negative pressure.
    c. The dressing that is used is either black or white foam that is cut to fit the wound.
    d. The transparent dressing should cover the wound, extend 3 to 5 cm beyond the wound edges, provide an occlusive seal, and be free of wrinkles.
30. For wound irrigation:
    a. Syringe size: 35 ml
    b. Needle size: 19 gauge
    c. psi: 8
    d. reduce the irrigating pressure and notify the health care provider.
31. a. Wound closed with staples
    b. Jackson-Pratt wound drainage system
32. The correct nursing interventions are statements a and d.
33. The steps in caring for a traumatic wound are:
    - Stabilize the patient's cardiopulmonary function
    - Promote hemostasis (stop any bleeding)
    - Cleanse the wound
    - Protect the site from further injury
34. a. Cold   c. Heat   e. Heat
    b. Heat   d. Cold
35. Application of heat is contraindicated in the presence of active bleeding or acute inflammation, and for patients with cardiovascular disease.

    Application of cold is contraindicated in the presence of edema at the site, decreased circulation, and shivering.
36. Heat and cold are usually applied for about 20 to 30 minutes.

37. The correct interventions for application of heat and cold are found in answers a, c, and g.
38. Total Score = 13 points
Patient Risk = "at risk" status

39.	1	45.	3	51.	1
40.	3	46.	3	52.	3
41.	3	47.	2	53.	1
42.	4	48.	2	54.	2
43.	2	49.	1	55.	4
44.	4	50.	4	56.	2

CHAPTER 36: Sensory Alterations

Case Studies

1. For this patient, you may implement the following interventions:
    - Assist in arranging the environment so that the patient knows where everything is and that clutter is out of the way
    - Recommend/assist in obtaining books with larger print, audiotaped books, and music
    - Allow time for discussion of feelings, needs, and concerns
    - Refer the patient to community agencies (e.g., Foundation for the Blind)
    - Instruct/assist in improvement of lighting in halls and stairways and use of color-coding (edges of stairs, medication bottles, and appliance dials, for example)
    - Instruct in importance of follow-up visits to the ophthalmologist
    - Investigate family and social contacts
2. A patient in an intensive care unit (ICU) may experience sensory overload from the intensity of sounds and activity and/or sensory deprivation from restricted visits of family and friends. The nurse should try to organize care so that the patient is allowed opportunity for uninterrupted rest, whenever possible. Monitors at patient's bedside may have volume controls so that they can be turned down to a lower level. The nurse also should take time to sit with the patient, either quietly or for verbal stimulation. Visits from family members and friends should be encouraged but not to the point of patient fatigue. The environment may be arranged so that the patient has a different or more pleasant view, and personal items (e.g., photos) may be placed within the patient's field of vision. It may be a challenge for the nurse in this setting to adapt the patient's sensory input, so creativity, within realistic limits, is recommended.

Chapter Review

1. a. Visual
   b. Auditory
   c. Gustatory
   d. Olfactory
   e. Tactile
   f. Kinesthetic
2. Diseases that may lead to visual impairment include age-related macular degeneration, glaucoma, cataracts, and diabetic retinopathy.
3. a. Sensory deprivation is an inadequate quantity or quality of stimulation that impairs perception (e.g., prolonged bed rest or hearing loss).
   b. Sensory overload occurs when the individual receives multiple stimuli and the brain is not able to disregard or selectively ignore some of the stimuli (e.g., health care units and activities).
4. a. Cerumen accumulation
   b. Presbycusis
   c. Cataract
   d. Xerostomia
   e. Meniere's disease
5. a. Age—older adulthood:
    - Decreased hearing acuity, speech intelligibility, and pitch discrimination
    - Increased dryness of cerumen, with obstruction of the auditory canal
    - Reduced visual fields; increased glare sensitivity; impaired night vision; reduced accommodation, depth perception, and color discrimination
    - Reduced sensitivity to odors and diminished taste discrimination
    - Difficulty with balance, spatial orientation, and coordination
    - Diminished sensitivity to pain, pressure, and temperature

   b. Medications—may cause ototoxicity or optic nerve irritation (chloramphenicol) or may reduce sensory perception (analgesics, sedatives, antidepressants)
   c. Smoking—may cause atrophy of taste buds and interference with olfactory function
   d. Environment—excessive stimuli, frequent activities, noise, TV, bright lights, pain, confinement
6. Assessment of vision and hearing:
   - Ask the patient to read
   - Observe the performance of ADLs (activities of daily living)
   - Observe the patient's use of glasses, magnifiers, or hearing aids
   - Observe patient's conversation/ interaction with others
7. Trauma is the leading cause of blindness in children, usually as the result of flying objects or penetrating wounds.

   Child eyesight safety includes avoiding toys with long, pointed handles or sharp edges; keeping the child from running with a pointed object; and keeping pointed objects and tools out of reach.
8. Chronic middle ear infections and exposure to loud noise contribute to hearing loss in children.
9. Sensory stimulation may be modified in the acute care environment by:
   - Increasing the patient's view outside and within the room
   - Arranging decorations, plants, photos, greeting cards, and the patient's personal items
   - Providing audio books and large-print reading material
   - Spending time with the patient; listening to and conversing with the patient
   - Playing pleasant music or turning on television shows that the patient enjoys
   - Providing attractive meals at the correct temperature
   - Providing a variety of textures and aromas to enhance the patient's appetite
10. The nurse may communicate with a hearing-impaired patient by:
    - Making sure that a hearing aid, if needed, is in place and in working order
    - Approaching the patient from the front to get his or her attention
    - Facing the patient on the same level, with adequate lighting
    - Making sure that glasses, if needed, are worn and are clean
    - Speaking slowly and articulating clearly, using a normal tone of voice
    - Rephrasing, rather than repeating information that is not heard
    - Using visible expressions and gestures
    - Talking toward the patient's better ear
    - Using written information to reinforce spoken words
    - Not restricting the hands of deaf patients
    - Avoiding eating, chewing, or smoking while speaking with the patient
    - Avoiding speaking while walking away, in another room, or from behind the patient
11. Ototoxicity may be caused by:
    - Antibiotics—aminoglycosides, vancomycin, minocycline, polymyxin B/C, erythromycin
    - Diuretics—ethacrynic acid, furosemide, torsemide, bumetanide
    - Analgesics—indomethacin, aspirin, ibuprofen, naproxen
    - Cardiac drugs—class Ia antidysrhythmics, quinidine, procainamide, disopyramide
    - Antineoplastic agents—bleomycin, displatin, dactinomycin, mechlorethamine
12. a. Hearing deficit—amplify low-pitch sounds, use lamps with sound activation, use assistive devices for telephones, and obtain closed captioning for the television
    b. Diminished sense of smell—use smoke and carbon monoxide detectors, take special care with disposal of matches and cigarettes, and check the expiration dates on foods
    c. Diminished sense of touch—lower the temperature of the water heater and use caution when checking the bath or shower water

13. Nursing diagnoses for a patient with a sensory deficit include:
    - *Disturbed body image*
    - *Fear*
    - *Hopelessness*
    - *Risk for injury*
    - *Powerlessness*
    - *Self-care deficit, bathing/hygiene*
    - *Self-care deficit, dressing/grooming*
    - *Risk for situational low self-esteem*
    - *Disturbed sensory perception*
    - *Impaired social interaction*
    - *Social isolation*
    - *Disturbed thought processes*
14. General screenings include examinations for congenital blindness and visual impairment in infants and young children, routine vision and hearing tests of school-age and adolescent children, regular medical eye/ear exams every 2 to 4 years for individuals older than age 40 and every 1 to 2 years for those older than age 65.
15. The appropriate actions for promotion of sensory stimulation in the home are answers a, d, and e.

16.	2	19.	1	22.	2
17.	2	20.	3	23.	1
18.	3	21.	4	24.	2

CHAPTER 37: Surgical Patient

Case Studies

1. Explain and demonstrate coughing and deep-breathing exercises with splinting of the abdominal incision. Assist in and encourage turning and positioning every 2 hours. Reinforce the use of the incentive spirometer. Explain and demonstrate range-of-motion exercises. Provide prescribed analgesia before activities, keeping in mind the action and dosage of the medication and its possible effect on the patient.

2. Preoperative teaching for the patient who is having ambulatory surgery may be done when the patient comes for preoperative tests and physical assessment. There also may be telephone contact with the patient on the evening before the surgery, as well as a 24-hour resource line for the patient to use for questions. Additional teaching may be conducted immediately before the procedure and before the patient's discharge. Information provided to the patient usually includes instructions specific to the surgery and anesthesia (e.g., dressings, activity and dietary restrictions), signs and symptoms of complications, and time frame for follow-up visits.

3. Any significant change in the patient's status should be reported to the surgeon and/or anesthesiologist immediately. Because of the effects of general anesthesia, temperature alterations are especially critical before surgical procedures. Surgery may be postponed until the patient's temperature has returned to normal.

4. The patient should be informed that, under usual circumstances, all loose items are removed before surgery. If the patient will be adversely affected by the removal of his "lucky" medallion, it may be pinned inside of the patient's gown or surgical cap, depending on the type of surgery. It is very important, however, that the operating room personnel be informed that the patient has the medallion in place before the surgery. It may be the policy of the agency that the patient will have to sign a form stating that he has kept the medallion (or other jewelry) on his person in case of a loss.

Chapter Review

1.	g	4.	f	7.	d
2.	c	5.	h	8.	b
3.	a	6.	e		

9. The patient who smokes cigarettes is at a greater risk for bronchospasm or laryngospasm. Aggressive pulmonary hygiene should be instituted for this patient, including frequent turning, coughing and deep breathing, incentive spirometry, and chest physiotherapy.
10. The following medical conditions may increase a patient's surgical risk: bleeding disorders, diabetes mellitus, heart disease, upper respiratory tract infection, cancer, liver disease, fever, chronic respiratory

disease, immunological disorders, and abuse of street drugs.

11. a. Cardiovascular—changes in structure and function reduce cardiac reserve and predispose the patient to postoperative hemorrhage, increased blood pressure, and clot formation
    b. Pulmonary—changes in structure and function reduce vital capacity, increase the volume of residual air left in the lungs, and reduce blood oxygenation
    c. Renal—changes in structure and function increase the possibility of shock with blood loss, limit the ability to metabolize drugs/toxic substances, increase the frequency of urination and the amount of residual urine, and reduce the sensation of the need to void
    d. Neurological—changes in function reduce the ability to respond to warning signs of complications and may lead to confusion after anesthesia
12. Obesity places a patient at greater risk as a result of diminished ventilatory capacity and higher risk of aspiration. There may also be other issues relating to circulation, endocrine function, and musculoskeletal integrity.
13. a. Insulin—a diabetic patient's need for insulin is reduced preoperatively because of NPO status. Dose requirements may increase postoperatively because of stress response and IV administration of glucose solutions
    b. Antibiotics—potentiation of anesthetics, possible respiratory depression from depressed neuromuscular transmission
    c. NSAIDs—inhibited platelet aggregation and prolonged bleeding time
14. General information in preoperative teaching includes:
    - Preoperative and postoperative routines
    - Expected sensations
    - Pain relief measures available (e.g., PCA)
    - Postoperative exercises
    - Activity and dietary restrictions
15. Routine preoperative screening tests include complete blood count, serum electrolyte analysis, coagulation studies, serum creatinine test, urinalysis, 12-lead electrocardiogram, and a chest x-ray.
16. Commonly used preoperative medications include:
    - Sedatives—used for relaxation and decrease in nausea
    - Tranquilizers—used to decrease anxiety and relax skeletal muscles
    - Narcotic analgesics—used to sedate, decrease pain and anxiety, and reduce the amount of anesthesia needed
    - Anticholinergics—used to decrease mucous secretions in the oral and respiratory passages and prevent laryngospasm
17. Nursing diagnoses that may be formulated include:
    - *Anxiety*
    - *Deficient knowledge*
18. NPO criteria:
    a. 2 hours before
    b. 8 to 12 hours before
19. The uses and side effects of the types of anesthesia are:
    a. General anesthesia—Used for major procedures that require extensive tissue manipulation. Side effects include cardiovascular depression or irritability, respiratory depression, and liver and kidney damage.
    b. Regional anesthesia—Used when operating on a specific body area. Side effects include a sudden decrease in blood pressure and respiratory paralysis.
    c. Local anesthesia—Used for minor procedures, especially in ambulatory surgery, and after general anesthesia for postoperative pain relief. Side effects include local irritation and inflammation.
    d. Conscious sedation—Used for procedures that do not require complete anesthesia. Respiration is maintained and the patient can

respond to stimuli. Side effects include respiratory depression and decreased level of consciousness.

20. Preoperative interventions include completion of a bowel prep (a), provision of an antimicrobial soap (c), removal of a wig (d), and removing the hearing aid when the patient gets to the OR area (f).
21. Verification in the PSCU includes the right patient, right procedure, right body part, right data in the chart, and right frame of mind for the patient.
22. Circulating nurse: a, c, d, and f
    Scrub nurse: b, e, and g
23. For intraoperative patient care:
    a. To prevent injury—sterile drapes, sponge and instrument counts, careful positioning, eye protection, grounding of electrical devices, availability of emergency equipment
    b. To maintain body temperature—warm room, warm irrigating solutions, warm blanket after surgery
    c. To prevent infection—standard precautions, sterile asepsis, skin scrubs
24. a. Pulmonary stasis— turning every 1 to 2 hours, coughing, deep breathing, incentive spirometry, chest physiotherapy
    b. Venous stasis—JROM exercises, turning, antiembolitic stockings, sequential compression device, adequate fluids
    c. Wound infection—sterile technique for dressing changes, standard precautions, adequate nutrition (proteins for wound healing)
25. The patient is qualified to be discharged based on options a, d, f, h, and i.
26. The patient should void within 8 hours of the procedure.
27. The first oral intake is usually a clear liquid diet.
28. Appropriate care for an operative incision includes answers b, c, and f.
29. The patient in the illustration is demonstrating the use of an incentive spirometer.

30.	3	37.	4	44.	2
31.	1	38.	3	45.	2
32.	3	39.	3	46.	4
33.	1	40.	2	47.	2
34.	2	41.	1	48.	3
35.	2	42.	3	49.	4
36.	2	43.	4